PUBLIC HEALTH ETHICS

THEORY, POLICY, AND PRACTICE

Edited by
Ronald Bayer
Lawrence O. Gostin
Bruce Jennings
Bonnie Steinbock

UNIVERSITY PRESS

2007

OXFORD
UNIVERSITY PRESS

Oxford University Press, Inc., publishes works that further
Oxford University's objective of excellence
in research, scholarship, and education.

Oxford   New York
Auckland   Cape Town   Dar es Salaam   Hong Kong   Karachi
Kuala Lumpur   Madrid   Melbourne   Mexico City   Nairobi
New Delhi   Shanghai   Taipei   Toronto

With offices in
Argentina   Austria   Brazil   Chile   Czech Republic   France   Greece
Guatemala   Hungary   Italy   Japan   Poland   Portugal   Singapore
South Korea   Switzerland   Thailand   Turkey   Ukraine   Vietnam

Published by Oxford University Press, Inc.
198 Madison Avenue, New York, New York 10016

www.oup.com

Oxford is a registered trademark of Oxford University Press

Library of Congress Cataloging-in-Publication Data
Public health ethics : theory, policy, and practice /
edited by Ronald Bayer . . . [et al.].
p. ; cm.
Rev. ed. of: New ethics for the public's health /
edited by Dan E. Beauchamp, Bonnie Steinbock. 1990.
Includes bibliographical references.
ISBN-13 978-0-19-518084-8; 978-0-19-518085-5 (pbk.)
ISBN 0-19-518084-4; 0-19-518085-2 (pbk.)
1. Public health—Moral and ethical aspects.
2. Medical policy—Moral and ethical aspects.
[DNLM: 1. Public Health—ethics—Collected Works.
2. Communicable Disease Control—Collected
Works.   3. Environmental Health—Collected Works.
4. Ethics, Medical—Collected Works.
5. Health Policy—Collected Works.   6. Social Problems—Collected Works.
WA 21 P9752 2006]
I. Bayer, Ronald. II. New ethics for the public's health.
RA427.25.P82 2006
174'.2—dc22   2006004331

9 8 7 6 5 4 3 2 1

Printed in the United States of America
on acid-free paper

For Ethan Stapleford and Max Bayer

To my father, Joseph Gostin, who rode his bicycle on his 90th birthday. And to Jean, Bryn, and Kieran, who provide a loving environment every day—an active life and nurturance are at the heart of public health

To my son, Andrew M. Jennings, for the future

And for Dan Beauchamp

Acknowledgments

For their support, guidance, and intellectual generosity, we thank Stephen Barbour, Alison Bateman-House, Daniel Callahan, Auburn Daily, Lance Gable, Nora Groce, Will Hutchinson, Eric Juengst, Ann Mellor, Stacy Sanders, Mark Schlesinger, Lesley Stone, and Micah Thorner.

Contents

About the Editors

Ronald Bayer is Professor at the Mailman School of Public Health, Columbia University. He is an elected Member of the Institute of Medicine. His books include *Private Acts, Social Consequences: AIDS and the Politics of Public Health*, *Mortal Secrets: Truth and Lies in the Age of AIDS* (with Robert Klitzman), *Unfiltered: Conflicts over Tobacco Policy and Public Health* (with Eric Feldman, co-editor), and the forthcoming *Searching Eyes: Privacy, the State, and Disease Surveillance in America* (with Amy Fairchild, James Colgrove, and Daniel Wolfe).

Lawrence O. Gostin is Associate Dean and Professor, Georgetown University Law Center; Professor of Public Health, the Johns Hopkins University; Fellow, Oxford University; and Director of the Center for Law and the Public's Health (Collaborating Center for the World Health Organization and Centers for Disease Control and Prevention). He is an elected Member of the Institute of Medicine. His books include *Public Health Law: Power, Duty, Restraint* and *Public Health Law and Ethics: A Reader*.

Bruce Jennings is Director of the Center for Humans and Nature; Senior Consultant at the Hastings Center; and Lecturer at the Yale School of Public Health. He has written widely on ethics and health policy and serves as an ethics consultant to the Centers for Disease Control. His books include *The Perversion of Autonomy: Coercion and Constraints in a Liberal Society* (co-authored with Willard Gaylin) and *Ethics and Public Health: Model Curriculum* (co-edited with Jeffrey Kahn, Anna Mastroianni, and Lisa S. Parker).

Bonnie Steinbock is Professor of Philosophy at the University of Albany, specializing in the ethics of reproduction and genetics. She is a Fellow of the Hastings

Center and a member of the Ethics Committee of the American Society of Reproductive Medicine. She is the author of *Life Before Birth: The Moral and Legal Status of Embryos and Fetuses* and is editor of *Legal and Ethical Issues in Human
Reproduction* and the *Oxford Handbook of Bioethics.* She is the co-editor (with
Alastair Norcross) of *Killing and Letting Die*; (with Dan Beauchamp) of *New Ethics
for the Public's Health*; and (with John Arras and Alex London) of *Ethical Issues
in Modern Medicine.*

PUBLIC HEALTH ETHICS

Introduction: Ethical Theory and Public Health

The Rise of Public Health Ethics

About 30 years ago, professional philosophers began to become interested in "bio-ethics" and other forms of "applied ethics." This was a major shift in academic philosophy. In the 1920s and 1930s, logical positivism taught that ethics did not permit reasoned analysis and debate because ethical statements could not be true or false but were at most expressions of feeling. During the 1950s, if philosophers did not reject the study of ethics altogether, they mainly approached it as a study of the way moral terms, such as *duty, right,* and *ought,* were used rather than as a substantive discussion of ethical and social problems. These discussions were best left to professionals, policy makers, and other experts.

A sea change occurred beginning in the 1960s. Partly this came as a result of demand by a generation of students affected by the civil rights movement and the Vietnam War for education that was "relevant." At the same time, the professions themselves were becoming more scientifically and technically oriented and were losing touch with their own older ethical codes and traditions. A new kind of bio-ethics began to arise in place of traditional medical ethics when a broad-based patient's rights movement, led by feminists concerned with women's health, began to question physician paternalism and to demand disclosure of medical information, informed consent, and active participation by the individual in personal health care. With the legacy of the Nuremberg trials of Nazi doctors in mind, as well as the Tuskegee Syphilis Study mentioned below and other scandals involving medical experimentation on human beings, this new area of practical ethics turned its attention to the regulation of medical research. Technological advances in medicine and biomedical

3

science, from psychosurgery and behavioral control to in vitro fertilization, to the use of life-sustaining treatments, also raised new ethical questions and dilemmas. Similar issues were discussed in other professions and in more general public policy issues such as foreign policy and warfare, equality and poverty, racial and gender discrimination and affirmative action, capital punishment, and the like.

Amid the social turmoil and conflict during the period from roughly 1965 to 1975, it was no longer possible to say, as the newly elected President John Kennedy had in 1960, that our society largely agrees about its ethical ends and goals, and that the only remaining questions to solve were technical questions about the means to achieve these goals. Clearly, fundamental debates about social goals, human rights, and justice were taking place, and our ethical ends were yet to be determined. Technical knowledge about means would not suffice. The study of ethics and the notion that ethics could contribute in a practical way to the conduct of life and the governance of society returned to the forefront of attention. Those with special training in ethics, including philosophers, began to come out of the academy and into the public square to join in the larger conversation.

The result of all this activity has been an extensive body of literature in applied and practical ethics, especially in the largest subfield within this domain, bioethics. Bioethicists have written on a wide range of issues, including the doctor-patient relationship, confidentiality, informed consent, medical experimentation, the definition of death, euthanasia and physician-assisted suicide, genetic testing and manipulation, abortion, assisted reproduction, and many others. Some of these issues, such as genetic screening and assisted reproduction, can be examined from a public health perspective as well as from the more individualistic perspective typical of biomedical ethics. Some issues, such as alcohol and drug policy or domestic violence, are unlikely to be represented in medical ethics texts.

Indeed, today there is rapidly growing interest within the field and profession of public health in those ethical issues and perspectives that may be said to be distinctive to public health and to set it apart from the perspective of clinical medicine.[1] This distinction is between ethical orientation focused on the interests and needs of an individual patient and an ethical orientation focused on the health of large numbers of people as they are affected not only by the biological processes of their own bodies but also by the social structures and environmental conditions that affect their health, as it were, from outside. Moreover, the physician-patient relationship is traditionally viewed as a private, contractual relationship. Public health practitioners, by contrast, are most often officials associated in some way with the government, and they exercise the authority and power of the state.

Because of the individualistic orientation of medical ethics, the concepts of autonomy and the negative rights of the person (the right not to be harmed) have tended to predominate in that field. In public health ethics, by the very nature of the problems and policies with which it deals, there will tend to be more emphasis on the interests and health of groups, the social justice of the distribution of social resources, and the positive or social/human rights of individuals. When social interests and the interests of individuals come into conflict, then there will be a conflict between medical ethics and public health ethics.

However, this theme of the proper balance between the public interest and the interests of individual persons, and the limits of state action in limiting the liberty of individuals—in a word, the theme of the proper relationship between the individual and society—go well beyond medicine and public health and form the framework of the tradition of political and ethical theory that is called *liberalism*. Much of public health ethics, indeed, arises in the context of liberalism, which is both a complex philosophical framework and the ideological framework that continues to be dominant in American political culture and throughout the world.

Of course, within the political culture of liberalism and in a pluralistic society, as one would expect, numerous ethical perspectives coexist on a matter of such widespread interest and importance as public health. In fact, in discussions of ethical issues in public health today one can discern several different styles or types of analysis.[2] Each of these orientations can be found reflected in the selections contained in this book. Complex and skillful discussions of public health ethics often blend or synthesize these styles, and each might be appropriate for any specific ethical problem. We review them here briefly before turning to discuss in more detail the substance of ethical analysis and ethical theory as they may be brought to bear on public health issues and policies.

Professional Ethics

The study of professional ethics tends to seek out the values and standards that have been developed by the practitioners and leaders of a given profession over a long period of time and to identify those values that seem most salient and inherent in the profession itself. Applied to public health, this perspective entails identifying the central mission of the profession (e.g., protection and promotion of the health of all members of society) and building up a body of ethical principles and standards that would protect the trust and legitimacy the profession should maintain.

Applied Ethics

As noted, another approach to public health ethics comes from the field that has emerged in recent years as applied or practical ethics, especially bioethics. The applied ethics perspective differs from the professional ethics perspective principally in that it adopts a point of view from outside the history and values of the profession. From this more general moral and social point of view, applied ethics seeks to devise general principles that can then be applied to real-world examples of professional conduct or decision making. These principles and their application are designed to give professionals guidance and to give those clients affected by professional behavior and the general public standards to use in assessing the professions. Thus, in applied ethics there is a tendency to reason abstractly and to draw from general ethical theories rather than from the folkways and knowledge base of the professions. The emphasis tends to be on professional conduct rather than on the virtues of professional character.

Advocacy Ethics

If there is a characteristic ethical orientation within the field of public health today, it is probably less theoretical or academic than either professional ethics or applied ethics. While on occasion this can be difficult for civil servants, the ethical persuasion liveliest in the field is a stance of advocacy for those social goals and reforms that public health professionals believe would enhance the general health and well-being, especially of those least well off in society. Such advocacy is in keeping with the natural priorities of those who devote their careers to public health. It has a strong orientation toward equality and social justice. Much of the research and expertise in public health throughout its history has shown how social deprivation, inequality, poverty, and powerlessness are directly linked to poor health and the burden of disease. In recent years, a growing international movement in support of human rights has exerted an important influence in public health as well.

These distinctions, of course, are useful for heuristic purposes only; in the actual ethical discourse that takes place both within public health and in the broader society about public health issues, one finds a blending and merger of these three perspectives. And, perhaps even philosophically it is best to attempt to combine the strengths of these three approaches for, at the end of the day, no one ethical perspective or theory is sufficient to capture the richness and complexity of public health. Ethical thinking in public health must be historically informed and practically oriented. It should also bring larger social values and historical trends to bear in its understanding of the current situation of public health and the moral problems faced. Public health ethics must be able to focus simultaneously on biological and chemical factors in the body and the natural environment, on individual behavior, and on the health effects of institutional arrangements and prevailing structures of cultural attitudes and social power.

Each of these orientations in public health ethics draws on a common set of conceptual tools, principles, ideals, and ethical theories. It is to them that we now turn. There are many different ethical theories. The aim of this Introduction is not to provide a thorough depiction or analysis of all of them. The intention is rather to provide students of public health or public policy who have not had courses in ethical theory with enough background to be able to understand and evaluate the ethical arguments made in this book.

What Is Ethics?

We start with some terminology. The word *ethics* can be used to refer to the set of rules, principles, values, and ideals of a particular group of people. This is called its descriptive sense. Thus, we might contrast the ethics of the Puritans with the ethics of the Hawaiian Islanders. The word *ethics* can also be used to refer to the systematic study of moral concepts and theories, typically in departments of philosophy. Some philosophers use the term *morality* to refer to ethics in its descriptive sense, that is, concerning the beliefs of particular groups of people about right and wrong, reserving the term *ethics* (or *moral philosophy* or *ethical theory*) for the subject taught in departments of philosophy. However, this usage is not universal, and we use the terms *ethics* and *morality* interchangeably. Students will have to examine the context to determine whether the subject is a group's beliefs about right and wrong or the theoretical study of moral beliefs and concepts.

Ethics in the philosophical or secular sense is distinguished from two other closely related sources of normative discourse, that is, discussion of what should be done or should be the case, not simply what is the case. These are religion and law.

Ethics and Religion

For many people, morality is identified with religion. The reasons for this are fairly obvious: All major religions—Judaism, Christianity, Islam, Hinduism, and Buddhism—have ethical teachings associated with them, and the fundamental ethical tenets of virtually all societies are based on religious teachings. Moreover, many people receive their moral training in religious institutions, such as church, synagogue, or Sunday school. This may lead them to think that ethics *must* be based in religious teaching. However, there is no necessary connection between religion and ethics. A person can be ethical and a nonbeliever. A completely secular ethics is perfectly possible, although it undoubtedly will coincide with the teachings of most religions in certain respects.

Moreover, religious tenets themselves can be subjected to moral assessment. For example, the doctrine of purgatory in Christianity was developed in response to the feeling of many Christians that it was cruel and unfair to commit unbaptized infants to eternal damnation. More recently, some Christian churches have rejected, based on moral arguments, the traditional teachings of Christianity regarding homosexuality or the ordination of women. Such moral evaluations of religious teachings would be literally impossible if morality were merely a function of religion.

Ethics and Law

Another source of guidance regarding how we should behave is the law. The law may reflect a society's moral consensus on issues such as abortion, surrogate motherhood, or physician-assisted suicide. Interpretation of what the law is often requires normative ethical analysis, as evidenced by legal writings, such as judicial decisions, amicus briefs, and articles by law professors. For example, in the landmark case of *Brown v. Board of Education* (347 U.S. 483, 1954), the Supreme Court was faced with the question of whether racially segregated public schools are constitutionally permissible. The Supreme Court decided that segregated schools violate the Constitution, even if the facilities in white and black schools are (as they never were in fact) equal. They are inherently unequal and so violate the equal protection cause of the Fourteenth Amendment because the intention and effect of racial segregation is to degrade, stigmatize, and deny equal opportunity to Negro children. The Court's decision was not a narrowly legalistic one but was based on substantive moral analysis of the concept of equality as it has evolved in the context of American institutions, traditions, and history.

The law may also be viewed as providing limits on what can and cannot be done. For example, federal rules governing medical experiments forbid the use of human subjects without their informed consent or that of a court-appointed surrogate. The rules settle the question of whether an experiment may be done; any study that uses people without their informed consent is impermissible. However, although legal considerations sometimes determine what may or may not be done, and legal considerations are often relevant to moral decisions, the law, no more than religion, does not determine morality. For one thing, just as religious teachings can be criticized on moral grounds, so can the law. Sometimes, this results in changes in the laws. For another, it may sometimes be right to violate the law, although determining when this would be justified is obviously a complex ethical issue.

Faced with complex ethical issues, students often wonder how justification in ethics is possible, given that different people and different societies apparently have different and conflicting moral views. In the next section, we examine some challenges to ethics that seek to cast doubt on the whole enterprise of moral justification and the possibility of arriving at rational resolutions to moral questions.

Challenges to Ethics

Nihilism

One source of cynicism about moral philosophy comes from the conviction—or suspicion—that there is no such thing as moral reality. This is known as *ethical nihilism,* and it can take several forms. One version of ethical nihilism maintains that morality is simply an illusion, like religion, and something we should get over. This implies that there is nothing really wrong with raping, torturing, and murdering a child. Although it is difficult to know how to go about disproving this extreme nihilistic claim, it is so far from the experience of virtually everyone that it is even more difficult to take it seriously.

A more plausible version of nihilism claims that morality simply reflects the interest of those in power. This view, originally stated by Thrasymachus in Plato's *Republic,* is also reflected in Marxist theory, as well as in contemporary critical legal theory and postmodernism. It must be admitted that not only the laws and institutions of society but also its moral beliefs are typically formulated and propagated by people in positions of power. They may impose what promotes their own self-interest on the downtrodden masses while hoodwinking the masses into believing that they are morally required to do what they are told to do. This sort of cynicism about morality seems most plausible in totalitarian regimes. However, even if power is more widely dispersed, as in a democracy, a variation of the criticism can be made. That is, it can be objected that what is claimed to be "objective morality" is nothing but disguised self-interest. Thus, people with well-paying jobs or other sources of income—the haves—may view their economic status as something they have worked for and therefore morally deserve, while the have-nots may regard the more fortunate as beneficiaries of an unjust economic system that profits from the existence of an underclass.

There is no objectively correct moral answer according to this version of moral nihilism but only the self-interest of the respective parties.

We can certainly acknowledge the ability of those in power to control behavior, ideology, and even the interpretation of history. We can also recognize that self-interest may skew people's moral beliefs. It does not follow, however, that morality is *nothing but* the expression of the interest of those in power. An important distinction can be drawn between *conventional morality*, the rules and values currently accepted and promulgated, and *critical* or *ideal* morality, which can be used to assess conventional morality. If morality were just the interests of the powerful, as Marxist theory alleges, then it would be literally impossible to condemn on moral grounds the behavior and policies of those in power. Yet, this is exactly what Marxist and other critics of capitalism attempt to do. The very existence of intelligible social criticism rests on the possibility of a critical or ideal morality that is not identified with the interests of those in power.

Relativism

Another challenge to the viability of ethics is *ethical relativism.* Ethical relativism does not say that morality is merely an illusion or something to get over or identify morality with the interests of the powerful. Rather, it claims that morality is relative to the mores, values, standards, or rules of a particular culture. What is right for one culture may be wrong for another. Thus, in one culture, premarital sex may be regarded as normal or healthy, and in another it may be regarded as sinful. There is no way to determine which culture is correct about the morality of premarital sex. Indeed, the question does not even make sense because morality is always relative to a particular culture. There is no right or wrong independent of culture.

A major advantage of ethical relativism is its ability to explain the variation in moral beliefs and customs throughout the world. Ethical relativism seems superior to an absolutist conception of morality that maintains there is one true moral code and any divergence from that code is immorality. Such a view seems arrogant and presumptuous in the face of the moral diversity of different cultures. Another point in favor of relativism is its recognition that moral beliefs and practices can only be understood within the context of a culture. A practice that at first sight appears irrational or abhorrent may come to make sense when we understand both the material conditions in which it occurs and its symbolic significance. The more we understand a culture, the less likely we are to misinterpret its moral beliefs.

At the same time, ethical relativism has consequences that are difficult to accept. For example, the Nazis thought that Aryans were a superior people, and that certain groups—Jews, gypsies, Slavs, and so on—should be deported, enslaved, or exterminated. If ethical relativism is true, then the fact that they believed that it is morally right to exterminate Jews makes it morally right—for them. Ethical relativism rules out the possibility of saying that their behavior was immoral, wicked, and wrong. Is there a way to acknowledge legitimate variations in moral beliefs without proclaiming that whatever people think is right is right—for them?

A first step might be to challenge the seemingly obvious claim that morality differs among cultures. Although this may be true in relation to views about (permissible) sex and marriage arrangements, it is less clear that such variation exists regarding basic or fundamental principles of morality, such as the wrongness of lying, stealing, assault, and murder. These acts seem to be universally condemned, undoubtedly because no group can continue to exist where distrust and aggression are the norm. Thus, despite initial appearances, there may be some universal norms because of the very nature of morality as a mechanism enabling people to live together in groups. A second important point is that it does not follow from the mere fact that people in different cultures have different beliefs about morality that their beliefs are correct or justifiable, any more than it follows from the fact that people have different beliefs about the physical world, that all their beliefs are equally correct. The mere fact that some people think the world is flat or that disease is caused by devils does not make it so (or even "true for them"). It means only that they sincerely (and mistakenly) believe it.

However, ethical relativists may argue that this is precisely the point. Although we can offer objective evidence that the world is round, not flat, or that disease is caused by microorganisms, not devils, it is impossible to offer objective evidence about morality. But is this in fact the case? Consider the nineteenth-century claim that slavery was morally justified. This rested in part on a belief in the intrinsic inferiority of the Africans who were captured and enslaved. It was said that they were incapable of taking care of themselves, incapable of learning, and incapable of the emotions their masters felt (such as anguish at the sale of their spouses or children). Not only is this clearly nonsense in hindsight but also it seems that at some level even those who made the claims must have known them to be false. After all, why make teaching a slave to read illegal if slaves are incapable of learning to read?

The point here is that objective, scientific facts play a significant role in moral judgments and constitute a basis for accepting or rejecting moral beliefs. The practice of "clitoridectomy" or female circumcision provides a good example. This practice, common to certain groups in Africa, is usually performed at puberty, although it may be done on very young children. The girl is held down by older women while her clitoris, or a portion of it, is removed. In the more radical versions of the procedure, the entire genitalia are removed. The lips of the vulva are sewn up, with only a small hole for urination and menstrual blood. Most often, no form of anesthesia is used, and the procedure is done with unsterilized razor blades or knives. The purpose of clitoridectomy is to reduce sexual pleasure and remove the temptation to sexual activity; the vulva is sewn up to ensure that the young women will remain a virgin until her marriage. In cultures in which the practice is widespread, it may be difficult or impossible for an uncircumcised girl to find a man who is willing to marry her.

Public health professionals and women's health activists around the world have condemned the practice. Not only is it extremely painful when performed but also it can have repercussions throughout the woman's life, especially for those subjected to the radical surgery in which the entire external genitalia are cut off. Intercourse is more difficult and painful, and childbirth more dangerous. Ironically, those who engage in the practice believe that it is necessary for cleanliness and conducive to fertility. In fact, circumcised women are more susceptible to infection and sexually transmitted diseases and are often rendered infertile. Insofar as the justification for the practice rests on incorrect factual beliefs, it can be rejected without challenging the moral beliefs of those who accept it.

However, the objection to female circumcision is not solely based on its adverse health consequences. Feminists and others using ethical perspectives now widespread around the world also reject the set of beliefs that underlie the practice: It is wrong for women to experience sexual pleasure; female virginity must be preserved; women's bodies are the property of their husbands; and it is permissible to mutilate the bodies of women to keep them meek, submissive, and sexually pure. Such beliefs are inconsistent with the recognition of women as full human persons entitled to equality and justice.

To summarize, ethical relativism has something to teach us, namely, that human cultures have diverse moral beliefs, many of which are equally valid. Moreover, to understand beliefs that differ from our own, it is necessary to understand them in the context of an entire culture and belief system. But, it does not follow that *whatever* people believe is right or immune from moral criticism. Moreover, our own cherished beliefs can also be challenged, something that ethical relativism rules out on principle. In fact, it is only if we *reject* relativism that we can learn from other cultures. To do so requires an objective, nonrelativistic standpoint from which we can critically examine our own attitudes and habits, as well as those other cultures.

In the final analysis, we believe, neither nihilism nor relativism is a persuasive or sustainable philosophical position. Yet, the question remains, How can ethical disagreements be resolved? If ethical progress is possible, how is it possible? On what basis can we arrive at solutions to the problems we face?

An obvious component of understanding and resolving ethical issues in public health is factual information. Facts—scientifically based evidence—are crucial to determining good public policy, but facts by themselves cannot indicate which policies should be implemented. Facts can influence policy only when the goals to be achieved are delineated. Despite the fact that goals may differ in different cultures and different communities, there are some goals and principles that have widespread acceptance. These include benefiting individuals (for example, by decreasing disease and improving their health), respect for self-determination, equality, and justice. Of course, the interpretation of these goals and principles is varied, as are beliefs about which policies are most likely to promote them.

Moreover, sometimes goals and principles can conflict. When they do, a strategy for prioritizing them is useful. This is a major reason for the appeal to ethical theory.

Ethical Theories

The study of ethics and morality can be divided roughly into two branches. *Normative ethics* is primarily concerned with providing a theoretical or foundational basis for how people ought to behave; *metaethics* is primarily concerned with analyzing the meanings of central ethical terms like *good, right, duty,* and *obligation.* The two are not as rigidly separate as it might at first seem because normative issues often turn on our interpretation of difficult concepts. For example, an issue in population policy is whether coercive means of reducing population growth are permissible. Clearly, forced abortions and the mandatory imposition of contraception on unwilling women are coercive means. But is coercion limited to threats of inflicting harm, or can offers and incentives in some contexts also be coercive? For example, it has been charged that laws increasing the welfare payments of women who agree to have Norplant (a long-acting contraceptive) implanted are a form of coercion. Others reject this label, saying that women who prefer to have more children are not deprived of any payments they would have received anyway. Therefore, they are not harmed or made worse off because of their choice, and they are not forced to choose the higher welfare payments. The critics of such statutes respond that the "choice" to receive higher payments or have more children is really "no choice" given the poverty in which welfare recipients live. This issue cannot be resolved without a persuasive analysis of the concept of coercion. (Of course, even if incentives are determined not to be coercive, they may be objectionable on a number of other grounds. By the same token, the mere fact that a policy is coercive is not a conclusive reason for regarding it as morally impermissible. Most laws are coercive, but they are not for that reason wrong.)

We see, then, that conceptual analysis is part of ethical and policy analysis. Equally important are normative ethical theories: theories about what makes right actions right (and wrong actions wrong). Generally speaking, normative theories fall into two broad types. One type is *consequentialist theory.* These are theories that base moral justification (the rightness or wrongness of an action; the goodness or badness of a state of affairs) on the consequences, effects, or outcomes that are produced. The consequences that are relevant for the purposes of moral justification can pertain to virtually anything, all sentient beings, for example, or even nonliving things (such as the destruction of a natural landscape or of a great work of art), but most commonly morally relevant consequences are linked to the effects an action or state of affairs has on human beings. So, consequentialist theories (sometimes also called *teleological* or *perfectionist* theories) will often include some general account of human (or animal) flourishing or the human good. One of the most well developed and influential examples of a consequentialist ethical theory is called *utilitarianism.* It was developed by philosophers such as Jeremy Bentham and John Stuart Mill and more recently by a large number of social reformers and economists. Many of the pioneering figures in modern public health, in the sanitarian and immunization movements, for example, were closely associated with and strongly influenced by utilitarianism.

The second main type of ethical theory is often called *deontological theory* (sometimes called *duty-based* or *rights-based* theory). These theories postulate ethical imperatives (moral rights and duties or obligations) that are binding independent of the consequences that follow at any given time as a result of following them. Ethical justification, therefore, comes from the obedience to moral rules, and their status as moral rules comes from their intrinsic reasonableness or rightness (or from divine command), not from their consequential effect on interests or welfare. Many theologically or religious ethical theories are of the deontological type (i.e., the Ten Commandments). Historically important philosophical versions of deontological ethical theories were developed by Immanuel Kant and by other thinkers from John Locke to John Rawls, who are known as *contractarian* theorists.

In the framework of philosophical liberalism that we mentioned, utilitarianism and contractarianism are two of the predominant ethical theories. Proponents of such theories also array themselves along a spectrum of how much emphasis and moral importance is given to the freedom of the individual and the limitation of social or governmental regulation at one end and to the common good and the obligations of the individual to society at the other. Three important points along this spectrum play a role in the ethical landscape of public health and so deserve our attention here. They are libertarian liberalism, egalitarian or welfare liberalism, and communitarianism.

Such theories are not simply descriptions of what is conventionally considered right or wrong behavior in a particular society or group. Instead, normative ethics attempts to identify and justify basic moral principles and to derive from them guidance for what we ought to do and what kind of people we should strive to become. The basic principles, values, character traits, and so forth can be applied to specific ethical issues, such as whether there should be mandatory acquired immunodeficiency syndrome (AIDS) testing in hospitals, when to begin population screening for genetic diseases, and what sort of alcohol and drug policies we should have.

Philosophers are often interested in ethical theory as providing a single key to morality. Classical utilitarians regard the maximization of happiness or pleasure as the ultimate goal, and everything else as reducible to happiness. Kantians regard happiness as relatively insignificant morally and in any event deny that principles like justice or respect for autonomy can be reduced to happiness. Virtue theorists maintain that there has been an overemphasis on right actions and too little attention paid to the kinds of people we should strive to become; feminists and Marxists claim that power relations are essential to an adequate moral theory. Communitarians deplore the excessively individualistic turn in modern moral philosophy, whether utilitarian or Kantian, and emphasize the importance of shared traditions, values, and goals, as well as the impact of actions and policies on the community considered as a whole rather than as a collection of individuals with separate interests.

Our aim here is not to determine the "correct" moral theory. Indeed, we are dubious that any one moral theory has a monopoly on truth. Probably all of them have something to contribute to the understanding of something as complex and multifaceted as morality. Two of them, utilitarianism and Kantian moral theory, have been dominant in both moral thinking and public policy. At least rudimentary acquaintance with these theories is essential for understanding the readings in this anthology. However, a third, communitarianism, is particularly appropriate for the aggregate approach to policy exemplified by public health.

Utilitarianism

Classical utilitarianism was formulated in the nineteenth century by Jeremy Bentham and John Stuart Mill, although it built on ideas that go back at least as far as the ancient Greeks. The heart of utilitarianism is "the greatest happiness principle," which holds that actions are right insofar as they tend to promote the greatest happiness of the greatest number, wrong as they tend to promote the reverse.[3]

The first thing to note about the utilitarian tradition is its emphasis on the likely consequences of whatever is under consideration. Actions, policies, motives, and so forth are all judged to be right or wrong, good or bad in terms of their expected consequences. Thus, utilitarianism is a form of consequentialism. Not all consequentialists are utilitarians, but since utilitarianism is the most familiar and influential consequentialist theory, it is the one on which we will focus. Second, the overarching goal to be achieved is pleasure or happiness, with pleasure and happiness understood not as transient states of mind or feelings, but rather as total well-being. The theory of value that maintains that pleasure or happiness is the ultimate good is known as *hedonism*. According to hedonism, pleasure is the only thing that is intrinsically good; all other good things—health, friendship, love, for example—are desirable because of the happiness they bring. Pain is intrinsically bad, although pain may be good if the experience of pain ultimately brings more pleasure or avoidance of pain. Thus, vaccination is good, even though it hurts, because it avoids the greater harm of serious disease.

Contemporary utilitarians have by and large rejected hedonism for several reasons. First, happiness is hard to define and even harder to measure. If it is equated to pleasure, considered as episodic sensations, then happiness can be quantified, but it is hard to believe that a life of pleasant sensations is the ultimate good. Happiness is more plausible as the ultimate end if we conceive of it as not limited to pleasure sensations but more globally as the satisfaction of goals contributing to well-being. However, this conception makes quantification and interpersonal comparison, which are essential to utilitarianism, extremely difficult.

Another reason for the rejection of hedonism is that the reduction of all goals and values to happiness, even on the broader interpretation of happiness, is implausible. Knowledge, art, and meaningfulness are all values, and it is far from clear either that these reduce to an aspect of happiness or that these things are valued because they contribute to happiness. They may be valued for themselves, independent of how happy they make people. For these reasons, contemporary utilitarians are more likely to think of the ultimate end not as happiness or pleasure but rather as the satisfaction of individual preferences.

An important question for any moral theory is how it determines which individuals or entities are entitled to moral consideration or moral status. Utilitarians generally consider *sentience,* or the ability to experience pain and pleasure, to be the important feature in deciding who counts or who has moral status. Given a hedonist theory of value, the emphasis on sentience is not surprising. But even preference utilitarians tend to consider sentience an important marker for moral status. This is because nonsentient beings (plants, rocks, buildings) do not have preferences and cannot be happy or unhappy. Thus, sentience is a necessary condition for inclusion in the utilitarian calculus. It is also considered a sufficient condition. That is, if a being suffers, then there is no justification for ignoring that suffering, whatever other characteristics it may have or lack. As Bentham said, "The question is not can they reason? Nor can they talk? But can they suffer?"[4] The principle of utility is to be applied not only to all human beings but also, as Mill said, to all sentient creation, as far as is possible.[5] (Some contemporary utilitarians think that it is a good deal more possible than Bentham or Mill were willing to acknowledge. Peter Singer, for example, has argued not only that animals count but also that they count as much as human beings.[6])

The third point about utilitarianism is that it is a maximizing theory. That is, the right action or policy is the one that achieves the greatest happiness possible. There is only one right action in any situation: the one that maximizes happiness or welfare. Fourth, utilitarianism is an egalitarian theory insofar as it insists that everyone's happiness is to be considered equally.

There are several features that make utilitarianism an attractive theory. One is that it provides a method for deciding which is the right action or policy, namely, the one that produces more good (however this is defined) than other alternatives. Another is that its goals are clearly important ones. What is the point of morality, it may be asked, if not to promote happiness and reduce misery? Surely, rules have no intrinsic value unless they achieve good results. Even someone who bases his or her conception of right and wrong on what God wants must ask *why* God wants us to do certain things and abstain from others. Following the Ten Commandments and the Golden Rule is likely to result in a happier world; this certainly was the way Mill regarded it.[7]

The possibility remains, however, that certain situations that maximize happiness could conflict with other values, such as honesty and fairness. A major objection to utilitarianism is that it could countenance great injustice, such as knowingly condemning an innocent person to prevent mob violence that would result in the deaths of many more innocent persons. Utilitarians respond by saying that this objection fails to consider the total, long-term effects of unjust or dishonest actions. Mill emphasized the destructive effects lying has on trust, saying that these bad effects could rarely, if ever, be outweighed by the good effects to be achieved by deception.[8] Moreover, the temptation to lie is often motivated by self-interest rather than a dispassionate and accurate assessment of the general utility. Recognition of this tendency requires us to adhere in most cases to what Mill called *secondary principles,* such as the rule against lying, as our best bet for achieving the greatest happiness. At the same time, Mill acknowledged that there may be rare instances in which it is justified to break a moral rule—for example, to lie to save a life.

In creating social policy, we often rely on utilitarian reasoning and the notion of the greatest good for the greatest number. For example, a policy requiring that all persons be immunized, with few exceptions, is likely to be most effective in combating communicable diseases. At the same time, it might expose a few, rare, susceptible individuals to vaccine-related damage or even death. Most people would find this acceptable because the good of universal vaccination outweighs the harm to a few. Nevertheless, the idea that the good of the majority can cancel out the welfare of the few has led to the criticism that utilitarianism devalues individuals and individual rights.

Resistance to utilitarian reasoning can be seen in other examples. Should society compel people to participate in genetic screening or even abortion to reduce the number of people born with genetic defects? Such a policy would reduce the costs of caring for such individuals and might be rational from a utilitarian standpoint. There is widespread agreement that even if such a policy did promote "the greatest happiness of the greatest number," it would nonetheless be morally unacceptable. As the President's Commission said in *Screening and Counseling*:

The chief objection to this agreement is that is rests upon a general principle that few, if any, would wish to see consistently implemented—namely, that a person's freedom to make the most intimate choices and even a person's very existence, depends upon the degree to which social utility is maximized. . . . Rather than finding utilitarianism particularly appropriate in determining social policy on genetics programs, the contrary appears to be the case, in light of the especially strong reasons to preserve individual liberty on matters of medical treatment and reproduction.[9]

It is likely that most utilitarians would also opt for a principle of voluntariness regarding reproductive decisions and try to justify such a principle on utilitarian grounds. Their argument would be that a society in which people's most intimate choices were regulated by state interference would be unlikely to be one that promoted the greatest happiness. Mill himself argued in *On Liberty* that a society that allowed for the greatest amount possible of individual liberty would be the happiest. However, there is no guarantee that this coincidence between the greatest liberty and the greatest happiness will obtain. Policies that are justified on grounds of social utility might conflict with other equally important principles, such as liberty, autonomy, equality, or justice.

Kantian Ethics

Although Immanuel Kant (1724–1804) lived before the classical utilitarians, Kantian ethics is best understood as a critique of the utilitarian approach (which was prefigured in the work of David Hume and others whom Kant had studied and so was not entirely new with Bentham and Mill).[10] Kant rejected both the theory of value associated with utilitarianism (hedonism) and its consequentialism. In contrast to the utilitarian emphasis on sentience as the basis for moral status, Kant regards the capacity for experiencing pain and pleasure as morally fairly insignificant. Instead, he emphasizes the connection between morality and reason. Reason is what separates man (human beings) from the rest of the animals and what makes us subject to the moral law. Our capacity for rational thought both entitles us to treatment and rights to which animals are not entitled and imposes on us obligations that animals do not have. Animals are not morally required to refrain from murder, theft, and deception. Indeed, these concepts cannot even be applied to animal behavior. Only rational creatures, capable of knowing the difference between right and wrong, can be responsible moral agents.

Of course, the fact that normal adult human beings are capable of rational thought (and thus are moral agents) does not entail that they will always behave morally, that is, in a morally correct fashion. To call people moral agents is not to deny that they may be immoral but rather to say that they are *responsible for* their behavior, that they can be blamed for acting wrongly. By contrast, infants, severely retarded individuals, and most animals are not capable of understanding the difference between right and wrong. Whether some primates, such as gorillas and chimpanzees, and perhaps other mammals, such as dolphins, have a moral sense is a debatable point. Nevertheless, even if these animals behave altruistically and reciprocally, it is unlikely that they can be considered moral agents in the way that most humans are. Certainly, most animals, like babies and very young children, are not responsible, and it would not be appropriate to blame them for any harm they might cause. Animals can often be trained to act in certain ways by rewards and punishments, but they are not capable of motivation by moral reasons (such as "You wouldn't like it if he did that to you").

Kant also objected to consequentialism. It is not the consequences of an act that make it right or wrong, for what happens as the result of what you do is not wholly within your control. It is perfectly possible that doing the right thing will have disastrous consequences, and that wrong actions may result in unexpected good results. Basing morality on the consequences makes it altogether too contingent, depriving it of the necessity that Kant regarded as essential to the possibility of morality and a moral law.

Does this mean that Kantian ethics tells us to ignore consequences? If that were the case, we would have to reject Kantian ethics as absurd. In deciding which course of action to take, of course we need to think about the impact on others. Rather, consequences are relevant for Kant only if the proposed action is morally permissible. And the permissibility of an action is not determined by the consequences.

If the permissibility of an action is not determined by its consequences, how is it determined? Or, to put the question another way, what makes right actions right and wrong actions wrong? There is widespread agreement that certain actions, such as lying, stealing, cheating, and harming others, are wrong. The fundamental question for Kant is *why* these things are wrong. The utilitarian answer is that such actions predictably lead to human misery. Kant considers this answer to be inadequate. He would say that even if no one gets hurt by a wrong action, even if it promotes more happiness than unhappiness, that does not make it right. Lying, stealing, and murder are intrinsically wrong; they cannot be made right by their creation of happiness.

Take cheating on examinations, for example. The utilitarian objection is based on the expected bad consequences. Would you want someone who graduated from law school or medical school by cheating to be your lawyer or doctor? Of course not. In addition, cheating quickly becomes insidious and demoralizes those who do not cheat. If "everyone is doing it" and getting away with it, then why put the effort into actually learning the material? The negative consequences of cheating are easily demonstrated.

However, these utilitarian objections to cheating could be met in certain circumstances. What if only a few people cheat while most remain honest? It is far from obvious that an isolated instance of cheating will necessarily have more bad effects than good. It is not always the case that successful cheating results in an unqualified person posing a risk to others. Imagine, for example, a very good student in a college with an honor code; this student accidentally comes across the answers to his physical anatomy exam. This gives him the opportunity to "ace" what will certainly be a very difficult exam and improve considerably his chances of getting into a top medical school. Should he use the answers? It seems obvious that this would be wrong, but it is not clear that the wrongness stems from the consequences. It cannot be said that cheating in this situation will enable an unqualified student to go on to practice medicine since we are assuming that the student is qualified.

Yet, this will not guarantee him a place in medical school, given the competition for admission. Of course, there is the chance that he will be found out, in which case he may be expelled. But, what if the chances of anyone finding out that he has seen the answers are extremely low? If no one finds out, then the subsequent demoralization and widespread cheating that are often alleged to be consequences of particular acts of cheating will not occur.

From a consequentialist perspective, the likelihood of the bad effects actually occurring is all-important. Yet, most of us do not base the judgment that he should not use the answers on how probable it is that he will be caught, or what the effect on other students will be, or whether he will go on to a brilliant medical career. Instead, if asked *why* it is wrong for him to use the answers, even if none of these bad consequences will occur, then we are likely simply to say, "It's still cheating." This captures the Kantian idea that the morally relevant consideration is not the consequences of the act but the *kind* of act it is. An act can have the best consequences—for example, save the most lives, make the greatest number of people happiest—and still be morally wrong.

If consequences do not determine the rightness or wrongness of actions, what then is the mark of right and wrong for Kant? Kant suggests that when we want to know if a proposed action (like cheating on an exam) is morally permissible, the question to ask ourselves is not "What are the likely consequences of doing this act?" but rather "Can I, as a rational agent, consistently will that everyone should act as I am now proposing to act?" If we turn this question into an action-guiding principle (what Kant calls a *command* or an *imperative*), we get "Act only on the maxim of an action that you can consistently will universally." Kant calls this principle the *categorical imperative*. What does it mean?

The intuitive idea is that morality requires us not to make exceptions of ourselves. We are not morally permitted to do things that we would regard as wrong if done by others. It does not matter that no one gets hurt as a result. An action is wrong if you cannot consistently will that everyone in this situation act in the way you propose to act.

How is this applied to the example of cheating? A typical misunderstanding is that universalizing the maxim (from "I should cheat" to "Everyone should cheat") would have bad results. If everyone cheated, then exams would be useless, and that would be unfortunate since exams are a good way to determine who is most qualified. However, this interpretation is not Kantian, but utilitarian, specifically rule-utilitarian, since it is based on the advantage to society of having exams. Kant's point is importantly different. The wrongness of cheating is not based on the social utility of having an examination system. Rather, it is literally impossible for cheating to be adopted openly as a universal policy. It is this feature that makes it impossible for a rational agent to will such a policy.

Someone who refrains from cheating, not out of fear of getting caught, and not even because he or she thinks that cheating will have bad consequences for everyone, but simply because the person's recognition that it is wrong (that is, that it contravenes the categorical imperative), acts from the motive of duty. For Kant, only those acts done from the motive of duty have genuine moral worth. Acts done out of sympathy, for example, lack real moral worth, although they are certainly not wrong and indeed should be encouraged.

This is perhaps the hardest aspect of Kantian ethics to understand. Why should not feelings be a source of moral behavior? Why should not an action that derives from sympathy be as morally praiseworthy as one done out of a sense of duty? Kant's answer is that our feelings are not something we can control, and therefore they are not something for which we can be held responsible. Rational agents can be expected to act rightly (that is, consistently with the categorical imperative) but not to have certain feelings. Indeed, doing the right thing (sharing one's possessions, helping others) is more praiseworthy if one does it even when one is feeling antisocial and misanthropic.

A central Kantian idea is that persons are ends in themselves, who have values and goals and make choices and decisions. As rational agents, persons have dignity and are entitled to respect. To treat individuals as persons is to respect their values and choices insofar as these are morally permissible. This means that people must never be treated merely as the means to others' ends.

Communitarian Ethics

Despite their differences, utilitarianism and Kantian ethics share some presuppositions. Both regard the individual as the focal point of moral concern. Although utilitarianism seeks to promote the greatest happiness of the greatest number, it determines what that is by reference to individual preferences. Kantian ethics also focuses on individuals in its insistence that the rights and dignity of the individual should never be sacrificed for the welfare of the whole. Both ethical approaches also share the central liberal idea that since different individuals have different values and different conceptions of the good life, society should remain neutral between these conceptions and not adopt any particular conception to the exclusion of others. The categorical imperative, for example, is consistent with many different ways of life. It gives very little positive guidance on how best to live. And while the principle of utility instructs us to maximize welfare, it leaves the determination of what constitutes an individual's welfare up to the individual. Mill was particularly insistent that the individual is best positioned to know what is in his or her own interest.

Recently, there has been a reaction to the emphasis on the individual in the dominant ethical theories by somewhat disparate groups of theorists who can be labeled *communitarians*. Communitarians reject the notion of timeless, universal ethical truths based on reason. Instead, they maintain that our moral thinking has its source in historical traditions of particular communities. Communities are not simply collections of individuals who happen to inhabit the same geographical area. Rather, they are composed of people who share customs, institutions, and values. These provide the starting point from which attempts to solve ethical problems must begin.

Perhaps the most important feature of communitarian ethics for our purposes is its idea of a *common good*. Whereas utilitarianism seeks to promote the welfare of all individuals taken together, communitarianism looks to the *shared* values, ideals, and goals of a community. It asks what kind of community we want to live in and uses this, rather than individual welfare exclusively, as guidance in determining social policy.

A problem for communitarians is that the individuals who make up communities may have very different ideas of what the community should be like. Which vision of "the good life" or "the good society" should prevail? Does not communitarianism, like utilitarianism, threaten a "tyranny of the majority"? In response, communitarians argue that even people with very different values will have shared values. Education is a good example of a shared value. That is, over and above each person's interest in becoming educated, the community as a whole has an interest in seeing that its citizens are educated. This is essential if the society is to be healthy economically and if democracy (another shared value of our community) is to operate. Undoubtedly, different individuals and groups will have different ideas about what and how the schools should teach, and these differences will have to be worked out in democratic fashion, which includes issues related to private schools, religious schools, and home schooling. Nevertheless, the commitment of the society to educating the young is a shared value.

The health of the public is another shared value. Not only does each individual have an interest in staying healthy but also all of us together share an interest in having a healthy population. Again, we may disagree about the best ways to promote the public's health and how to weigh individual liberty against the welfare of the whole. Nevertheless, reducing disease, saving lives, and promoting good health are shared values, part of the common good. As public health is fundamentally an effort to promote these shared goals, public health is a species of communitarianism.

Communitarianism challenges the libertarian or market model, which places the highest value on liberty. Liberty here means the absence of restraint, not the liberty to accomplish certain goals, which is often called *positive liberty*. Libertarians see the government as the biggest threat to liberty in the modern state because government controls the means of violence and coercion. They regard the market as the most efficient way to expand liberty for all citizens.

Like libertarians, liberals also place a high value on individual liberty. However, liberty is not the sole value for liberals: Social and economic equality is also a desirable end. Furthermore, liberals do not embrace the market with the same enthusiasm as libertarians. Liberals believe that the government has a significant role to play in regulating the market and offering some form of social safety net that includes health care for the needy, employment and education programs, and pensions to protect the elderly.

Communitarians share with liberals the view that the market needs to be controlled and regulated to protect people. But where liberals tend to think solely in terms of harms and benefits to individuals and to insist that individuals determine their own ends and goods, communitarians stress goods that are held or enjoyed in common: clean air and water, the environment, education, and the public's health and safety. These goods cannot be achieved by individual effort alone but must be obtained by collective action and new institutions. Moreover, such collective action and new institutions not only promote the common good but also can strengthen the allegiance of individuals to the community.

Theory and Practice

Different ethical theories provide different basic principles for deciding what is right or wrong, what should be done or avoided. However, ethical decision making is almost never a matter of automatically applying principles and generating an answer. There are several reasons why this is so. One reason is that the right thing to do often depends on the facts of the case, and these may be difficult to ascertain. For example, at the beginning of the human immunodeficiency virus/acquired immunodeficiency syndrome (HIV/AIDS) epidemic there was much discussion about whether public health officials should close gay bathhouses. Those who argued in favor said that the bathhouses, which were places where men could engage with dozens of partners, were breeding grounds for the spread of disease. Those who opposed said that closing the bathhouses would not change behavior. Men would continue to have multiple partners in more private settings, and the opportunity to educate people about safe sex would be lost. Both sides made a plausible case, and it was not obvious which strategy would reduce the spread of AIDS.

Another reason why principles cannot be used to generate solutions in any straightforward way is that they sometimes conflict with one another as well as with other values or goals. For example, an important principle or goal of public health is to reduce the incidence of disease. Genetic diseases can be prevented by screening people to find out who are carriers and then attempting to influence them not to reproduce and thereby pass on genes that cause disease. But it can be argued that any attempt to influence individuals' reproductive decision making violates another important principle, namely, self-determination or autonomy. Which value—the reduction of disease or respect for autonomy—should take precedence? The answer is not obvious. Thus, even if we could decide which ethical theory is the correct one, the application of that theory to specific practical issues will often be indeterminate or controversial. In any event, there is no consensus about the right ethical theory. This fact is often discouraging to students, who may become cynical about the value of studying moral philosophy. What's the point, if no one can say whether utilitarianism is superior to Kantian ethics, or if both are superseded by contractarianism, virtue ethics, or feminist approaches?

We maintain that this disillusionment is unwarranted. The purpose of studying moral philosophy is not to discover which ethical theory "has it right"; rather, different ethical theories provide insight into a range of important considerations. Utilitarians are right to insist on the relevance of consequences and the importance of securing happiness and well-being, but their critics (nonconsequentialists) are equally right in insisting that there are other important values, such as justice and self-determination, that cannot be reduced to happiness. It seems increasingly likely that no one moral theory is the whole story. Rather, each represents a partial contribution to an extraordinarily complex moral reality.

Recall our discussion of the Kantian principle that human beings should be treated as ends in themselves and never as mere means. This notion is the basis of the notion, growing out of the Nuremberg trials, that it is ethically mandatory to obtain informed consent from patients and human subjects used in medical and scientific experiments. One of the most blatant examples of the violation of the principle of informed consent occurred in the Tuskegee syphilis experiment.

To some extent, utilitarianism can explain the horrific wrongness of the Tuskegee syphilis experiment: Men who could have been cured of a devastating disease were allowed to go blind and mad and ultimately die. However, even if no cure was available, and therefore none of the subjects were harmed or made worse off by being in the study, it was still wrong, starting at its inception. This judgment is best explained in Kantian terms. It is wrong to conduct medical experiments, regardless of their potential social value and independent of the harm that may be inflicted, on persons who have not given their free and informed consent. To use people in this way is to treat them as mere means, rather than ends in themselves.

Public health has a clear utilitarian or consequentialist component. It aims to promote human welfare and reduce human misery and is solidly based on factual evidence. At the same time, it is limited by Kantian or deontological considerations, such as respect for persons and their rights. The hard questions arise when individual rights clash with the general welfare. Rights theorists maintain that rights "trump" consideration of the general welfare, but surely this depends on the nature and significance of the right claimed as well as the magnitude of risk to the general population. This issue may be traced like a leitmotif through the chapters to follow.

Many philosophers have seen the principal issue of public health as that of paternalism or the intrusion of the state on individual liberty to promote health and safety, such as with requirements that individuals wear seat belts while using automobiles. These kinds of issues were not seen as inherently exciting or as illuminating of the future that was coming for medicine and ethics. Yet, the ethical disputes in public health are far more extensive than the debates over paternalism would suggest. What is the nature of the population? Of the community? Does the community share a common good? Who bears the burdens of prevention? Should public health turn away from moralism, the use of the law to promote a specific morality, altogether, even when that morality might reduce the risks of contracting a dread disease? What do all Americans deserve when it comes to health care, and can the market provide affordable health care for all? Should we provide health care for all in a way that recognizes its character as a common good and in a way that promotes a sense of sharing something in common? What is the ethical relevance of emergent new epidemics and ecological threats, worldwide? These are the issues we turn to in the readings that follow.

Notes

1. Nancy E. Kass, "An Ethics Framework for Public Health," *American Journal of Public Health* 91(11): November 2002, 1776–1782. James F. Childress, Ruth R. Faden, Ruth D. Garre, Lawrence O. Gostin, Jeffrey Kahn, Richard J. Bonnie, Nancy E. Kass, Anna C. Mastroianni, Jonathan D. Moreno, and Phillip Nieburg, "Public Health Ethics: Mapping the Terrain," *Journal of Law, Medicine, and Ethics* 30: 2002, 170–178.

2. This typology is drawn from Daniel Callahan and Bruce Jennings, "Ethics and Public Health: Forging a Strong Relationship," *American Journal of Public Health* 92(2): February 2002, 169–176.

3. John Stuart Mill, *Utilitarianism* (1861), ed. George Sher (Indianapolis, IN: Hackett, 1979), p. 7.

4. Jeremy Bentham, "An Introduction to the Principles of Morals and Legislation," chapter 17, paragraph 4 in J. H. Burns and H. L. A. Hart, eds., *The Collected Works of Jeremy Bentham* (London: Oxford University Press, 1970), p. 283.

5. Mill, *Utilitarianism*, p. 11.

6. Peter Singer, *Animal Liberation* (New York: Avon Books, 1975).

7. Mill, *Utilitarianism*, p. 17.

8. Ibid., p. 22.

9. President's Commission for the Study of Ethical Problems in Medicine and Biomedical and Behavioral Research, *Screening and Counseling for Genetic Conditions* (Washington, DC: Government Printing Office, 1983), chapter 2, pp. 47–48.

10. Kant's best-known work on ethics is *Groundwork (or Foundations) of the Metaphysic of Morals* (originally published 1785; repr. Immanuel Kant, *Foundations of the Metaphysics of Morals with Critical Essays*, ed. Robert Paul Wolff, trans. Lewis White Beck [Indianapolis: Bobbs-Merrill, 1969]).

Further Reading

Bayer, Ronald, and Amy L. Fairchild, "The Genesis of Public Health Ethics," *Bioethics* 18(6): November 2004, 473–492.

Beauchamp, Dan E., *The Health of the Republic: Epidemics, Medicine, and Moralism as Challenges to Democracy* (Philadelphia: Temple University Press, 1988).

Childress, James F., Ruth R. Faden, Ruth D. Gaare. Lawrence P. Gostin, Jeffrey Kahn, Richard J. Bonnie, Nancy E. Kass, Anna C. Mastroianni, Jonathan D. Moreno, and Phillip Nieburg, "Public Health Ethics: Mapping the Terrain," *Journal of Law, Medicine & Ethics* 30(2): Summer 2002, 170–178.

Goodman, Richard A., Mark A. Rothstein, Richard E. Hoffman, Wilfredo Lopez, and Gene W. Matthews, eds., *Law in Public Health Practice* (Oxford: Oxford University Press, 2002).

Gostin, Lawrence O., *Public Health Law* (Berkeley: University of California Press, 2001).

Gostin, Lawrence O., ed., *Public Health Law and Ethics: A Reader* (Berkeley: University of California Press, 2002).

Gostin, Lawrence O., ed., "Symposium: Public Health Law and Ethics," *Journal of Law, Medicine & Ethics* 30(2): Summer 2002.

Jennings, Bruce, "Frameworks for Ethics in Public Health," *Acta Bioethica* 9(2): 2003, 165–176.

Jennings, Bruce, Jeffrey Kahn, Anna Mastroianni, and Lisa S. Parker, eds., *Ethics and Public Health: Model Curriculum* (Washington, DC: Association of Schools of Public Health, 2003). Also available online at http://www.asph.org/document.cfm?page=782.

Kass, Nancy E., "Public Health Ethics: From Foundations and Frameworks to Justice and Global Public Health," *Journal of Law, Medicine, & Ethics* 32(2): Summer 2004, 232–242.

Lappé, Marc, "Ethics and Public Health," in John M. Last, ed., *Maxcy-Rosenau Public Health and Preventive Medicine,* 12th ed. (Norwalk, CT: Appleton-Century-Crofts, 1986), pp. 1867–1877.

Mann, Jonathan M., "Medicine and Public Health, Ethics and Human Rights," *Hastings Center Report* 27(3): May/June 1997, 6–13.

Mann, Jonathan M., Sofia Gruskin, Michael A. Grodin, and George J. Annas, eds., *Health and Human Rights: A Reader* (New York: Routledge, 1999).

Morone, James A., "Enemies of the People: The Moral Dimension to Public Health," *Journal of Health Politics, Policy, & Law* 22(4): August 1997, 993–1020.

Singer, Peter, ed., *A Companion to Ethics* (Oxford: Blackwell, 1993).

PART I

THE PUBLIC HEALTH PERSPECTIVE

Introduction

A book that seeks to inform readers about public health ethics, a concept that overlaps with but is distinct from biomedical ethics, must begin with an explanation of the public health perspective. It is helpful, therefore, to explore the meaning of *public health* and how it differs from medicine and health care. Public health, like medicine, is not fixed or static, but rather is richly informed by history, culture, politics, and law. Throughout part I, and this volume itself, we draw attention to the sociopolitical dimensions of public health. In many ways, public health cannot be separated from society and politics because public health requires the allocation of resources, the exercise of the state's authority, and the judgments of officials elected and appointed.[1]

Perhaps the single most important feature of public health is that it strives to improve the functioning and longevity of populations. The field's purpose is to monitor and evaluate the health status of populations, as well as to devise strategies and interventions designed to ease the burden of injury, disease, and disability. Public health interventions save statistical lives and reduce rates of injury and disease within populations. These savings are of real lives, but the savings cannot be linked to specific persons. This creates a political problem because public health officials cannot claim credit for rescuing identifiable persons—credit that has a powerful appeal in a culture of individualism.[2]

Public health differs from medicine, which has a primary focus on the individual patient. The physician diagnoses disease and offers medical treatment to ease symptoms and, if possible, to cure. Access to high-quality medical care is one of many conditions necessary for good health. Public health, on the other hand, seeks to understand the conditions and causes of ill-health (and good health) in the populace as a whole. It seeks to ensure a favorable environment in which people can maintain their health. Public health is, of course, concerned about individuals because of their inherent worth and because a population is healthy only if its constituents (individuals) are relatively free from injury and disease. Indeed, many public health agencies offer medical care for the poor, particularly for conditions that have "spillover" effects for the wider community, such as treatment for sexually transmitted diseases (STDs), tuberculosis (TB), and HIV/AIDS.

For public health, though, prevention is preeminent. Public health historians often tell a classic story of the power of prevention. In September 1854, John Snow wrote, "The most terrible outbreak of cholera which ever occurred in this Kingdom, is probably that which took place in Broad Street, Golden Square [Soho, London], and the adjoining streets, a few weeks ago." Snow, a celebrated epidemiologist, linked the cholera outbreak to a single source of polluted water, the Broad Street pump. He convinced the Board of Guardians of St. James's Parish, in whose parish the pump fell, to remove the pump handle as an experiment. Within a week, the outbreak was all but over, with the death toll standing at 616 Sohoites.[3]

Typical of public health interventions are vaccination against infectious diseases, health education to reduce risk behavior, fluoridation to avert dental caries, and seat belts or motorcycle helmets to avoid injuries. Medicine, by contrast, is often focused on the amelioration or cure of injuries or diseases after they have occurred. But prevention and amelioration, of course, are not mutually exclusive. Medicine is also concerned with prevention, as physicians often counsel patients to avoid risk behaviors such as smoking, consumption of high-fat foods, unprotected sex, or excessive use of alcoholic beverages. At the same time, public health is attentive to the claims of amelioration. As noted, health departments frequently offer health care for the poor. The goals of medicine and public health are especially intertwined in the field of infectious diseases, in which medical treatment can dramatically reduce contagiousness. The individual benefits from treatment, and society benefits from reduced exposure to disease.

Inherent in public health is a deep theoretical, historical, and constitutional relationship to government. Individuals acting alone can accomplish a great deal to achieve health protection, particularly if they have the means to purchase the necessities of life (e.g., medical care, housing, and nutritious food). However, only the state can truly safeguard the public's health and well-being.

The legal maxim *salus populi est suprema lex* (the welfare of the people is the supreme law) demonstrates the close connection between state power and the public's well-being. From a constitutional perspective, the "police power" provides the historic wellspring of authority to protect the common welfare. The linguistic origins of the concept of *police* demonstrate the close association between public health and governmental authority: *politia* (the state), *polis* (the city), and *politeia* (citizenship).[4] The seminal Supreme Court case of *Jacobson v. Massachusetts* explains the jurisprudential rationale behind the police power:

> A fundamental principle of the social compact [is] that the whole people covenants with each citizen, and each citizen with the whole people, that all shall be governed by certain laws for the "common good. . . ." [G]overnment is instituted . . . "for the protection, safety, prosperity and happiness of the people, and not for the profit, honor or private interests of any one man, family or class of men."[5]

But however extensive the authority of the state to protect the public's health and safety, there are limits.[6] Indeed, the tensions between agency power and restraints on power are central to the study of public health. When government acts to promote the common good, it often diminishes individual interests in autonomy, privacy, and liberty. The exercise of police powers also affects economic interests, particularly when agencies regulate businesses and professionals. The study of public health ethics requires students to conceptualize and carefully evaluate the inevitable tensions between individual rights and collective interests.[7] These issues are compounded by controversies about the legitimate scope of public health.[8] Contemporary public health embraces a broad approach, addressing the socioeconomic and cultural foundations of morbidity, mortality, and well-being.[9] Public health advocates have ventured into policies ranging from poverty, homelessness, and social inequalities, to racism, gender discrimination, homophobia, violence, and war.[10] Their claim is that significant health improvement at the population level can occur only by addressing root determinants of health.

Critics of this broad conception of public health prefer a targeted and by definition narrower approach that focuses on discrete governmental interventions to prevent the immediate causes of morbidity and premature mortality.[11] Traditional infectious disease measures, for example, include screening, reporting, partner notification, directly observed therapy, and isolation. Opponents of the broad conceptualization of the public health mandate claim that, by overreaching, public health will lose its authoritative status, its special mission. They may acknowledge the empirical evidence demonstrating the impact of social inequalities on health and the insights of demographers like Thomas McKeon,[12] who demonstrated the impact of nutritional status on the decline of tuberculosis. However, adherents of a focused public health mission cite immunization as one of but many examples of how carefully defined public health interventions can have profound impacts. Further, they note that the outbreak of tuberculosis at the end of the 1980s and early 1990s, as well as the threat of drug-resistant tuberculosis, was brought to an end by effective tuberculosis control measures, including directly observed therapy. It was not a change in the fundamental social conditions of those at risk for tuberculosis that could account for this important public health achievement. Finally, critics of the broad approach have argued that public health officials lack the expertise and authority to tackle so many diverse topics, from socioeconomic conditions in society to global issues like war, racism, and sexism.

Public health in many respects is caught in a dilemma. On the one hand, public health professionals have deep intuitions that the population's health is significantly affected by the social, economic, and cultural contexts in which people live. On the other hand, the more public health officials advocate for structural change and redistribution of resources within societies, the greater the risk of alienation from elected officials and the public at large.

There may be a deeper level of tension here. Public health is by definition an arm of the state and a profession of public service. It must work within the bounds of the law and respect the judgments of elected officials. Yet, public health often functions as a voice of social conscience and a champion for the disadvantaged, who disproportionately suffer from injury, disability, and disease. It is not always easy for public health officials to "speak truth to power."

The four selections for part I offer insights into the public health perspective as well as its scope. The first selection is the classic article by the British epidemiologist Geoffrey Rose, "Sick Individuals and Sick Populations." Rose makes the simple, but insightful, observation that a "preventive measure which brings much benefit to the population offers little to each participating individual." This is a "prevention paradox" because populations are made up of individuals; how, then, can one benefit a population without benefiting the individuals who compose it? The fact is that improving the health of populations results in disappointingly small improvements to the health of any *given* individual.

In the second selection, Dan Beauchamp explores the aforementioned tension between the preeminence of individualism in American culture and the collective goals of public health. After describing the history of public health regulatory authority, which flows from the idea that government is charged with protecting both private *and* group interests, he concludes by highlighting the risk in ignoring the "communitarian language of public health."

Chapter 3 turns to a selection written by members of the influential Institute of Medicine (IOM) Committee on the Future of the Public's Health in the Twenty-first Century. This report provides an important account of the all-encompassing perspective of public health. Lawrence O. Gostin, Jo Ivey Boufford, and Rose Marie Martinez explain the key IOM proposals and go further by suggesting concrete ways to raise the standards of public health agencies and hold them accountable.

Many of the critiques of the broad public health perspective are informed by a conservative perspective resistant to the expansion of government programs.[13] Mark A. Rothstein's critique, in the final selection, is sympathetic to public health. Yet, he still places boundaries on the legitimate scope of public health action: "public health officials taking appropriate measures pursuant to specific legal authority, after balancing private rights and public interests. . . ."

Notes

1. Bayer, Ronald, and Jonathan D. Moreno, "Health Promotion: Ethical and Social Dilemmas of Government Policy," *Health Affairs* 5: Summer 1986, 72–85.

2. Burris, Scott, "The Invisibility of Public Health: Population-Level Measures in a Politics of Market Individualism," *American Journal of Public Health* 87: 1997, 1607–1610.

3. Summers, Judith, *Soho—A History of London's Most Colourful Neighborhood* (London: Bloomsbury, 1989), pp. 113–117.

4. Novak, William J., *The People's Welfare: Law and Regulation in Nineteenth-Century America* (Chapel Hill: University of North Carolina Press, 1996).

5. 197 U.S. 11, 26–27 (1905).

6. For a systematic examination of governmental public health power and limits on that power, see Lawrence O. Gostin, *Public Health Law: Power, Duty, Restraint* (Berkeley and New York: University of California Press and Milbank Memorial Fund, 2nd ed. forthcoming, 2007).

7. Callahan, Daniel, and Bruce Jennings, "Ethics and Public Health: Forging a Strong Relationship," *American Journal of Public Health* 92: 2002, 169–176.

8. Beaglehole, Robert, and R. Bonita, *Public Health at the Crossroads: Achievements and Prospects* (New York: Cambridge University Press, 1997).

9. Pearce, Neil, "Traditional Epidemiology, Modern Epidemiology, and Public Health," *American Journal of Public Health* 86: 1996, 678–683.

10. Rothman, Kenneth J., Hans-Olov Adami, and Dimitrios Trichopoulos, "Should the Mission of Epidemiology Include the Eradication of Poverty?" *Lancet* 352: 5 September 1998, 810–813.

11. Satel, Sally L., *PC MD: How Political Correctness Is Corrupting Medicine* (New York: Basic Books, 2000).

12. McKeon, Thomas, *The Role of Medicine: Dream, Mirage or Nemesis?* (London: Nuffield Provincial Hospital Trust, 1976).

13. Epstein, Richard A., "Let the Shoemaker Stick to His Last: A Defense of the 'Old' Public Health," *Perspectives in Biology and Medicine* 46(3) Suppl.: Summer 2003, S138–S159.

1

Sick Individuals and Sick Populations

Geoffrey Rose

The Determinants of Individual Cases

In teaching epidemiology to medical students, I have often encouraged them to consider a question which I first heard enunciated by Roy Acheson: "Why did *this* patient get *this* disease at *this* time?" It is an excellent starting point because students and doctors feel a natural concern for the problems of the individual. Indeed, the central ethos of medicine is seen as an acceptance of responsibility for sick individuals.

It is an integral part of good doctoring to ask not only, "What is the diagnosis, and what is the treatment?" but also, "Why did this happen, and could it have been prevented?" Such thinking shapes the approach to nearly all clinical and laboratory research into the causes and mechanisms of illness. Hypertension research, for example, is almost wholly preoccupied with the characteristics which distinguish individuals at the hypertensive and normotensive ends of the blood pressure distribution. Research into diabetes looks for genetic, nutritional, and metabolic reasons to explain why some people get diabetes and others do not. The constant aim in such work is to answer Acheson's question, "Why did *this* patient get this disease at this time?"

The same concern has continued to shape the thinking of all of us who came to epidemiology from a background in clinical practice. The whole basis of the case-control method is to discover how sick and healthy individuals differ. Equally the basis of many cohort studies is the search for "risk factors," which identify certain individuals as being more susceptible to disease, and from this we proceed to test whether these risk factors are also causes, capable of explaining why some individuals get sick while others remain healthy, and applicable as a guide to prevention.

To confine attention in this way to within-population comparisons has caused much confusion (particularly in the clinical world) in the definition of normality. Laboratory "ranges of normal" are based on what is common within the local population. Individuals with "normal blood pressure" are those who do not stand out from their local contemporaries and so on. What is common is all right, we presume.

Applied to etiology, the individual-centered approach leads to the use of relative risk as the basic representation of etiological force, that is, "the risk in exposed individuals relative to risk in non-exposed individuals." Indeed, the concept of relative risk has almost excluded any other approach to quantifying causal importance. It may generally be the best measure of etiological force, but it is no measure at all of etiological outcome or of public health importance.

Unfortunately this approach to the search for causes, and the measuring of their potency, has to assume a heterogeneity of exposure within the study population. If everyone smoked 20 cigarettes a day, then clinical, case-control, and cohort studies alike would lead us to conclude that lung cancer was a genetic disease, and in one sense that would be true since if everyone is exposed to the necessary agent, then the distribution of cases is wholly determined by individual susceptibility.

Within Scotland and other mountainous parts of Britain (figure 1.1, left section),[1] there is no discernible relation between local cardiovascular death rates and the softness of the public water supply. The reason is apparent if one extends the enquiry to the whole of the United Kingdom. In Scotland, everyone's water is soft, and the possibly adverse effect becomes recognizable only when study is extended to other regions which have a much wider range of exposure ($r = -0.67$). Even more clearly, a case-control study of this question within Scotland would have been futile. Everyone is exposed, and other factors operate to determine the varying risk.

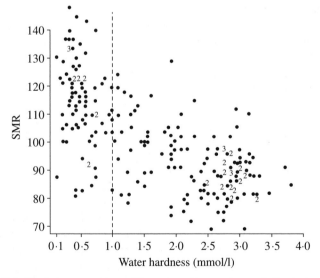

Figure 1.1 Relation between water quality and cardiovascular mortality in towns of the United Kingdom.

   Epidemiology is often defined in terms of study of the determinants of the distribution of the disease, but we should not forget that the more widespread is a particular cause, the less it explains the distribution of cases. The hardest cause to identify
is the one that is universally present, for then it has no influence on the distribution
of disease.

The Determinants of Population
Incidence Rate

I find it increasingly helpful to distinguish two kinds of etiological question. The first
seeks the causes of cases, and the second seeks the causes of incidence. "Why do
some individuals have hypertension?" is a quite different question from "Why do
some populations have much hypertension, while in others it is rare?" The questions
require different kinds of study, and they have different answers.

   Figure 1.2 shows the systolic blood pressure distributions of middle-aged men in
two populations—Kenyan nomads[2] and London civil servants.[3] The familiar question, "Why do some individuals have higher blood pressure than others?" could be
equally well asked in either of these settings, since in each the individual blood pressures vary (proportionately) to about the same extent, and the answers might well be
much the same in each instance (that is, mainly genetic variation, with a lesser component from environmental and behavioral differences). We might achieve a complete understanding of why individuals vary, and yet quite miss the most important
public health question, namely, "Why is hypertension absent in the Kenyans and
common in London?" The answer to that question has to do with the determinants of
the population mean, for what distinguishes the two groups is nothing to do with the
characteristics of individuals, it is rather a shift of the whole distribution—a mass
influence acting on the population as a whole. To find the determinants of prevalence and incidence rates, we need to study characteristics of populations, not characteristics of individuals.

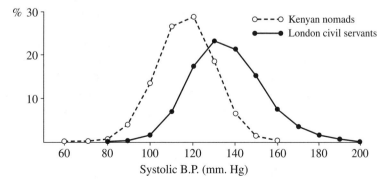

Figure 1.2 Distributions of systolic blood pressure in middle-aged men in two
populations.

A more extreme example is provided by the population distributions of serum cholesterol levels[4] in East Finland, where coronary heart disease is very common, and Japan, where the incidence rate is low: The two distributions barely overlap. Each country has men with relative hypercholesterolemia (although their definitions of the range of "normal" would no doubt disagree), and one could research into the genetic and other causes of these unusual individuals; but if we want to discover why Finland has such a high incidence of coronary heart disease we need to look for those characteristics of the national diet which have so elevated the whole cholesterol distribution. Within populations it has proved almost impossible to demonstrate any relation between an individual's diet and his serum cholesterol level; and the same applies to the relation of individual diet to blood pressure and to overweight. But at the level of populations it is a different story: It has proved easy to show strong associations between population mean values for saturated fat intake versus serum cholesterol level and coronary heart disease incidence, sodium intake versus blood pressure, or energy intake versus overweight. The determinants of incidence are not necessarily the same as the causes of cases.

How Do the Causes of Cases Relate to the Causes of Incidence?

This is largely a matter of whether exposure varies similarly within a population and between populations (or over a period of time within the same population). Softness of water supply may be a determinant of cardiovascular mortality, but it is unlikely to be identifiable as a risk factor for individuals because exposure tends to be locally uniform. Dietary fat is, I believe, the main determinant of a population's incidence rate for coronary heart disease, but it quite fails to identify high-risk individuals.

In the case of cigarettes and lung cancer, it so happened that the study populations contained about equal numbers of smokers and nonsmokers, and in such a situation case-control and cohort studies were able to identify what was also the main determinant of population differences and time trends.

There is a broad tendency for genetic factors to dominate individual susceptibility but to explain rather little of population differences in incidence. Genetic heterogeneity, it seems, is mostly much greater within than between populations. This is the contrary situation to that seen for environmental factors. Thus migrants, whatever the color of their skin, tend to acquire the disease rates of their country of adoption.

Most noninfectious diseases are still of largely unknown cause. If you take a textbook of medicine and look at the list of contents, you will still find, despite all our etiological research, that most are still of basically unknown etiology. We know quite a lot about the personal characteristics of individuals who are susceptible to them, but for a remarkably large number of our major noninfectious diseases we still do not know the determinants of the incidence rate.

Over a period of time we find that most diseases are in a state of flux. For example, duodenal ulcer in Britain at the turn of the century was an uncommon condition affecting mainly young women. During the first half of the century the incidence rate rose steadily, and it became very common, but now the disease seems to be disappearing, and yet we have no clues to the determinants of these striking changes in incidence rates. One could repeat that story for many conditions.

There is hardly a disease whose incidence rate does not vary widely, either over time or between populations at the same time. This means that these causes of incidence rate, unknown though they are, are not inevitable. It is possible to live without them, and if we knew what they were it might be possible to control them. But, to identify the causal agent by the traditional case-control and cohort methods will be unsuccessful if there are not sufficient differences in exposure within the study population at the time of the study. In those circumstances all that these traditional methods do is to find markers of individual susceptibility. The clues must be sought from differences between populations or from changes within populations over time.

Prevention

These two approaches to etiology—the individual and the population based—have their counterparts in prevention. In the first, preventive strategy seeks to identify high-risk susceptible individuals and to offer them some individual protection. In contrast, the "population strategy" seeks to control the determinants of incidence in the population as a whole.

The "High-Risk" Strategy

This is the traditional and natural medical approach to prevention. If a doctor accepts that he is responsible for an individual who is sick today, then it is a short step to accept responsibility also for the individual who may well be sick tomorrow. Thus screening is used to detect certain individuals who hitherto thought they were well but who must now understand that they are in effect patients. This is the process, for example, in the detection and treatment of symptomless hypertension, the transition from healthy subject to patient being ratified by the giving and receiving of tablets. (Anyone who takes medicines is by definition a patient.)

What the "high-risk" strategy seeks to achieve is something like a truncation of the risk distribution. This general concept applies to all special preventive action in high-risk individuals—in at-risk pregnancies, in small babies, or in any other particularly susceptible group. It is a strategy with some clear and important advantages (table 1.1).

Its first advantage is that it leads to intervention which is appropriate to the individual. A smoker who has a cough or who is found to have impaired ventilatory function has a special reason for stopping smoking. The doctor will see it as making sense to advise salt restriction in the hypertensive. In such instances the intervention makes sense because that individual already has a problem which that particular measure may possibly ameliorate. If we consider screening a population to discover those with high serum cholesterol levels and advising them on dietary change, then that intervention is appropriate to those people in particular: They have a diet-related metabolic problem.

Table 1.1 Prevention by the High-Risk Strategy: Advantages

1. Intervention appropriate to individual
2. Subject motivation
3. Physician motivation
4. Cost-effective use of resource
5. Benefit:risk ratio favorable

The high-risk strategy produces interventions that are appropriate to the particular individuals advised to take them. Consequently it has the advantage of enhanced subject motivation. In our randomized controlled trial of smoking cessation in London civil servants we first screened some 20,000 men and from them selected about 1,500 who were smokers with, in addition, markers of specially high risk for cardiorespiratory disease. They were recalled and a random half received antismoking counseling. The results, in terms of smoking cessation, were excellent because those men knew they had a special reason to stop. They had been picked out from others in their offices because, although everyone knows that smoking is a bad thing, they had a special reason why it was particularly unwise for them.

There is, of course, another and less reputable reason why screening enhances subject motivation, and that is the mystique of a scientific investigation. A ventilatory function test is a powerful enhancer of motivation to stop smoking: an instrument which the subject does not quite understand, that looks rather impressive, has produced evidence that he is a special person with a special problem. The electrocardiogram is an even more powerful motivator, if you are unscrupulous enough to use it in prevention. A man may feel entirely well, but if those little squiggles on the paper tell the doctor that he has got trouble, then he must accept that he has now become a patient. That is a powerful persuader. (I suspect it is also a powerful cause of lying awake in the night and thinking about it.)

For rather similar reasons the high-risk approach also motivates physicians. Doctors, quite rightly, are uncomfortable about intervening in a situation where their help was not asked for. Before imposing advice on somebody who was getting on all right without them, they like to feel that there is a proper and special justification in that particular case.

The high-risk approach offers a more cost-effective use of limited resources. One of the things we have learned in health education at the individual level is that once-only advice is a waste of time. To get results we may need a considerable investment of counseling time and follow-up. It is costly in use of time and effort and resources, and therefore it is more effective to concentrate limited medical services and time where the need—and therefore also the benefit—is likely to be greatest.

A final advantage of the high-risk approach is that it offers a more favorable ratio of benefits to risks. If intervention must carry some adverse effects or costs, and if the risk and cost are much the same for everybody, then the ratio of the costs to the benefits will be more favorable where the benefits are larger.

Unfortunately the high-risk strategy of prevention also has some serious disadvantages and limitations (table 1.2). The first centers around the difficulties and costs of screening. Supposing that we were to embark, as some had advocated, on a policy

Table 1.2 Prevention by the High-Risk Strategy:
Disadvantages

1. Difficulties and costs of screening
2. Palliative and temporary, not radical
3. Limited potential for (a) individual, (b) population
4. Behaviorally inappropriate

of screening for high cholesterol levels and giving dietary advice to those individuals at special risk. The disease process we are trying to prevent (atherosclerosis and its complications) begins early in life, so we should have to initiate screening perhaps at the age of 10. However, the abnormality we seek to detect is not a stable lifetime characteristic, so we must advocate repeated screening at suitable intervals.

In all screening one meets problems with uptake and the tendency for the response to be greater among those sections of the population who are often least at risk of the disease. Often there is an even greater problem: Screening detects certain individuals who will receive special advice, but at the same time it cannot help also discovering much larger numbers of "border-liners," that is, people whose results mark them as at increased risk but for whom we do not have an appropriate treatment to reduce their risk.

The second disadvantage of the high-risk strategy is that it is palliative and temporary, not radical. It does not seek to alter the underlying causes of the disease but to identify individuals who are particularly susceptible to those causes. Presumably in every generation there will be such susceptibles, and if prevention and control efforts were confined to these high-risk individuals, then that approach would need to be sustained year after year and generation after generation. It does not deal with the root of the problem, but seeks to protect those who are vulnerable to it, and they will always be around.

The potential for this approach is limited—sometimes more than we could have expected—both for the individual and for the population. There are two reasons for this. The first is that our power to predict future disease is usually very weak. Most individuals with risk factors will remain well, at least for some years; contrariwise, unexpected illness may happen to someone who has just received an "all clear" report from a screening examination. One of the limitations of the relative risk statistic is that it gives no idea of the absolute level of danger. Thus the Framingham Study has impressed us all with its powerful discrimination between high- and low-risk groups, but when we see (figure 1.3)[5] the degree of overlap in serum cholesterol level between future cases and those who remained healthy, it is not surprising that an individual's future is so often misassessed.

Often the best predictor of future major disease is the presence of existing minor disease. A low ventilatory function today is the best predictor of its future rate of decline. A high blood pressure today is the best predictor of its future rate of rise. Early coronary heart disease is better than all the conventional risk factors as a predictor of future fatal disease. However, even if screening includes such tests for early disease, our experience in the Heart Disease Prevention Project (table 1.3)[6] still points to a very weak ability to predict the future of any particular individual.

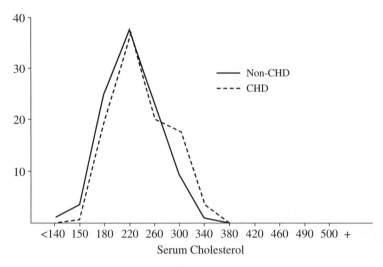

Figure 1.3 Percentage distribution of serum cholesterol levels (mg/dL) in men aged 50–62 who did or did not subsequently develop coronary heart disease (CHD) (Framingham Study).

This point came home to me only recently. I have long congratulated myself on my low levels of coronary risk factors, and I joked to my friends that if I were to die suddenly, I should be very surprised. I even speculated on what other disease—perhaps colon cancer—would be the commonest cause of death for a man in the lowest group of cardiovascular risk. The painful truth is that for such an individual in a Western population the commonest cause of death—by far—is coronary heart disease! Everyone, in fact, is a high-risk individual for this uniquely mass disease.

There is another, related reason why the predictive basis of the high-risk strategy of prevention is weak. It is well illustrated by some data from Alberman and Berry[7] which relate the occurrence of Down syndrome births to maternal age (table 1.4). Mothers under 30 years are individually at minimal risk, but because they are so numerous, they generate half the cases. High-risk individuals aged 40 and above generate only 13 percent of the cases.

The lesson from this example is that *a large number of people at a small risk may give rise to more cases of disease than the small number who are at a high risk*. This

Table 1.3 Five-Year Incidence of Myocardial Infarction (MI) in the U.K. Heart Disease Prevention Project

Entry Characteristic	% of Men	% of MI Cases	MI Incidence Rate, %
Risk factors alone	15	32	7
Ischemia	16	41	11
Ischemia + risk factors	2	12	22
All men	100	100	4

Table 1.4 Incidence of Down Syndrome According to Maternal Age

Maternal Age (years)	Risk of Down Syndrome per 1000 Births	Total Births in Age Group (as % of all ages)	% of Total Down Syndrome Occurring in Age Group
< 30	0.7	78	51
30–34	1.3	16	20
35–39	3.7	5	16
40–44	13.1	0.95	11
> 45	34.6	0.05	2
All ages	1.5	100	100

situation seems to be common, and it limits the utility of the high-risk approach to prevention.

A further disadvantage of the high-risk strategy is that it is behaviorally inappropriate. Eating, smoking, exercise, and all our other lifestyle characteristics are constrained by social norms. If we try to eat differently from our friends it will not only be inconvenient, but we risk being regarded as cranks or hypochondriacs. If a man's work environment encourages heavy drinking, then advice that he is damaging his liver is unlikely to have any effect. No one who has attempted any sort of health education effort in individuals needs to be told that it is difficult for such people to step out of line with their peers. This is what the high-risk preventive strategy requires them to do.

The Population Strategy

This is the attempt to control the determinants of incidence, to lower the mean level of risk factors, to shift the whole distribution of exposure in a favorable direction. In its traditional "public health" form it has involved mass environmental control methods; in its modern form it is attempting (less successfully) to alter some of society's norms of behavior.

The advantages are powerful (table 1.5). The first is that it is radical. It attempts to remove the underlying causes that make the disease common. It has a large potential—often larger than one would have expected—for the population as a whole. From Framingham data one can compute that a 10 mm Hg lowering of the blood pressure distribution as a whole would correspond to about a 30 percent reduction in the total attributable mortality.

The approach is behaviorally appropriate. If nonsmoking eventually becomes "normal," then it will be much less necessary to keep on persuading individuals. Once

Table 1.5 Prevention by the Population Strategy: Advantages

1. Radical
2. Large potential for population
3. Behaviorally appropriate

a social norm of behavior has become accepted and (as in the case of diet) once the supply industries have adapted themselves to the new pattern, then the maintenance of that situation no longer requires effort from individuals. The health education phase aimed at changing individuals is, we hope, a temporary necessity, pending changes in the norms of what is socially acceptable.

Unfortunately the population strategy of prevention has also some weighty drawbacks (table 1.6). It offers only a small benefit to each individual since most of them were going to be all right anyway, at least for many years. This leads to the *prevention paradox*.[8] "A preventive measure which brings much benefit to the population offers little to each participating individual." This has been the history of public health—of immunization, the wearing of seat belts, and now the attempt to change various lifestyle characteristics. Of enormous potential importance to the population as a whole, these measures offer very little—particularly in the short term—to each individual, and thus there is poor motivation of the subject. We should not be surprised that health education tends to be relatively ineffective for individuals and in the short term. Mostly people act for substantial and immediate rewards, and the medical motivation for health education is inherently weak. Their health next year is not likely to be much better if they accept our advice or if they reject it. Much more powerful as motivators for health education are the social rewards of enhanced self-esteem and social approval.

There is also in the population approach only poor motivation of physicians. Many medical practitioners who embarked with enthusiasm on antismoking education have become disheartened because their success rate was no more than 5 or 10 percent: In clinical practice one's expectation of results is higher. Grateful patients are few in preventive medicine, where success is marked by a nonevent. The skills of behavioral advice are different and unfamiliar, and professional esteem is lowered by a lack of skill. Harder to overcome than any of these, however, is the enormous difficulty for medical personnel to see health as a population issue and not merely as a problem for individuals.

In mass prevention, each individual has usually only a small expectation of benefit, and this small benefit can easily be outweighed by a small risk.[8] This happened in the World Health Organization clofibrate trial,[9] where a cholesterol-lowering drug seems to have killed more than it saved, even though the fatal complication rate was only about 1/1,000 per year. Such low-order risks, which can be vitally important to the balance sheet of mass preventive plans, may be hard or impossible to detect. This makes it important to distinguish two approaches. The first is the restoration of biological normality by the removal of an abnormal exposure (e.g., stopping smoking, controlling air pollution, moderating some of our recently acquired dietary deviations); here there can be some presumption of safety. This is not true for the other

Table 1.6 Prevention by the Population Strategy: Disadvantages

1. Small benefit to individual (prevention paradox)
2. Poor motivation of subject
3. Poor motivation of physician
4. Benefit:risk ratio worrisome

kind of preventive approach, which leaves intact the underlying causes of incidence and seeks instead to interpose some new, supposedly protective intervention (e.g., immunization, drugs, jogging). Here, the onus is on the activists to produce adequate evidence of safety.

Conclusions

Case-centered epidemiology identifies individual susceptibility, but it may fail to identify the underlying causes of incidence. The high-risk strategy of prevention is an interim expedient, needed in order to protect susceptible individuals, but only for so long as the underlying causes of incidence remain unknown or uncontrollable; if causes can be removed, susceptibility ceases to matter.

Realistically, many diseases will long continue to call for both approaches, and fortunately competition between them is usually unnecessary. Nevertheless, the priority of concern should always be the discovery and control of the causes of incidence.

References

1. Pocock SJ, Shaper AG, Cook DG, et al. British Regional Heart Study: geographic variations in cardiovascular mortality and the role of water quality. *Br Med J* 1980;283: 1243–1249.

2. Shaper AG. Blood pressure studies in East Africa. In: Stamler J, Stamler R, Pullman TN, eds. *The Epidemiology of Hypertension*. New York: Grune and Stratten; 1967: 139–145.

3. Reid DD, Brett GZ, Hamilton PJS, et al. Cardiorespiratory disease and diabetes among middle-aged male civil servants. *Lancet* 1974;1:469–473.

4. Keys A. *Coronary Heart Disease in Seven Countries*. American Heart Association Monograph Number 29. New York: American Heart Association; 1970.

5. Kannel WB, Garcia MJ, McNamara PM, et al. Serum lipid precursors of coronary heart disease. *Human Pathol* 1971;2:129–151.

6. Heller RF, Chinn S, Tunstall Pedoe HD, et al. How well can we predict coronary heart disease? Findings in the United Kingdom Heart Disease Prevention Project. *Br Med J* 1984;288:1409–1411.

7. Alberman E, Berry C. Prenatal diagnosis and the specialist in community medicine. *Community Med* 1979;1:89–96.

8. Rose G. Strategy of prevention: lessons from cardiovascular disease. *Br Med J* 1981;282:1847–1851.

9. Committee of Principal Investigators. A co-operative trial in the primary prevention of ischaemic heart disease. *Br Heart J* 1978;40:1069–1118.

2

Community

The Neglected Tradition of Public Health

Dan E. Beauchamp

What are the limits of government in protecting the health and safety of the public? As more and more states regulate personal behavior to protect the public health and safety, this question again becomes central. Can there be good reasons for public health paternalism in a democracy? Are health and safety individual interests, or also common and shared ends? . . .

The Meaning of the Common Good

In one version of democratic theory, the state has no legitimate role in restricting personal conduct that is substantially voluntary and that has little or no direct consequence for anyone other than the individual. This strong antipaternalist position is associated with John Stuart Mill. In his essay "On Liberty," which has deeply influenced American and British thought for over 100 years, Mill wrote: "[t]he only purpose for which power can be rightfully exercised over any member of a civilized community, against his will, is to prevent harms to others."[1] Mill restricts paternalism to children and minors. In this view the common good consists in maximizing the freedom of each individual to pursue his or her own interests, subject to a like freedom for every other individual. In the words of Blackstone, "The public good is . . . essentially interested [in] . . . the protection of every individual's private rights."[2]

In a second version, health and safety remain private interests, but some paternalism is accepted, albeit reluctantly. As Joel Feinberg argues, common sense makes us reject a thoroughgoing antipaternalism.[3] Many restrictions on liberty are relatively minor and the savings in life and limb extremely great. Further, often voluntary choices are not completely so; many choices are impaired in some sense. But, as Dennis Thompson contends, even where choices are not impaired, as in the choice not to wear seatbelts or to take up smoking, paternalism might still be accepted because the alternative would be a great loss of life and a society in which each citizen was, for many important decisions, left alone with the consequences of his or her choice.[4]

This reluctant acceptance of paternalism leaves many democrats uneasy. Another alternative is to redefine voluntary risks to an individual as risks to others. Indeed, many argue that all such risks have serious consequences for others, and that the state may therefore limit such activities on the basis of the harm principle.[5] Others challenge the category of voluntariness head on, arguing that most such risks, like cigarettes and alcohol use, have powerful social determinants.[6]

The constitutional basis for the protection of the public health and safety has largely been ignored in this debate. This tradition, and particularly the regulatory power (often called the police power), flows from a view of democracy that sees the essential task of government as protecting and promoting *both* private and group interests. Government is supposed to defend both sets of interests through an evolving set of practices and institutions, and it is left to the legislatures to determine which set of interests predominates when conflicts arise.

In the constitutional tradition, the common good refers to the welfare of individuals considered as a group, the public or the people generally, the "body politic" or the "commonwealth" as it was termed in the early days of the American republic.[7] The public or the people were presumed to have an interest, held in common, in self-protection or preservation from threats of all kinds to their welfare. The commonwealth idea was widely influential among New England states during the first half of the nineteenth century.[8]

The commonwealth doctrine helped shape the regulatory power in Massachusetts and throughout the United States. The central principles underlying the police or regulatory power were the treatment of health and safety as a shared purpose and need of the community and (aside from basic constitutional rights such as due process) the subordination of the market, property, and individual liberty to protect compelling community interests.

This republican image of democracy was a blending of social contract and republican thought, as well as Judeo-Christian notions of covenant. In the republican vision of society, the individual has a dual status. On the one hand, individuals have private interests and private rights; political association serves to protect these rights. On the other hand, individuals are members of a political community—a body politic.

This common citizenship, despite diversity and divergence of interests, presumes an underlying shared set of loyalties and obligations to support the ends of the political community, among which public health and safety are central. In this scheme, public health and safety are not simply the aggregate of each private individual's interests in health and safety, interests which can be pursued more effectively through collective action. Public health and safety are community or group interests (often referred to as "state interests" in the law), interests that can transcend and take priority over private interests if the legislature so chooses.

The idea of democracy as promoting the common or group interest is captured in Joseph Tussman's classic work on political obligation: "Familiar as it is, there is something fundamentally misleading about the slogan that the aim of government is 'welfare of the individual.' . . . [T]he government's concern for the individual is not to be understood as a special concern for *this* or *that* individual but rather as concern for all individuals. Government, that is to say, serves the welfare of the community."[9]

This emphasis on the *public's* health has never meant that the state's power to protect health and safety is unlimited. It has meant that individual liberty and the institutions of the market and private property, operating in the public world, are subject to a developing set of practices designed to defend the common life and the community. Although we call markets "private," all markets operate within the public or common world shared by individual members of the community.

Beyond this public world, which includes the market and collective spheres, there is the private or personal sphere where each individual is devoted to his own. As Hannah Arendt noted, "Throughout his life man moves constantly within what is his *own,* and he also moves in a sphere that is *common* to him and his fellow men. The 'public good,' the concerns of the citizen, is indeed the common good because it is localized in the *world* which we have in common *without* owning it."[10]

It is the private sphere that is problematic for public health. Public health sometimes intrudes into this private sphere in the interest of the health and safety of the community. But, as we shall see in the development of the regulatory or police power, the main thrust has been to focus on the controlling conditions in the public world, particularly by shaping the institutions of the market and private property.

Emergence of Police Power

In 1850, the Massachusetts Sanitary Commission presented its *Report* to the state legislature. Lemuel Shattuck, a member of the legislature, was the chief author.[11] The guiding definition of public health was set out in the opening pages:

> The condition of perfect *public health* requires such laws and regulations, as will secure to man associated in society, the same sanitary enjoyments that he would have as an isolated individual; and as will protect him from injury from any influences connected with his locality, his dwelling-house, his occupation, or those of his associates or neighbors, or from any other social causes. It is under the control of public authority, and public administration; and life and health may be saved or lost, and they are actually saved or lost, as this authority is wisely or unwisely exercised.

Shattuck's report clearly accepts the existence of a public realm that is the legitimate object of government intervention to protect the public health and that requires the alteration of the existing system of property rights and the regulation of the marketplace for its protection.

In Massachusetts, during the same period when the Sanitary Commission's *Report* was issued, a parallel development in legislation and in law sought to alter the system of rights surrounding private property. The goal was to facilitate rapid economic development on the one hand and at the same time to permit the state to control and monitor that development in order to protect the public's health and safety.

The commonwealth idea was a direct legacy of eighteenth-century American and English radical opposition to the Crown, a body of political thought that powerfully shaped the American revolutionary tradition.[12] The primacy of the public or the common good over private interests and the use of the powers of legislation to regulate the economy and protect the health and safety of the community were central to this body of republican thought.

Our root ideas about health and safety policy can be traced to these early state policies. As a leading constitutional scholar, Leonard Levy has argued: "[T]he police power may be regarded as the legal expression of the Commonwealth idea, for it signifies the supremacy of public over private rights. To call the police power a Massachusetts doctrine would be an exaggeration, though not a great one. [I]t is certainly no coincidence that in Massachusetts, with its Commonwealth tradition, the police power was first defined and carried to great extremes from the standpoint of vested interests."

Apparently, Chief Justice John Marshall was the first to coin the term "police power" in referring to the powers of the states to regulate public health and safety matters in the classic case of *Gibbons v. Ogden* in 1824. Marshall was attempting to clarify the boundary between these powers and the powers of Congress over interstate commerce: "[Police] powers form a portion of that immense mass of legislation which embraces everything within the territory of the state, not surrendered to the general government; all which can advantageously be exercised by the states themselves. Inspection laws, quarantine laws, health laws of every description . . . are component parts of this mass."[13]

The classic definition of the police power was established in *Commonwealth v. Alger* (1851), a decision written by Chief Justice Shaw of the Massachusetts Supreme Court.[14] In this case, Shaw established the basic premises of the police power of the states. His broad definition of this power remains the most influential to this date: "The power we allude to is . . . the police power, the power vested in the legislature by the constitution, to make, ordain and establish all manner of wholesome and reasonable laws, statutes and ordinances, either with penalties or without, not repugnant to the constitution, as they shall judge to be for the good and welfare of the commonwealth, and of the subjects of the same."

In this decision Justice Shaw was ruling on what might seem a minor issue. The case involved a man who owned property on Boston Harbor and who built a wharf that extended beyond a boundary to the public right of way established by the legislature. When the state ordered him to take it down, he went to court, arguing that the legislature had interfered with his property, and that it had not been demonstrated or even argued that his wharf constituted a nuisance or a harm to anyone.

As Levy noted (in referring to another case), great principles are often decided in cases of little factual interest. In the *Alger* decision, Shaw set out the basic premise underlying the police power: "We think it is a settled principle, growing out of the nature of a well ordered civil society, that every holder of property, however absolute and unqualified may be his title, holds it under the implied liability that his use of it may be so regulated, that it shall not be injurious to the equal enjoyment of others having an equal right to the enjoyment of their property in this commonwealth."

To Shaw, the idea of the "common good" implied the health, safety, or welfare of the citizens of Massachusetts. This common interest in health and safety was not adequately protected by common law principles governing the use of property. The common interest in health and safety could only be adequately protected through legislation and regulations affecting the whole people. The common law doctrine regulating the use of property was *Sic utere tuo ut alienum non laedas* (Use your own property in such a manner as not to injure that of another).[15]

In *Alger,* Shaw greatly broadened this principle from a case-by-case investigation of whether each citizen had harmed the interest of another, to a broad instrument for the control of property potentially injurious to the interests of the community. As Shaw argued, "Things done may or may not be wrong in themselves, or necessarily injurious and punishable as such at common law, but laws are passed declaring them offenses, and making them punishable, because they tend to injurious consequences."

According to Levy, Shaw "believed that the general welfare required the anticipation and prevention of prospective wrongs from the use of private property." As Ernest Freund argued decades later, the common law of nuisance could deal with evils only after they came into existence: "The police power endeavors to prevent evil by checking the tendency towards it, and it seeks to place a margin of safety between that which is permitted and that which is sure to lead to injury or loss. This can be accomplished . . . by establishing positive standards and limitations which must be observed, although to step beyond them would not necessarily create a nuisance at law."[16]

In perhaps the second most influential police power decision of the nineteenth century, *Munn v. Illinois* (1876), the Supreme Court affirmed these basic principles. The case involved the state of Illinois and its regulation of grain operators' rates in Chicago.[17] Justice Field, arguing for the minority, stated that the market was essentially a private institution: "The business of a warehouseman was, at common law, a private business, and is so in its nature. It has no special privileges connected with it, nor did the law ever extend to it any greater protection than it extended to all other private business."

But Chief Justice Waite, arguing for the majority, disagreed: "Property does become clothed with a public interest when used in a manner to make it of public consequence, and affect the community at large. When, therefore, one devotes his property to a use in which the public has an interest, he, in effect, grants to the public an interest in that use, and must submit to be controlled by the public for the common good, to the extent of the interest he has thus created."

All authorities agree that the police power is very extensive and checked only by express grants of the Constitution to protect basic rights. There is still recurring disagreement on the underlying principle of the regulatory power. Some scholars argue that the basic principle of the regulatory power remains *sic utere.*[18] But other scholars reject this view. For example, Ernest Freund, in one of the most thorough studies of the regulatory power of any period, argues that "[N]o community confines its care of the public welfare to the enforcement of the principles of the common law . . . it exercises its compulsory powers for the prevention . . . of wrong by narrowing common law rights . . . and [through] positive regulations which are not confined to wrongful acts. It is this latter kind of state control which constitutes the essence of the police power."[19]

The Relevance of Community

This is a crucial issue because on it turns the relevance of the category of the community for the regulatory power. If the regulatory power is simply the enforcement—writ large—of the law that no one should use his or her property in a manner that offends another individual's interests, then the category of community is rendered meaningless. But as W. G. Hastings, another leading scholar of the police power, pointed out, if this power was limited only to prevent harms to others, this does not explain why courts uniformly supported the drastic regulation of alcohol by the states. Although judges often pointed to the evil that drinking causes for others than themselves (such as their families or their employers), it was plain to everyone that regulating the "liquor traffic" involved limiting actions that harmed mostly the drinkers themselves. The temperance and prohibition campaigns, first in the 1850s and later at the turn of the century, to control legally and even destroy the alcohol trade provided some of the strongest and clearest rulings of the courts on the police powers.[20] . . .

Perhaps the most significant case testing the constitutionality of state prohibition was *Mugler v. Kansas* (1887).[21] *Mugler* concerned a brewery owner charged with making beer after a state constitutional amendment forbade the manufacture, sale, and use of alcoholic beverages. Plaintiff's counsel argued that the Kansas constitutional amendment was an attempt to regulate purely personal conduct not subject to a compelling state interest. Counsel quoted Mill and the common law principles of *sic utere* as the basic founding principles of the English and American legal tradition. As counsel for the plaintiff argued: "If a state convention or legislature can punish a citizen for manufacturing beer . . . for his own use, then instead of civil liberty, we are living under the most unlimited and brutal despotism known in history. . . . Broad and comprehensive as this [police] power is, it cannot extend to the individual tastes and habits of the citizen, which are confined entirely to himself and have no effect upon others."

The Supreme Court ruled against the plaintiff and held for the state of Kansas. Justice Harlan, writing for the majority, had this to say:

> There is no justification for holding that the State under the guise merely of the police regulations, is aiming to deprive the citizen of his constitutional rights: for we cannot shut out of view the fact, within the knowledge of all, that the public health, the public morals, and the public safety, may be endangered by the general use of intoxicating drinks. . . . So far from such a regulation having no relation to the general end sought to be accomplished, the entire scheme of prohibitions, as embodied in the [state] constitution and laws of Kansas, might fail, if the right of each citizen to manufacture intoxicating liquors for his own use as a beverage were recognized. . . . Those rights are best secured in our government, by the observance,

upon the part of all, of such regulations as are established by competent authority, to promote the common good.

The Court did not, and could not, pass judgment on the *wisdom* of the state prohibition measures. This judgment, in a republican scheme of government, rests with the legislative body. But the Court did affirm the basic political principles underlying the powers of the states to control and limit the market and private property to protect the health and safety of the citizenry. During the last decades of the nineteenth century, the Supreme Court capitulated to corporate and extreme laissez-faire interests. During this period the Court sought to block the states' power to improve the working conditions for labor and to facilitate union organization against capital. Even so, the Court continued to uphold striking powers for the states to regulate property when the health and safety of the general citizenry was at stake.

Contemporary Public Health Problems

Several twentieth-century developments have obscured the philosophical roots of the regulatory power, especially as they work to protect the public health. Because the locus of action for protecting the health and safety of the public has swung to the federal government and because the justification for this federal power lies primarily with the commerce clause of the Constitution, the group principle behind public health has tended to be subordinated to the language of individual rights.

The political justification of public health has also tended to be ignored. Most contemporary legal scholars cite the 1905 Supreme Court decision *Jacobson v. Massachusetts* as the leading case underlying public health.[22] *Jacobson* dealt with a Cambridge, Massachusetts, ordinance requiring compulsory vaccination in a smallpox outbreak. The language of *Jacobson* contains an exemplary and classical defense of the regulatory power, but the facts of the case focus on the control of epidemics and the overriding necessity for requiring compulsory vaccination to prevent the spread of infection. This has encouraged many scholars to interpret the regulatory power for protecting the public health on the more narrow grounds of preventing injury to others and to overlook the use of this power to limit liberty in the market or other areas of the public realm, even if such restriction does not protect the interests of other specific individuals.

The two most recent constitutional controversies regarding public health policy and the police power are the fluoridation and the motorcycle helmet controversies.[23] Once again these controversies show the courts willing to accept public health paternalism. However, in the case of the helmet decisions, sometimes the broad principles of the regulatory power have tended to be replaced by spurious legal reasoning.

State supreme courts have unanimously upheld the constitutionality of both measures, and the U.S. Supreme Court has refused to review fluoridation cases, presumably because they pose no threats to constitutional rights. Plaintiffs have argued that fluoridation is an attempt to employ mass medication and constitutes a violation of individual autonomy in an area that is properly private. They have argued that the use of the regulatory power to control private rights was only justified in the past by the threat of contagious diseases. . . .

The courts have been less consistent on the question of helmet laws for motorcyclists. Although state supreme courts have unanimously supported the state's power to require helmet usage, the decisions have often introduced as additional justification the danger unhelmeted cyclists pose for others on the road or the possibility that unprotected cyclists may become wards of the state. . . .

The Language of Public Health

What are we to make of this constitutional tradition surrounding the development of the regulatory power for health and safety? What relevance does it have for the policy disputes of today, particularly those concerning the limitation of lifestyle risks?

The constitutional tradition for public health constitutes one of those "second languages" of republicanism that Robert Bellah and his coauthors speak of in their recent book *Habits of the Heart.*[24] In their book, the first language (or tradition of moral discourse) of American politics is political individualism. But there are "second languages" of community rooted in the republican and biblical tradition that limit and qualify the scope and consequences of political individualism.

Public health as a second language reminds us that we are not only individuals, we are also a community and a body politic, and that we have shared commitments to one another and promises to keep. As the Preamble to the Massachusetts Constitution puts it:

> The end of the institution, maintenance and administration of government is to secure the existence of the body politic; to protect; and to furnish the individuals who compose it, with the power of enjoying, in safety and tranquility, their natural rights, and the blessings of life. . . . The body politic is a social compact, by which the whole people covenants with each citizen, and each citizen with the whole people, that all shall be governed by certain laws for the common good.

The danger is that we can come to discuss public health exclusively within the dominant discourse of political individualism, relying either on the harm principle or a narrow paternalism justified on grounds of self-protection alone. By ignoring the communitarian language of public health, we risk shrinking its claims. We also risk undermining the sense in which health and safety are a signal commitment of the common life—a central *practice* by which the body politic defines itself and affirms its values.

In *Habits of the Heart,* practices are those shared activities that are not purely instrumental and that help shape and affirm the common life. Practices can be religious, esthetic, or ethical. Public health belongs to the realm of the political and the ethical. Public health belongs to the ethical because it is concerned not only with explaining the occurrence of illness and disease in society, but also with ameliorating them. Beyond instrumental goals, public health is concerned with integrative goals—expressing the commitment of the whole people to face the threat of death and disease in solidarity.

Public health is also a practical science. Spanning the world of science and practical action, it seeks reasonable and practical means of altering property arrangements or limiting liberty to promote the health of the public generally.

These two ideas, the ideas of second languages and of social practices, shed light on why paternalism—at least public health paternalism—plays an affirmative role in the republican tradition. In the constitutional categories for protecting the public health, the regulatory power is to protect not individual citizens, but rather citizens considered as a group, the public health. In this tradition, the public, as well as the community itself, has a reality apart from the citizens who comprise it. Fundamental constituents of the community and the common life are its practices and institutions.

Practices are communal in nature and concerned with the well-being of the community as a whole and not just the well-being of any particular person. Policy, and here public health paternalism, operates at the level of practices and not at the level of individual behavior. . . .

This distinction between practices and behavior should help us see the difference between public health paternalism aimed at the group and the "personal paternalism" of the doctor-patient, lawyer-client relationship. While there are public elements of these professional relationships—and while the state can (rightly or wrongly) structure these relationships in a paternalistic fashion—their essence is based on a personal encounter between a professional and a client. This is not the case with public health paternalism. Public health paternalism should also be kept separate from the legal doctrine of *parens patriae*, where the state assumes the role of parent in instances where parental supervision is absent or deemed deficient.

This suggests that public health paternalism and the language of community on which it is based fit the parent-child analogy very poorly. To Mill, all paternalism was wrong because the individual is best placed to know his own good: "He is the person most interested in his own well-being: the interest which any other person, except in cases of strong personal attachment, can have in it, is trifling."

But, precisely because public health paternalism is aimed at the group and its practices, and not the specific individual, Mill's point is wrong. The good of the particular person is not the aim of health policy in a democracy which defends both the community and the individual. In fact, Mill is wrong twice, because particular individuals are often very poorly placed to judge the effects that market arrangements and practices have on the population as a whole. This is the task for legislatures, for organized groups of citizens, and for other agents of the public, including the citizen as voter.

Mill's dichotomy of either the harm principle or self-protection is too limited; the world of harms is not exhausted by self-imposed and other-imposed injuries. There is a third and very large set of problems that afflicts the community as a whole and that results primarily from inadequate safeguards over the practices of the common life. Economists and others often refer to this class of harms as "summing up problems" or "choice-in-the-small versus choice-in-the-large."[25]

Creating, extending, or strengthening the practices of public health—and the collective goods principle that underlies it—ought to be the primary justification for our health and safety policy. Instead we usually base these regulations on the harm principle. We usually justify regulating the steel or coal industry on the grounds that workers and the general public have the risks of pollution or black lung visited on them, but consumers are not obliged to drink alcohol or smoke cigarettes. While this may be true, in the communitarian language and categories of public health, fixing blame is not the main point. We regulate the steel or coal industry because market competition undervalues collective goods like a clean environment or workers' safety. Using social organization to secure collective goods like public health, not preventing harms to others, is the proper rationale for health and safety regulations imposed on the steel or coal industry, or the alcohol or cigarette industry. . . .

The main lesson to learn from public health paternalism as it has developed in the constitutional tradition may well be that the second language of community and the virtues of cooperation and beneficence still exist, albeit precariously, alongside a tradition of political individualism. Strengthening the public health includes not only the practical task of improving aggregate welfare, it also involves the task of reacquainting the American public with its republican and communitarian heritage and encouraging citizens to share in reasonable and practical group schemes to promote a wider welfare of which their own welfare is only a part. In political individualism, seatbelt legislation, or signs on the beach restricting swimming when a lifeguard is not present restrict the individual's liberty for his or her own good. In this circumstance the appropriate slogan is: "The life you save may be your own." But in the second language of public health these restrictions define a common practice which shapes our life together, for the general or the common good. In the language of public health, the motto for such paternalistic legislation might be: "The lives we save together might include your own."

Notes

1. John Stuart Mill, "On Liberty," in M. Cohen, ed., *The Philosophy of John Stuart Mill* (New York: Modern Library, 1961), pp. 185–319. (Mill's essay was first published in 1859.)

2. Quoted in Leonard Levy, *The Law of the Commonwealth and Chief Justice Shaw* (Cambridge, Mass.: Harvard University Press, 1957), p. 310.

3. Joel Feinberg, *Social Philosophy* (Englewood Cliffs, N.J.: Prentice-Hall, 1973), pp. 45–52.

4. Dennis Thompson, "Paternalism in Medicine, Law, and Public Policy," in Daniel Callahan and Sissela Bok, eds., *Ethics Teaching in Higher Education* (New York: Plenum Press, 1980), pp. 245–72.

5. D. H. Regan, "Justification for Paternalism," in J. R. Pennock and J. W. Chapman, eds., *The Limits of Law* (New York: Lieber-Atherton, 1974), pp. 189–210. Another approach is to justify liberty-limiting for personal risks on grounds of cost-benefit, a variation of the harm principle. See T. Beauchamp, "The Regulation of Hazards and Hazardous Behavior," *Health Education Monographs* 6 (1976), 242–57.

6. My "Public Health as Social Justice," *Inquiry* 13 (1976), 3–14, comes close to this position. See also R. Crawford, "You Are Dangerous to Your Health," *Social Policy* 8 (1978), 11–20.

7. See Levy, pp. 303–21. See also Oscar Handlin and Mary Handlin, *Commonwealth. A Study of the Role of Government in the American Economy: Massachusetts, 1774–1861* (Cambridge, Mass.: Belknap Press, 1969), and Ronald M. Peters, Jr., *The Massachusetts Constitution of 1780—A Social Compact* (Amherst: University of Massachusetts Press, 1978).

8. The present work is heavily indebted to Ernest Freund, *The Police Power—Public Policy and Constitutional Rights* (Chicago: Callaghan & Company, 1904), and to Levy's classic study of Chief Justice Shaw. I have also relied on Scott M. Reznick's extensive study of the police power, "Empiricism and the Principle of Conditions in the Evolution of the Police Power: A Model for Definitional Scrutiny," *Washington University Law Quarterly*, no. 1 (1978), 1–90, as well as Rodney L. Mott, *Due Process of Law* (Indianapolis, 1926), and W. G. Hastings, "The Development of Law as Illustrated by the Decisions Relating to the Police Power of the State," *Proceedings of the American Philosophical Society* 39 (1900), 359–64.

9. Joseph Tussman, *Obligations and the Body Politic* (New York: Oxford University Press, 1960), pp. 27–28.

10. Hannah Arendt, "Public Rights and Private Interests," in Michael Mooney and Florian Stuber, eds., *Small Comfort for Hard Times: Humanists on Public Policy* (New York: Columbia University Press, 1977), p. 104.

11. Lemuel Shattuck, *Report of the Sanitary Commission of Massachusetts, 1850* (Cambridge: Harvard University Press, 1948), pp. 9–10.

12. See Gordon Wood, *The Creation of the American Republic, 1776–1787* (New York: W. W. Norton & Co., 1969), for the best discussion of the development of revolutionary thought, and especially the importance of the notion of the public or the common good to that body of thought.

13. Gibbons v. Ogden, 22 U.S. (9 Wheaton) 1 (1824). For . . . an interpretation of the police power along the lines suggested in this article, see Harry N. Scheiber, "Public Rights and the Rule of Law in American Legal History," *California Law Review* 72 (1984), 217–51. Scheiber's article is an excellent source for the growing literature in legal history on the importance of "the public" and of "public rights" and "community" in nineteenth-century American law. I am much in debt to Professor Scheiber's work and to his criticisms of an earlier draft of this article.

14. Commonwealth v. Alger, 61 Mass (7 Cushing) 53 (1851).

15. *Black's Law Dictionary*, 4th ed., 1968, p. 1551.

16. Freund, *The Police Power—Public Policy and Constitutional Rights*, pp. 25–26.

17. Munn v. Illinois, 94 U.S. 113 (1876).

18. The most influential nineteenth-century legal theorists holding this view were Thomas M. Cooley and Christopher G. Tiedeman. Cooley's most famous treatise is *A Treatise on the Constitutional Limitations Which Rest upon the Legislative Power of the State of the American Union* (Boston: Little, Brown, 1868). Tiedeman's best-known work on the police power is *A Treatise on the Limitations of Police Power in the United States*, 2 vols. (St. Louis: F. Thomas Law Book Co., 1900). See also E. Corwin, *Liberty against Government* (Baton Rouge: Louisiana State University Press, 1948). But Levy, Freund, and W. G. Hastings take the opposing view, as does W. W. Willoughby in *The Constitutional Law of the United States*, 2nd ed. (New York: Baker, Voorhis & Co., 1929).

19. Freund, *The Police Power—Public Policy and Constitutional Rights*, p. 6.

20. See Norman H. Clark, *Deliver Us from Evil* (New York: Norton, 1976); John Allen Krout, *The Origins of Prohibition* (New York: 1925); and Paul Aaron and David Musto,

"Temperance and Prohibition in America: An Overview," in Mark H. Moore and Dean R. Gerstein, eds., *Alcohol and Public Policy: Beyond the Shadow of Prohibition* (Washington, D.C.: National Academy Press, 1981), pp. 140–42.

21. Mugler v. Kansas, 123 U.S. 623 (1887).

22. Jacobson v. Massachusetts, 197 U.S. 11 (1905).

23. See, for example, "Limiting the State's Police Power: Judicial Reaction to John Stuart Mill," *University of Chicago Law Review* 37 (1970), 605–27; Robert E. Clark and Michael M. Sophy, "Fluoridation: The Courts and the Opposition," *Wayne Law Review* 13 (1967), 338–75; George A. Strong, "Liberty, Religion and Fluoridation," *Santa Clara Lawyer* 8 (1967), 37–58; Kenneth M. Royalty, "Motorcycle Helmets and the Constitutionality of Self-Protective Legislation," *Ohio State Law Journal* 30 (1969), 355–81; Notes, "Constitutional Law—Police Power—Michigan Statute Requiring Motorcyclists to Wear Protective Helmets Held Unconstitutional," *Michigan Law Review* 67 (1968), 360–73.

24. Robert N. Bellah, Richard Madsen, William M. Sullivan, Ann Swidler, and Steven M. Tipton, *Habits of the Heart* (Berkeley: University of California Press, 1985).

25. For the "summing up problem" see Thomas Schelling, *Micromotives and Macrobehavior* (New York: Norton, 1978). For the differences between choice-in-the-small and choice-in-the-large, see F. Hirsch, *Social Limits to Growth* (Cambridge, Mass.: Harvard University Press, 1978).

3

The Future of the Public's Health

Vision, Values, and Strategies

Lawrence O. Gostin, Jo Ivey
Boufford, and Rose Marie Martinez

The modern public health system is undergoing a remarkable transition, moving from discrete interventions to address infectious diseases to broad social, cultural, and economic reforms to address the root causes of ill health.[1] This transition is embodied in two foundational reports of the Institute of Medicine (IOM). The first, *The Future of Public Health* (1988), defined public health as the obligation of organized society to assure the conditions for people to be healthy. The second, *The Future of the Public's Health in the Twenty-first Century* (2002), went further by proposing the following ambitious strategies for health protection and promotion: (1) strengthen the governmental public health infrastructure; (2) encourage major private-sector actors to promote the health of their members and surrounding communities; and (3) improve the broad determinants of population health.[2] The vision of modern public health, then, is expansive: "healthy people in healthy communities," with public health agencies primarily responsible and accountable for assuring the health of the population.[3]

This broad vision is politically charged. Critics express strong objections: Why should health be a primary social undertaking when compared with other competing priorities? Why should private actors take responsibility for the public's health? Are public health agencies going beyond their legitimate scope by supporting fundamental changes in the socioeconomic environment? These are legitimate and challenging questions. The goals of public health are too often assumed or simply asserted, rather than cogently explained and justified.

This paper has several interrelated purposes and is intended to fill a gap in the literature. First, it sets out a framework for safeguarding and improving the public's health, with detailed recommendations. Second, it offers a justification for a broad public health vision, while acknowledging that the issues are complex and the appropriate social responses deserve robust political debate. Rather than simply asserting the salience of population health, we address, head-on, the major critiques posed by scholars and politicians who prefer a narrow scope for public health action. Our hope is to leave the reader with a robust conception of the public health enterprise, including governmental public health, public/private partnerships, and favorable conditions for healthy populations.

State of the Nation's Health

The health of the U.S. public continuously improved throughout the twentieth century. By every measure, Americans are now healthier, live longer, and enjoy lives that are less likely to be marked by injury, ill health, or premature death. During the past century, for example, infant mortality decreased, and the average life span rose from 45 years to nearly 80.[4] Public health achievements include safer foods, fluoridation of drinking water, control of infectious diseases, fewer deaths from heart disease and stroke, motor vehicle safety, and safer workplaces.[5]

The public's health still has room to improve. Although the United States has one of the highest levels of per capita gross domestic product (GDP) in the world, Americans' health status is poor compared with the health status of populations that have similar levels of economic development. Although the United States has the third-highest GDP of the 30 member countries of the Organization for Economic Cooperation and Development (OECD), it ranks 23rd in infant mortality (7.1 deaths per 1,000 live births) and 18th in life expectancy at birth (76.7 years for both sexes).[6] The World Health Organization (WHO) ranks the United States 37th among global health systems, reflecting concerns about access to and cost of health care, relatively poor health indicators, and sizable racial and socioeconomic disparities.[7]

The relatively poor U.S. health status is even more noteworthy because of high U.S. health spending—$4,373 per capita—which is the highest in the world and more than double the OECD median of $2,000.[8] Approximately 14 percent of U.S. GDP ($1.4 trillion in 2001) is directed toward health, compared with 9.2 percent in Canada, 7.4 percent in Japan, and 7.1 percent in the United Kingdom.[9]

Although identifying the pathways between investment and health outcomes requires further research, several trends appear important. More than 95 percent of U.S. federal and state health spending is directed toward personal health care and biomedical research; only 1–2 percent is directed toward prevention.[10] These governmental funding priorities, consistent for decades, do not reflect scientific understandings of population health. There is strong evidence that access to medical care is a less-important determinant of health than behavior and environment, which are responsible for more than 70 percent of avoidable deaths.[11] This history of investment skewed toward personal health care offers a political strategy that is unlikely to achieve a maximum impact on the public's health.

Strategies for Improving the Public's Health

If current policies do not ensure the highest attainable health for the U.S. population, then what strategies would be more effective? The IOM's 2002 report offers at least three core strategies. Here, we offer concrete proposals that go beyond this report.

Strengthen the Governmental Public Health Infrastructure

Government has primary authority and responsibility for assuring the conditions in which people can be healthy. Yet public health agencies are structurally weak in each of their core components, which led the IOM to conclude that the agencies are largely in disarray. Numerous other reports have drawn attention to the lack of public health preparedness.[12] The Centers for Disease Control and Prevention (CDC) concludes that despite recent improvements, the public health infrastructure "is still structurally weak in nearly every area."[13] Indeed, structural deficiencies exist in each of the major components of the public health system, including outdated statutes; a poorly prepared workforce; lack of state-of-the-art information and communications systems (to improve surveillance, outbreak investigations, program evaluations, and interventions); and inadequate laboratory capacity.[14]

The recent emphasis on bioterrorism preparedness and influx of federal funds could strengthen the public health system if the resources enabled agencies to protect against both bioterrorism and other health threats. Public health professionals, however, express concern about substitution effects, in which bioterrorism funds detract from ongoing programs.[15] An independent evaluation using major indicators such as response plans demonstrated continued lack of preparedness for public health emergencies.[16] Also, public health agencies face severe cuts because of the current state budget crisis, which may cause preparedness to deteriorate further.[17]

To address these weaknesses, we offer the following recommendations:

Recommendation 1: Congress should establish a national Public Health Council (PHC). The PHC, comprising the secretary of the Department of Health and Human Services (HHS) and state health commissioners, with representative local health officials and outside experts, would (1) collaborate on action to achieve national health goals as articulated in *Healthy People 2010;* (2) advise the HHS secretary on financing, policy, and regulations affecting the public's health; (3) develop a funding system to sustain the public health infrastructure; and (4) evaluate the impact of domestic policies on national health outcomes and reductions of health disparities. It would improve collaboration among levels of government, provide a forum for strategic planning and monitoring progress, and elevate the status of public health within government.

Recommendation 2: HHS should report annually to Congress on the state of the nation's health. The HHS secretary should be accountable for assessing the state of the nation's public health system and its capacity to provide the essential public health services to every community. The assessment should include a systematic evaluation of progress in meeting national health goals (for example, leading health indicators); funding and technical assistance for public health agencies to ensure sustainability; and identification of strengths and gaps in system capacity. Such assessments are needed to keep Congress and the public informed and would play an important role in policy development.

Recommendation 3: Congress should establish a stable funding mechanism, such as a "trust fund" to support state and local public health agencies. Agencies suffer from two interrelated problems: lack of adequate funding to support ongoing services and inflexible sources of funds. When the federal government does support public health services, it is frequently for specific purposes (for example, bioterrorism preparedness) or to serve specific constituencies (for example, people with HIV/AIDS), and funding streams are often time limited. This form of "silo" or "stovepipe" funding cannot sustain a permanent infrastructure and discourages evidence-based planning, policies, and programs.[18] The PHC should advise Congress about the level of financial support necessary for the trust fund and develop a formula to allocate resources that assures adequate state and local cost sharing.

Recommendation 4: Congress should set conditions for receipt of funds based on states' progress toward and adherence to quality standards. HHS, through the PHC, should establish national standards of quality and hold states accountable for meeting them. Innovative work is already taking place to establish objective measures of public health effectiveness and identify qualifications for the public health workforce.[19] If agencies are charged with improving the public's health and receive adequate funding, they should be held accountable under these quality standards.

Engage Nongovernmental Actors in Partnerships for Public Health

Although the duty to safeguard the public's health has been assigned historically to government, through the work of national, state, tribal, and local health agencies, no single agency can assure all of the conditions for the public's health.[20] Public health agencies can act as a catalyst for action by other government departments and nongovernmental actors. The intersectoral public health system includes many important entities, but the 2002 IOM report focused on five: health care institutions, the community, businesses, the media, and academe.

1. Institutions: Health care is important because personal health is a value in itself and contributes to population health.[21] However, health care services are not fully accessible to many people. Approximately 14.6 percent of the population, or 43 million people, lack health insurance; racial and ethnic minorities and the poor are disproportionately burdened.[22] Also, health plans often do not cover many services for prevention, mental health, substance abuse treatment, and dental health.[23] Health care providers can play an important role in promoting health through patient care, attention to the health of their own workers, and investments in promoting the health of the communities they serve.

2. Community: Although the term *community* is often imprecise, many local entities such as churches, civic organizations, and health advocacy groups can contribute to the health of their neighborhoods. Community involvement in and promotion of health action can be effective.[24] Community organizations are well placed to assess needs, inventory resources, formulate collaborative responses,

and evaluate outcomes for community health improvements. They can also promote healthy behavior and lifestyles and can facilitate social networks.

3. Businesses: Businesses play a major role in the health of their employees and the population through their effects on natural and built environments, workplace conditions, and relationships with communities. The cost-effectiveness of prevention and health promotion efforts for an employer's workforce and the value of corporate action to promote broader community health have been demonstrated.[25]

4. Media: The news and entertainment media shape public opinion and influence decision making, with potentially critical effects on population health. Yet public health activities often attract little media coverage, perhaps because journalists and public health officials do not understand each other's perspectives and methods. Ongoing dialogue and educational opportunities could improve media coverage of public health. In addition, the media should consider increased airtime for public health messages.

5. Academe: Academe provides degree programs and continuing education to the current and future public health workforce. However, changes are needed in curricular and financial incentives to link curricular content and teaching methods more closely to the practice needs of the public health workforce. New investments and academic reorganization are needed for community-based prevention research that evaluates the effects of interventions on population health.

To ensure that health system partners contribute to the public's health, we propose the following governmental programs and incentives:

Recommendation 5: The federal government should lead a national effort to achieve stable health care coverage for every person residing in the United States. This coverage should include age-appropriate preventive services and oral health, mental health, and substance abuse treatment. The uninsured have difficulty getting care, and the services they receive may not be timely, appropriate, or well coordinated.[26] Insurance coverage is associated with better health outcomes for children and adults.[27]

Recommendation 6: Federal and state governments should support community-led public health efforts. Community organizations are close to the populations they serve and therefore are a crucial part of the public health system. Public health agencies should provide adequate funding and technical assistance to, and engage in partnerships with, communities. This could enable communities to inventory resources, assess needs, formulate collaborative responses, and evaluate outcomes for community health improvement and reduction of health disparities.

Recommendation 7: Public health agencies should create incentives for (and, if necessary, regulate) businesses to strengthen health promotion and disease and injury prevention for their employees and communities. Government should provide incentives through the tax code and conditional spending to encourage the private sector to engage in health-promoting activities. Monetary incentives can greatly affect corporate behavior. There is also a role for governmental regulation to ensure that businesses act responsibly. Thus, the state must strengthen regulations relating to occupational health and safety, sanitary food and living conditions, and the environment, among other areas.

Recommendation 8: The media should increase the time devoted to public service announcements and contribute to a well-informed public on matters of health. An ongoing dialogue and collaborative efforts between public health agencies and the media would benefit the public's health. Consideration of stronger regulations regarding public service announcements (for example, more airtime in "prime time") is warranted, as is increased inclusion of health messages in popular entertainment media.

Recommendation 9: Academic institutions should increase interdisciplinary learning opportunities for public health students, strengthen and expand their training of the current public health workforce, and reward faculty for both basic and applied public health research. Academe is critically important in the education and training of the public health workforce and in providing a science base for public health policy. The federal government should increase funding for investigator-initiated research relating to public health prevention and practice.

Improve the Multiple Conditions for the Public's Health

Thus far we have made the case for strengthening the governmental public health infrastructure and forming public/private partnerships. However, much controversy persists as to the appropriate scope of public health action. We support a broad emphasis on the conditions in which people can be healthy. To achieve population health, it is necessary to transform national health policy, with its traditional dominant investments in personal health care and biomedical research to treat disease after it happens, to a more balanced policy that invests in the multiple determinants of societal health.

The multiple determinants of health encompass the physical or built environment, the natural environment, the informational environment, the social environment, the economic environment, and the work environment.[28] This finding is embedded within an influential ecologic theory that characteristics of places and even nations carry with them health risks for the people who live there.

Perhaps the two farthest-reaching, and therefore most controversial, determinants of health relate to the "built" and socioeconomic environments. Public health has a long history of designing the built environment to reduce injury (workplace safety, traffic calming, and fire codes), infectious diseases (sanitation, zoning, and housing codes), and environmentally associated harms (lead paint, asbestos, and toxic emissions). The United States is facing an epidemiological transition from infectious to chronic diseases such as cardiovascular disease, cancer, diabetes, asthma, and depression. The challenge is to enable communities to facilitate physical and mental well-being. Although research is ongoing, we know that environments can be designed to promote more active lifestyles, improve nutrition, decrease the use of harmful products (such as cigarettes and alcoholic beverages), reduce violence, and increase social interactions (helping neighbors and building social capital).[29]

A strong and consistent finding of epidemiological research is that socioeconomic status (SES) is correlated with morbidity, mortality, and functioning.[30] SES is a complex phenomenon based on income, education, and occupation. The relationship between SES and health often is referred to as a "gradient" because of the graded and continuous nature of the association; health differences are observed well into the middle ranges of SES. These empirical findings have persisted across time and cultures and remain viable today.[31]

Some researchers go further, suggesting that the overall level of socioeconomic inequality in a society affects health.[32] That is, societies with large disparities between the rich and poor tend to have inferior health status. The validity of these studies has been challenged recently.[33] However, some claim that from an ethical perspective, "social justice is good for our health."[34] Government can take active steps to improve the built and socioeconomic environments in several ways.

> *Recommendation 10: State and local governments should engage in land-use planning to encourage healthier lifestyles and habitats.* Government has available numerous tools to make the physical environment more conducive to healthy living: economic incentives to encourage green spaces and recreational facilities; building and housing codes to reduce toxic exposures; zoning to increase availability of wholesome foods and products; and school requirements to serve healthy foods and promote exercise among students. Scientific data on the kinds of designs and land-use arrangements that promote health would at least ensure that policymakers and planners carefully take account of the community's health and safety.
>
> *Recommendation 11: The federal government and the states should adopt more comprehensive strategies to reduce health disparities.* Health policymakers have documented major health disparities within the population and have set a goal of reducing them.[35] Federal and state governments should direct policies and programs designed to reduce health disparities.[36] Priority should be given to those with greatest need, such as the poor and racial minorities. Disparities can be reduced through targeted public health interventions to serve these populations and general improvements in access to essential services such as income support, education, and health care.

Justifications for an Expanded Vision of Public Health

Critics have argued powerfully against the foregoing proposals for achieving a healthier population.[37] In this section we respond to these challenges, recognizing that the questions posed are incisive and deserve careful scrutiny.

Why Should Health Be a Primary Social Undertaking?

Critics argue that population health should not necessarily be a primary social undertaking when compared with competing priorities for investment in transportation, energy, education, or national security. Although it is true that the political organs of government decide on national and state priorities, there are good reasons to give special attention to health.[38]

Every person understands, at least intuitively, why health is vital to well-being. If individuals have physical and mental health, they are better able to socialize, work, and engage in the activities of family and social life that bring meaning and happiness. Perhaps not as obvious, however, is that health is also essential for the functioning of populations. Without minimum levels of health, people cannot fully engage in social interactions, participate in the political process, exercise rights of citizenship, generate wealth, create art, and provide for the common security. Notably, evidence is emerging that direct investments in health can have positive effects on the economy.[39] A safe and healthy population builds strong roots for a country—its governmental structures, social organizations, cultural endowment, economic prosperity, and national defense. Understood in this way, then, population health becomes a transcendent value.

Are Fundamental Changes in Physical, Social, and Economic Conditions Warranted?

Critics argue that public health agencies overreach and lose their legitimacy when they address the broad determinants of health.[40] There are, to be sure, political dangers in straying too far from what many consider public health's traditional mandate.[41] Despite these political risks, addressing the broad determinants of health leads to more effective social policy. Discrete interventions cannot create the conditions to promote and protect the public's health because they do not attend to the underlying causes.[42] Public health agencies must act on scientific research, and a growing body of evidence suggests the importance of physical, social, and economic conditions for the population's health.[43] As the main proponent of population health in society, the public health community must call attention to the "upstream" causes of morbidity and premature death and must propose a broad range of social, economic, and behavioral tools needed to make populations healthier.[44]

Critics often dispute the evidence demonstrating a causal relationship between low SES and poor health outcomes and reject social policies designed to lift people out of poverty.[45] The explanatory variables for the relationship between SES and health are not entirely understood. However, waiting for researchers to definitively find the causal pathways would be difficult and time-consuming, given the multiple confounding factors involved. This would indefinitely delay policies that could powerfully affect people's health and longevity.

Critics similarly offer a stinging assessment of public health efforts to alter the built environment: "The anti-sprawl campaign is about telling [people] how they should live and work, about sacrificing individuals' values to the values of their politically powerful betters. It is coercive, moralistic, [and] nostalgic."[46] Critiques such as this one fail to take account of history, norms, and evidence.[47] Historically, government has been actively involved in land-use planning.[48] It is not a matter of whether the state should plan cities and towns, but how. The evidence demonstrates that organized societies have a remarkable capacity to plan, shape the future, and help populations gain health and well-being.[49] History, theory, and empirical evidence do not make it inevitable that the state will, or always should, prefer health-enhancing policies. However, government does have an obligation to carefully consider the population's health in its land-use policies.

Assuring the Public's Health: Future Challenges

We are acutely aware that key obstacles await the strategies we have enumerated. Achieving a highly functioning governmental public health system is difficult; the necessary tasks are technically within our reach but require political will. There are many reasons to question the political commitment to population health—a history of underinvestment, silo funding, and a culture of individualism. In matters of funding, standard setting, and accountability, federalism poses another problem. Which government—federal, tribal, state, or local—holds the power and duty to devote resources and create policy?

The challenges to achieving effective partnerships in public health are equally apparent. The private and voluntary sectors possess no duty to act for the public good, and there is little political consensus about creating incentives and requirements to do so. The government's role vis-à-vis the private sector has always been controversial. Those who support limited government and a broad sphere of economic freedom may oppose partnerships that go beyond the purely voluntary, but the potential value of closer cooperation is becoming more clear.

Finally, and self-evidently, there are deep challenges in creating policy to improve the socioeconomic conditions of health. Socioeconomic determinants evoke images of redistribution of wealth and status, which are unpopular in many circles. However, this is not merely a question of ideology but one of science. The task will be to demonstrate an evidence-based way to reduce socioeconomic disparities and to show that this improves health outcomes.

Given these challenges, we understand that our aspirations for "healthy people in healthy communities" need to compete in the marketplace of ideas. Yet we think that population health does deserve a special place in national debates and priorities, and it has taken a backseat to other political interests for too long.

The authors are on the Institute of Medicine (IOM) Board on Health Promotion and Disease Prevention (Gostin and Martinez) and Committee for Assuring the Health of the Public (Gostin and Boufford). This paper does not necessarily represent the views of either group.

Notes

1. F. Baum, *The New Public Health* (New York: Oxford University Press, 2002).

2. Institute of Medicine, *The Future of the Public's Health in the Twenty-first Century* (Washington, DC: National Academies Press, 2002).

3. U.S. Department of Health and Human Services (DHHS), *Healthy People 2010* (Washington: DHHS, 2000).

4. DHHS, *Health, United States, 2001, with Urban and Rural Health Chartbook* (Washington, DC: DHHS, 2002).

5. J. P. Koplan and D. W. Fleming, "Current and Future Public Health Challenges," *Journal of the American Medical Association* 284, no. 13 (2000): 1696–1698.

6. Organization for Economic Cooperation and Development, *National Accounts of OECD Countries, Volume 1, 1989–2000,* main aggregates (Geneva: OECD, 2002); OECD, "OECD Health Data 2002," Press Release, 24 June 2002; and U. E. Reinhardt, P. S. Hussey, and G. F. Anderson, "Cross-National Comparisons of Health Systems Using OECD Data, 1999," *Health Affairs* 21, no. 3 (2002): 168–191.

7. A. Tandon et al., "Measuring Overall Health System Performance for 191 Countries," WHO Global Programme on Evidence for Health Policy Discussion Paper Series no. 30 (Geneva: World Health Organization, 2003).

8. OECD, "OECD Health Data 2002."

9. K. Levit et al., "Inflation Spurs Health Spending in 2000," *Health Affairs* 21, no. 1 (2000): 172–181; WHO, *World Health Report 2002* (Geneva: WHO, 2002); and U.S. Centers for Disease Control and Prevention, "Highlights: Major Findings from *Health, United States, 2003*," August 2003, http://www.cdc.gov/nchs/products/pubs/pubd/hus/highlits.pdf (accessed 8 April 2004).

10. J. I. Boufford and P. R. Lee, *Health Policies for the Twenty-first Century: Challenges and Recommendations for the U.S. Department of Health and Human Services* (New York: Milbank Memorial Fund, 2001); and K. W. Eilbert et al., *Measuring Expenditures for Essential Public Health Services* (Washington, DC: Public Health Foundation, 1996).

11. J. M. McGinnis and W. H. Foege, "Actual Causes of Death in the United States," *Journal of the American Medical Association* 270, no. 18 (1993): 2207–2212.

12. IOM, *Public Health Systems and Emerging Infections: Assessing the Capabilities of the Public and Private Sectors: Workshop Summary* (Washington, DC: National Academies Press, 2000).

13. DHHS, "Public Health's Infrastructure: A Status Report" (prepared for the Senate Appropriations Committee, 2001).

14. Regarding statutes, see, for example, L. O. Gostin, "Public Health Law Reform," *American Journal of Public Health* 91, no. 9 (2001): 1365–1368; and L. O. Gostin, "Public Health Law in an Age of Terrorism: Rethinking Individual Rights and Common Goods," *Health Affairs* 21, no. 6 (2002): 79–93. Regarding the workforce, see Trust for America's Health (TFAH), *Public Health Preparedness: Progress and Challenges since September 11th, 2001* (Washington, DC: TFAH, 2002); and IOM, *Who Will Keep the Public Healthy? Educating Public Health Professionals for the Twenty-first Century* (Washington, DC: National Academies Press, 2002). Regarding technology, see Association of State Public Health Laboratories, "Core Functions and Capabilities of State Public Health Laboratories," *Morbidity and Mortality Weekly Report* 51, no. RR-14 (2002): 1–8.

15. L. K. Altman and A. O'Connor, "Health Officials Fear Local Impact of Smallpox Plan," *New York Times,* 5 January 2003.

16. TFAH, *Ready or Not? Protecting the Public's Health in the Age of Bioterrorism* (Washington, DC: TFAH, 2003).

17. A. Cohen, "What Alabama's Low-Tax Mania Can Teach the Rest of the Country," *New York Times,* 20 October 2003.

18. Turning Point Performance Management National Excellence Collaborative,

"From Silos to Systems: Using Performance Management to Improve the Public's Health" (Washington, DC: Public Health Foundation, 2003).

19. IOM, *Improving Health in the Community: A Role for Performance Monitoring* (Washington, DC: National Academies Press, 1997); IOM, *Using Performance Monitoring to Improve Community Health: Exploring the Issues* (Washington, DC: National Academies Press, 1996); and Task Force on Community Preventive Services, "Introducing the *Guide to Community Preventive Services:* Methods, First Recommendations, and Expert Commentary," *American Journal of Preventive Medicine* 18(1S) (2000): 1–142.

20. IOM, *Healthy Communities: New Partnerships for the Future of Public Health* (Washington, DC: National Academies Press, 1996).

21. E. M. Kennedy, "Quality, Affordable Health Care for All Americans," *American Journal of Public Health* 93, no. 1 (2003): 14.

22. R. J. Mills, *Health Insurance Coverage: 2001* (Washington, DC: U.S. Bureau of the Census, 2002); IOM, *Unequal Treatment: Confronting Racial and Ethnic Disparities in Health Care* (Washington, DC: National Academies Press, 2002); and Kaiser Commission on Medicaid and the Uninsured, "Health Insurance Coverage in America, 2002 Data Update," December 2003, http://www.kff.org/uninsured/4154.cfm (accessed 8 April 2004).

23. G. Solanki, H. H. Schauffler, and L. S. Miller, "The Direct and Indirect Effects of Cost-Sharing on the Use of Preventive Services," *Health Services Research* 34, no. 6 (2000): 1331–1350.

24. M. Gibbon, R. Labonte, and G. Laverack, "Evaluating Community Capacity," *Health and Social Care in the Community* 10, no. 6 (2002): 485–491.

25. D. M. Hashimoto, "The Future Role of Managed Care and Capitation in Workers' Compensation," *American Journal of Law and Medicine* 22, nos. 2 and 3 (1996): 234.

26. U.S. House Committee on Education and the Workforce, "House Passes Bipartisan Bill to Give Uninsured Americans Access to Affordable Health Care," 19 June 2003, http://edworkforce.house.gov/press/press108/06jun/ahpsph061903.hhtm (accessed 8 April 2004); and U.S. Congress Office of Technology Assessment, "Does Health Insurance Make a Difference?—Background Paper" (Washington, DC: U.S. Government Printing Office, 1992).

27. IOM, *The Future of the Public's Health.*

28. IOM, *Rebuilding the Unity of Health and the Environment: A New Vision of Environmental Health for the Twenty-first Century* (Washington, DC: National Academies Press, 2001); N. Kunzli, "The Public Health Relevance of Air Pollution Abatement," *European Respiratory Journal* 20, no. 1 (2002): 198–209; F. van Poppel and C. van der Heijden, "The Effects of Water Supply on Infant and Childhood Mortality: A Review of Historical Evidence," *Health Transition Review* 7, no. 2 (1997): 113–148; R. E. Rice and C. K. Atkin, eds., *Public Communication Campaigns,* 2nd ed. (Newbury Park, CA: Sage, 2000); N. Pearce and G. Davey Smith, "Is Social Capital the Key to Inequalities in Health," *American Journal of Public Health* 93, no. 1 (2003): 122–129; IOM, *Unequal Treatment;* and R. Karasek and T. Theorell, *Healthy Work* (New York: Basic Books, 1990).

29. S. Srinivasan, A. Dearry, and L. R. O'Fallon, "Creating Healthy Communities, Healthy Homes, Healthy People: Initiating a Research Agenda on the Built Environment and Public Health," *American Journal of Public Health* 93, no. 9 (2003): 1446–1450; R. Ewing et al., "Relationship between Urban Sprawl and Physical Activity, Obesity, and Morbidity," *American Journal of Health Promotion* 18, no. 1 (2003): 47–57; R. Jackson and C. Kochitzky, *Creating a Healthy Environment: The Impact of the*

Built Environment on Public Health, Sprawl Watch Clearinghouse Monograph Series, http://www.sprawlwatch.org/health.pdf (accessed 9 April 2004); and WHO, "Diet, Nutrition, and the Prevention of Chronic Diseases," WHO Technical Report Series, 2003, http://www.who.int/ nut/documents/trs-916.pdf (accessed 9 April 2004).

30. E. Rogot et al., eds., *A Mortality Study of 1.3 Million Persons by Demographic, Social, and Economic Factors: 1979–1985 Follow-Up* (Bethesda, MD: National Institutes of Health, 1992).

31. E. M. Kitagawa and P. M. Hauser, *Differential Mortality in the United States: A Study of Socio-economic Epidemiology* (Cambridge, MA: Harvard University Press, 1973); M. G. Marmot et al., "Health Inequalities among British Civil Servants: The Whitehall II Study," *Lancet* 337, no. 8754 (1991): 1387–1393; and D. Acheson, *Independent Inquiry into Inequalities in Health* (London: Stationery Office, 1998).

32. R. G. Wilkinson, *Unhealthy Societies: The Afflictions of Inequality* (London: Routledge, 1996).

33. J. Lynch et al., "Is Income Inequality a Determinant of Population Health? Part 1: A Systematic Review," *Milbank Quarterly* 82, no. 1 (2004): 5–99.

34. N. Daniels, B. Kennedy, and I. Kawachi, "Justice Is Good for Our Health," *Boston Review* 25, no. 1 (2000): 6–15; and D. E. Beauchamp, "Public Health as Social Justice," *Inquiry* 13, no. 1 (1976): 3–14.

35. IOM, *Unequal Treatment;* IOM, *Guidance for the National Healthcare Disparities Report* (Washington, DC: National Academies Press, 2002); and Agency for Healthcare Research and Quality, *National Healthcare Disparities Report* (Washington, DC: DHHS, 2003).

36. H. Graham, "Social Determinants and Their Unequal Distribution: Clarifying Policy Understandings," *Milbank Quarterly* 82, no. 1 (2004): 101–124.

37. N. Eberstadt and S. Satel, *Health and the Income Inequality Hypothesis: A Doctrine in Search of Data* (Washington, DC: AEI Press, 2004).

38. L. O. Gostin, "Law and Ethics in Population Health," *Australian and New Zealand Journal of Public Health* 28, no. 1 (2004): 7–12.

39. J. Sachs, ed., *Report of the Commission on Macroeconomics and Health* (Geneva: WHO, 2001).

40. R. A. Epstein, "Let the Shoemaker Stick to His Last: A Defense of the 'Old' Public Health," *Perspectives in Biology and Medicine* 46, no. 3 Suppl. (2003): S138–S159.

41. L. O. Gostin, *Public Health Law and Ethics: A Reader* (Berkeley and New York: University of California Press and Milbank Memorial Fund, 2002).

42. J. M. McGinnis and W. H. Foege, "Actual Causes of Death in the United States," *Journal of the American Medical Association* 270, no. 18 (1993): 2207–2212.

43. M. Marmot and R. G. Wilkinson, eds., *Social Determinants of Health* (New York: Oxford University Press, 1999).

44. J. M. McGinnis, P. Williams-Russo, and J. R. Knickman, "The Case for More Active Policy Attention to Health Promotion," *Health Affairs* 21, no. 2 (2002): 78–93.

45. J. M. Mellor and J. D. Milyo, "Income Inequality and Health Status in the United States," *Journal of Human Resources* 37, no. 3 (2002): 510–539; and A. Garber, "Pursuing the Links between Socioeconomic Factors and Health," in *Pathways to Health: The Role of Social Factors,* ed. D. S. Gomby and B. H. Kehrer (Menlo Park, CA: Kaiser Family Foundation, 1989), 271–315.

46. V. Postrel, "The Pleasantville Solution: The War on 'Sprawl' Promises 'Livability' but Delivers Repression, Intolerance—and More Traffic," *Reason* 30, no. 10 (1999): 4.

47. W. C. Perdue, L. A. Stone, and L. O. Gostin, "The Built Environment and Its Relationship to the Public's Health: The Legal Framework," *American Journal of Public Health* 93, no. 9 (2003): 1390–1394.

48. W. C. Perdue, L. A. Stone, and L. O. Gostin, "Public Health and the Built Environment: Historical, Empirical, and Theoretical Foundations for an Expanded Role," *Journal of Law, Medicine, and Ethics* 31, no. 4 (2003): 557–566.

49. R. J. Jackson, "The Impact of the Built Environment on Health: An Emerging Field," *American Journal of Public Health* 93, no. 9 (2003): 1382–1383.

4

Rethinking the Meaning
of Public Health

Mark A. Rothstein

Public health is a dynamic field. Outbreaks of new diseases, as well as changing patterns of population growth, economic development, and lifestyle trends all may threaten public health and thus demand a public health response. As the practice of public health evolves, there is an ongoing need to reassess its scientific, ethical, legal, and social underpinnings. Such a reappraisal must consider the disagreement among public health officials, public health scholars, elected officials, and the public about the proper role of public health and the distinctions, for example, between public health and clinical care, and public health and health promotion.

In this article I will attempt to characterize the main points of contention as well as offer my own views regarding the proper scope of public health. Greater clarity and consensus on the meaning of public health are likely to lead to more efficient and effective public health interventions as well as increased public and political support for public health activities.

Alternative Definitions of "Public Health"

Human Rights as Public Health

There is a growing trend to include within the sphere of public health all the societal factors that affect health. This is a very long list, including war, violence, poverty, economic development, income distribution, natural resources, diet and lifestyle, health care infrastructure, overpopulation, and civil rights.[1] There is much to recommend viewing the sources of health broadly—in other words, considering health as more than the absence of illness and disease. Yet the conceptual value of considering the health of a population in light of a wide array of factors does not necessarily translate into a practical framework for implementing policy. The term *public health* is a legal term of art, and it refers to specifically delineated powers, duties, rights, and responsibilities. Even beyond its legal usage, public health applies to specific institutions and individuals, such as public health departments and public health officials.

The "human rights as public health" definition has been applied both internationally and domestically. According to Morris Schaefer: "The health of most people in the world depends less on access to medical services than on efficient farming, distributive justice, ensuring 'domestic tranquility,' and broad-based, sustainable development of natural and built environments."[2] Similarly, on a national level, William R. Breakey has written: "We should be as much concerned about the thousands of people who are homeless in American cities and the thousands of children in residentially unstable families as we are when there is an epidemic of an infectious disease affecting a few hundred people, and we should respond with the same urgency."[3] Schaefer and Breakey are certainly right in their assessments. Nevertheless, just because war, crime, hunger, poverty, illiteracy, homelessness, and human rights abuses interfere with the health of individuals and populations does not mean that eliminating these conditions is part of the mission of public health.

It is understandable why knowledgeable and caring health professionals would want to improve the health of individuals and communities by focusing on the root causes of illness and disease. Analyzing political, economic, and social issues in a scientific manner is appealing by providing essential data and more rigorous methodology. It also seems to help make the concerns more objective and their remediation more achievable. Unfortunately, labeling so many activities as public health does little if anything to eliminate the problem of poor health. "Even if we claimed that poverty is the root cause of all disease, which it surely is not, we would hardly be closer to solving the problem—just as we were no closer to eliminating the threat of nuclear war after pointing out that Armageddon would interfere with physicians' treatment of their patients."[4]

Ilan H. Meyer and Sharon Schwartz refer to the transformation of social issues into health issues as the "public healthification" of social problems, which they consider analogous to the medicalization of individual social problems.[5] In their view, public health provides too narrow a perspective to be effective. "In the case of many social problems, public health research questions as currently conceptualized are less complex than the social and political issues (conflicting interest groups, conflicting value systems, power relationships) that need to be resolved for interventions to be successfully applied."[6]

In a recent article, Larry Gostin describes three main reasons the all-inclusive notion of public health is not only ineffective but counterproductive.[7] First, the field of public health lacks precision if it includes such disparate areas of concern that have as their only commonality causing adverse effects on health. Second, as the field of public health expands well beyond its core area of expertise, it can claim no special abilities to end wars, modernize agriculture, or restructure economies. Third, by becoming involved with economic redistribution and social restructuring, the field becomes highly politicized.

The human rights definition of public health also raises practical problems. What curriculum could possibly train public health professionals on all the various root causes of poor health? What political system or public health budget will support far-ranging interventions by those charged with protecting public health? What effect will such seemingly quixotic activities have on the ability of public health professionals to combat traditional public health problems, such as infectious diseases and poor sanitation, as well as new threats, such as bioterrorism?

Individuals trained in public health should not give up the noble struggle to ensure that every person has a minimum standard of living to support a healthy life. But this battle must be fought together with people from all disciplines and all walks of life and without using the self-defeating strategy of annexing human rights into the public health domain.

Population Health as Public Health

A somewhat less-expansive, but still broad definition is the one traditionally used in public health. Under the traditional conception, public health focuses on the health of entire populations rather than individual patients. According to Dan Beauchamp and Bonnie Steinbock: "Whereas in medicine, the patient is an individual person, in public health, the 'patient' is the whole community or population. The goal of public health is to reduce disease and early death in populations."[8]

One of the most commonly cited definitions of public health in this vein comes from the Institute of Medicine (IOM) report *The Future of Public Health:* "Public health is what we, as a society, do collectively to assure the conditions for people to be healthy."[9] Although I would place this definition in the traditional category, it is a vague definition that fails to indicate the primary objective or scope of public health. Unlike most other definitions of public health, it does not explicitly state that public health is concerned with the health of the population rather than individuals.

The IOM report also makes public health the responsibility of everyone, although it gives primacy to government efforts: "The mission of public health is addressed by private organizations and individuals as well as by public agencies. But the governmental public health agency has a unique function: to see to it that vital elements are in place and that the mission is adequately addressed."[10] In contrast to this government-centered approach, a more expansive definition of public health cited in, but not necessarily endorsed by, the IOM report is the following: "It's anything that affects the health of the community on a mass basis."[11] Under such a view, efforts to improve access to health care as well as more general measures to prevent injury and illness and reduce morbidity and mortality, such as advice to use sunscreen and eat healthy foods, would be considered public health. I term this conception of public health the "population health as public health" model.

There are three important characteristics of the population health as public health model. Each characteristic, however, raises concerns. First, this version of public health is the province of both the public and private sectors. Thus, public health would include the efforts of nonprofit organizations, commercial entities, and private citizens to promote healthy lifestyles. A beer company's "drink with moderation" campaign, a cigarette company's program to discourage underage smoking, and a religious organization's promotion of abstinence to reduce teen pregnancy would all be considered public health efforts. With such a broad approach, there is a risk that the urgency of public health will become diluted, and the public will have an increasingly difficult time in distinguishing public health from public relations.

Second, population health as public health fails to establish any meaningful lines of demarcation between individual health and public health. Under the population health as public health approach, when individual health measures are performed on or addressed to an unspecified but sufficient number of individuals, then this becomes public health. For example, when primary care physicians adopt as the standard of care a new type of screening test or treatment modality, the result may be to improve the health of numerous individuals. But it is unclear at what point cumulative individual health measures become population health. It is also unclear when responsibility for such a health measure shifts from the individual health care provider to a public health official.

Third, unlike traditional public health measures, such as infectious disease control, the failure to undertake population health measures, such as a treatment or preventive measure for a person who is sick or at risk, does not place the health of other individuals in jeopardy. Consequently, when population health is based on multiple individual health actions, it may not justify coercive measures on the part of the government. Responsibility for these interventions would lie with individual health providers, nongovernmental organizations, and government agencies acting in their noncoercive, population health role. The population health as public health approach is thus ill-defined, with diverse actors pursuing widely divergent strategies to deal with the same health problems, tackling health problems of varying severity, and often pursuing their own agendas with little coordination or accountability. Furthermore, it is ill-advised to adopt a definition of public health that mixes government with nongovernment initiatives, coercive with noncoercive measures, and harms that affect individual health with those that affect the health of the public.

Government Intervention as Public Health

The third conception of public health, and the one I advocate, is more limited in scope. "Government intervention as public health" involves public officials taking appropriate measures pursuant to specific legal authority, after balancing private rights and public interests, to protect the health of the public. These measures may be coercive. The existence of a public threat demands a public response, and in a representative political system it is the government that is authorized to act on behalf of the public.[12] The police power is the constitutional authority on which public health measures are based. According to the U.S. Supreme Court:

> According to settled principles, the police power of a state must be held to embrace, at least, such reasonable regulations established directly by legislative enactment as will protect the public health and the public safety. . . . There are manifold

restraints to which every person is necessarily subject for the common good. On any other basis organized society could not exist with safety to its members.[13]

The moral and political authority (and duty) of the government to mandate public health actions, including quarantine, isolation, immunization, contact tracing, property seizures, and environmental regulation, derives from one of the following three conditions. First, the health of the population is threatened. The paradigmatic public health threat is an infectious disease, where the threat to the public is through the horizontal transmission of infection. Other health threats may have a public health effect because they involve common resources and because the failure to control the problem at the source will lead to adverse health consequences to many people. Thus, person-to-person transmission is not necessary to have a public health threat. Food safety, sanitation, water fluoridation, insect and vermin control, and pollution control are examples of public health measures to address health threats to the public.

The second type of condition to justify a public health intervention occurs when the government has unique powers and expertise related to an essential aspect of public health. Disease reporting and surveillance illustrates this category. Legally mandated reporting of certain types of health conditions, such as some infectious diseases, occupational diseases, cancers, sexually transmitted diseases, gunshot wounds, child fatalities, and suspected cases of domestic violence, are all important to the collective health of the community. Reporting allows for data aggregation and analysis, as well as more direct intervention to prevent additional cases. Without mandatory reporting, important cases would be lost, and only the government has the authority to mandate reporting. Moreover, government public health agencies have access to the trained professionals needed to interpret the data.

The third type of condition to justify a public health intervention occurs when government action is more efficient or more likely to produce an effective intervention. An example would be newborn screening programs, which are mandated by law in every state. Public health programs to identify inborn errors of metabolism and other heritable disorders offer uniformity in standards and reporting. In addition, screening programs are often tied to publicly financed follow-up and treatment.

The key element of public health is the role of the government—its power and obligation to invoke mandatory or coercive measures to eliminate a threat to the public's health. Without a threat to the public, it is much more difficult to make a case for the use of coercive powers; in the absence of such legal authority, the participation of individuals in health-enhancing activities ordinarily must be voluntary. Applying these principles to the three sources of moral and political authority for governmental public health activity, the justification for activity goes in descending order from (1) population-wide health threat; to (2) unique governmental powers and expertise about an essential aspect of public health; to (3) the need for more efficient and effective governmental action in ensuring public health. Public health activities in this third category may overlap with population health measures. Consequently, newborn screening for phenylketonuria (PKU), congenital hypothyroidism, and other disorders; school-based medical screening for scoliosis, tuberculosis, vision and hearing problems, dental caries, and other conditions; and broad health promotion activities may be considered in varying degrees by different jurisdictions to lack the urgency and public health effects necessary to require universal participation.

Under this narrower definition of public health, a "public health clinic" providing primary care is *not* engaged in public health; it is a public entity providing individual health care. In the United States, because there is no guaranteed access to health care, the responsibility for providing health care to uninsured individuals often falls to public health agencies. One effect of this allocation of responsibility is that providing primary care services tends to be commingled with, and to crowd out, other public health functions. As a result, many health departments lack the resources to engage in core public health functions, such as epidemiology, disease surveillance, and environmental regulation.

Dr. Barry Levy, former president of the American Public Health Association, observed that 97 percent of those questioned in a Harris poll did not know what public health is, and that a substantial number of the respondents said that public health is health care for the indigent.[14] According to Dr. Levy: "It should therefore not surprise us that many of our elected officials believe that when you move so-called indigent people into private-sector managed care programs, there is no need for public health anymore."[15]

In Support of a Narrower Definition

There are five reasons I believe it is desirable to embrace a narrower definition of public health. First, health-related activities that trigger the coercive power of government raise the most serious and complex legal and ethical issues; only activities falling within a narrow definition of public health can justify the use of this power. Second, the narrow and more specific classification of public health activities indicates the outer limits of coercion for government programs. Third, the classification scheme helps in allocating responsibilities for public, population, and individual health among the private, public, and not-for-profit sectors. Fourth, classifying possible government activities according to public health roles helps in setting priorities. Fifth, because public health has been the justification for some overreaching or even reprehensible prior government activities, ranging from eugenics to unethical research on human subjects, a narrow definition of public health will help steer public health officials away from activities that are inappropriate for the government.

This last point is illustrated by the recent emphasis on public health genetics.[16] Public health involves government action, coercive powers, and societal interests taking precedence over individual rights. In genetics, the dominant values are autonomy, reproductive freedom, and privacy. Thus, public health genetics seems paradoxical, thereby strongly suggesting that any undertaking in the field must be approached with great care. Any government activity is of particular concern when applied to genetics and reproduction. After all, paternalistic, coercive, government efforts to improve the nation's health through genetic intervention were the hallmarks of the eugenics programs adopted in the first third of the twentieth century. Public policy in genetics has yet to recover from this debacle of mixing public health powers with the scientific means to achieve ostensibly desirable social objectives.

Accordingly, those who would advocate a broad view of public health genetics beyond proven measures, such as newborn screening, should have to demonstrate that government action is essential and that detailed measures have been taken to protect individual rights.

Public health genetics also must draw clear distinctions with clinical genetics and clinical medicine. For example, hereditary hemochromatosis is a recessively inherited disorder of iron overload. It can cause serious organ damage if undetected, but it is relatively easy to test for presymptomatically using a genetic test, and it is easy to treat through periodic phlebotomies. Is reducing the morbidity associated with hemochromatosis a public health issue or a clinical issue that can be resolved through genetic testing by primary care providers in the course of regular medical examinations? I would argue that it is an individual health issue that, collectively, may become a population health issue, but it is not a public health issue.

Public Health Professionals, Schools, and Agencies

The taxonomy I am proposing may seem threatening to some public health professionals who may view the classification scheme as unsupportive of their work, misguided, naive, dangerous, or callous. I believe that such views would reflect an inaccurate interpretation of my proposal. I unequivocally support all of the health-related activities under the categories of individual health, population health, and public health. I also support even the broadest aims of the human rights as public health model. What I oppose is the use of the term *public health* as an open-ended descriptor of widely divergent efforts to improve the human condition. It surely will not hasten the elimination of disparate forms of human privations to call them public health issues.

A return to a narrow definition of public health should not have any effect on the curricula of schools of public health, although it might be appropriate to change their names to schools of public and population health. Even though aspects of health promotion, health education, health policy, health services, health research, and health law may be outside the government intervention as public health model, these and similar subjects are an essential part of the public (and population) health curriculum. So, too, are epidemiology, biostatistics, toxicology, sanitation, occupational and environmental health sciences, and all of the other methodology and basic science disciplines on which public health is based. For educational purposes, it does not matter whether particular methods and skills belong to population health or public health, and it does not matter whether the students subsequently work in the public, nonprofit, or private sector.

The narrow definition of public health may have an effect on setting the priorities of public health agencies. The top priorities should be those matters requiring mandatory interventions and therefore falling within the narrow definition of public health. In theory, the issues described as population health, including health promotion and health research, would be the next priority. This allocation of responsibilities, however, assumes that the public health agency is not responsible for providing basic medical care, such as prenatal and well-baby care, and other services. To the extent that these are health department responsibilities, then they will need to be integrated into the second level of priorities, after those measures that directly and immediately affect the health of the population.

The Ethical Foundations of Public Health

According to the definition I have suggested, public health invariably involves a balancing of individual and group interests, or private and public interests. Viewed in terms of bioethics, the conflict is between autonomy and paternalism. Decisions about where to strike the balance are not static, and they are influenced by varied and often-changing value systems—on an individual, groupwide, and population-wide basis. This fact suggests several necessary responses by public health officials. First, public health interventions must be culturally sensitive and take into account a range of values on issues such as privacy, autonomy, liberty, and dignity. Second, because public attitudes change over time, public health officials must continually justify public health interventions, even long-standing measures of proven efficacy. Third, public health officials and their allies in the public and private sectors must be vigilant. For example, according to the Centers for Disease Control and Prevention report *Public Health's Infrastructure: A Status Report*: "Complacency about the need to maintain vigilance against public health threats has allowed the costly resurgence of many nearly eliminated diseases, including, most recently, tuberculosis and measles."[17]

A few examples will demonstrate the balancing of group versus individual and public versus private interests. Immunization requirements have been a keystone of public health practice since the early part of the twentieth century. Within the last 10 years, however, there have been a number of efforts in state legislatures to increase the statutory exemptions from mandatory immunization. In many states, parents have long been permitted to raise religious objections to immunizations. Some advocates would extend the grounds for exemption to include general personal beliefs about the safety or efficacy of immunization. Broad exemptions, however, raise the distinct possibility of a resurgence of vaccine-preventable disease.[18] Thus, in terms of public health policy, it is necessary to recognize the objections to immunization among growing segments of the population and to demonstrate the current safety, efficacy, and importance of mandatory immunization. Without such documentation, policy development in the legislative arena may afford greater weight to individual liberty interests and asserted parental rights than to public health.

In some instances, public health policy development involves the balancing of two competing private interests. For example, occupational and environmental health are traditional areas of public health activity. New research has established that individuals vary in their risk of illness from occupational exposure based on genetic factors. Should an employer be permitted to use genetic tests to exclude from hazardous exposures individuals who have a genetically increased risk of occupational illness?[19] From a scientific standpoint, numerous factors must be considered, including the absolute risk, the relative risk, the severity of the risk, the latency period, and whether the condition is treatable.[20] Assuming that it made sense from a scientific standpoint to reduce the exposure of at-risk individuals, this would only be a starting point for the policy analysis. The interests of the employer in productivity and profitability (as well as the public interest in preventing illness) would still need to be balanced against the privacy and economic interests of the individual. Here, the conflict between autonomy and paternalism involves primarily private interests, but the government's role in public health (as well as in civil rights and employment policy) is to strike the proper balance.

Conclusion

In common parlance, "public health" is now a general, descriptive term and not a term of art. It is incongruous to embrace the broadest meaning of public health at the same time that our legal system and public health infrastructure are based on a narrow definition of public health jurisdiction, authority, and remedies. Moreover, the boundless conception of public health now gaining in popularity not only may fail to achieve its goal of alleviating the economic and social roots of ill health, but it may actually impede the ability of public health officials to provide traditional public health services.

The moral and political power of governments to act in the realm of public health devolves from the existence of a serious threat to the public. Coercive public health measures are justified by the natural law principle of self-preservation applied on a societal basis. Indeed, modern public health traces its philosophical roots to nineteenth-century utilitarianism.[21] The broad power of government to protect public health includes the authority to supersede individual liberty and property interests in the name of preserving the greater public good. It is an awesome responsibility, and therefore it cannot and must not be used indiscriminately.

According to the definition I support, only public health officials can undertake public health actions because their coercive powers are firmly grounded in constitutional provisions and enabling legislation. In my view, public health does not include providing basic health services or population health measures, such as health promotion, and it does not include private actors undertaking similar individual or population health measures. The distinctions among the definitions of public health and their various applications are more than semantic. A clearer understanding of the role of public health helps to allocate responsibilities, set priorities, and avoid inappropriate government activities.

Gabriela Alcalde of the Institute for Bioethics, Health Policy and Law at the University of Louisville School of Medicine, contributed to this article.

Notes

1. See, e.g., B. C. Amick III et al., eds., *Society and Health* (New York: Oxford University Press, 1995); S. P. Marks, "Jonathan Mann's Legacy to the Twenty-first Century:

The Human Rights Imperative for Public Health," *Journal of Law, Medicine & Ethics,* 29 (2001): 131–138; M. Marmot and R. G. Wilkinson, eds., *Social Determinants of Health* (New York: Oxford University Press, 1999).

2. University of Washington School of Public Health and Community Medicine, Department of Health Services, *Public Health & Related Definitions,* at http:// depts.washington.edu/hserv/research/phdefinitions.shtml (last revised 13 April 1998) (statement of Morris Schaefer).

3. W. R. Breakey, "It's Time for the Public Health Community to Declare War on Homelessness," *American Journal of Public Health,* 87 (1997): 153–155, at 153.

4. K. J. Rothman, H.-O. Adami, and D. Trichopoulos, "Should the Mission of Epidemiology Include the Eradication of Poverty?" *Lancet,* 352 (1998): 810–813, at 812.

5. I. H. Meyer and S. Schwartz, "Social Issues as Public Health: Promise and Peril," *American Journal of Public Health,* 90 (2000): 1189–1191, at 1189.

6. Ibid. at 1191.

7. L. O. Gostin, "Public Health, Ethics, and Human Rights: A Tribute to the Late Jonathan Mann," *Journal of Law, Medicine & Ethics,* 29 (2001): 121–130, at 123.

8. D. E. Beauchamp and B. Steinbock, "Population Perspective," in D. E. Beauchamp and B. Steinbock, eds., *New Ethics for the Public's Health* (New York: Oxford University Press, 1999), at 25.

9. Committee for the Study of the Future of Public Health, Institute of Medicine, *The Future of Public Health* (Washington, DC: National Academy Press, 1988), at 19.

10. Ibid. at 7.

11. Ibid. at 37 (quoting unidentified interviewee).

12. See L. O. Gostin, "Public Health Law in a New Century Part I: Law as a Tool to Advance the Community's Health," *Journal of the American Medical Association,* 283 (2000): 2837–2841.

13. *Jacobson v. Massachusetts,* 197 U.S. 11, 25, 26 (1905).

14. B. S. Levy, "Creating the Future of Public Health: Values, Vision, and Leadership," *American Journal of Public Health,* 88 (1998): 188–192, at 189.

15. Ibid.

16. See M. A. Rothstein, "Genetics and Public Health in the Twenty-first Century: Using Genetic Information to Improve Health and Prevent Disease" [book review], *New England Journal of Medicine,* 343 (2000): 1580.

17. U.S. Department of Health and Human Services, Centers for Disease Control and Prevention, *Public Health's Infrastructure: A Status Report* (2001), at 12, available at http://www.phppo.cdc.gov/documents/phireport2_16.pdf (accessed March 21, 2002).

18. C. Feudtner and E. K. Marcuse, "Ethics and Immunization Policy: Promoting Dialogue to Sustain Consensus," *Pediatrics,* 107 (2001): 1158–1164.

19. See M. A. Rothstein, "Genetics and the Work Force of the Next Hundred Years," *Columbia Business Law Review,* 2000 (2000): 371–402.

20. See M. A. Rothstein, *Medical Screening and the Employee Health Cost Crisis* (Washington, DC: Bureau of National Affairs, 1989), at 132–140.

21. A. H. M. Kerkhoff, "Origin of Modern Public Health and Preventive Medicine," in S. Doxiadis, ed., *Ethical Dilemmas in Health Promotion* (New York: Wiley, 1987).

Further Reading

Beauchamp, Dan E., *The Health of the Republic: Epidemics, Medicine, and Moralism as Challenges to Democracy* (Philadelphia: Temple University Press, 1988).

Berkman, Lisa F., and Ichiro Kawachi, eds., *Social Epidemiology* (New York: Oxford University Press, 2000).

Gostin, Lawrence O., "Health of the People: The Highest Law?" *Journal of Law, Medicine & Ethics* 32(3): Fall 2004, 509–515.

Hardin, Garrett, "The Tragedy of the Commons," *Science* 162(3859): 13 December 1968, 1243–1248.

Institute of Medicine, *The Future of the Public's Health in the Twenty-first Century* (Washington, DC: National Academies Press, 2002).

PART II

AUTONOMY AND PATERNALISM

Introduction

In *Free to Be Foolish*, Howard Leichter asserts:

> There is now widespread agreement among both the general population and health professionals that a good deal of disease is self-inflicted, the product of our own imprudent behavior. The premise that individuals contribute significantly to their own ill health or premature death appears unassailable in view of the mounting evidence relating various personal habits and lifestyle choices, such as poor nutrition, smoking, alcohol and drug abuse, failure to wear seatbelts, and unsafe sexual practices, to major causes of morbidity and mortality. While it is generally accepted that each of us is, to a certain extent, "dangerous to our own health," there is far less agreement on what can or should be done about making people less foolish.[1]

The issues posed in this part of the book can be thought of in terms of the following questions: What are the appropriate limits of the state in a liberal society in regulating, restricting, or prohibiting behaviors that lead to premature morbidity and mortality; in shaping, molding, or influencing the preferences and desires of its citizens; in protecting citizens from commercial influences that may encourage or sustain patterns of behavior that are antiethical to the goals of public health? Does the focus on the behavior of individuals inevitably entail a shift in attention from the institutional and structural roots of disease to the most vulnerable? Does it represent a form of victim blaming?

Because of the profound influence of individualism on American culture and politics, a useful place to begin is with an oft-quoted passage from John Stuart Mill's essay *On Liberty,* in which we encounter a robust defense of the individual against intrusions by the state and society in general:

85

The only purpose for which power can be rightfully exercised over any member of the civilized community, against his will, is to prevent harm to others. His own good, either physical or moral, is not sufficient warrant. He cannot rightfully be compelled to do or forbear because it will be better for him to do so, because it will make him happier, because, in the opinions of others, to do so would be wise, or even right. These are good reasons for remonstrating with him, or reasoning with him, or persuading him, or entreating him, but not for compelling him, or visiting him with any evil in case he do otherwise. To justify that, the conduct from which it is desired to deter him, must be calculated to produce evil to some one else. The only part of the conduct of any one, for which he is amenable to society, is that which concerns others. In the part which merely concerns himself, his independence is, of right, absolute. Over himself, over his own body and mind, the individual is sovereign.[2]

The target of Mill's animus is paternalism—the attempt to impose limitations on someone or to require actions by someone for his or her own good. From his vantage, such impositions can be justified in two circumstances: (1) with children, because it is assumed that they are incapable of deciding on their own behalf, and (2) with those who, because of cognitive limitations, cannot choose on their own behalf.

By contrast, intervention is justified, for Mill, when one acts in a way that may pose harm to others. Other-regarding harms are the appropriate target of government regulation. The shorthand for this justification has come to be known as the "harm principle." We return to this issue in part V.

Conventionally put, the principle asserts "your freedom to swing your arm ends where my nose begins." This apparently straightforward formulation opens the way to a series of questions involving the nature of harms that may be prevented. While the bodily injury entailed in a blow to the nose is clearly a harm for Mill, what about an injury that is threatened; one that is possible, or only remotely so; one that is merely statistical, smoking in an open-air café, for example? What if the potential harm involves an annoyance, for example, the smell of smoke in an open-air stadium? What if an act is self-regarding in terms of injury but is other-regarding in terms of economic burdens imposed on others? The point here is to underscore the extent to which Mill's formulation can either serve to impose radical limits on what government can do in the name of public health or, if very broadly interpreted, open the way to the type of interventions that would for all practical purposes eliminate the distinction between the realm of the private and that of the social, between the self-regarding and other regarding. After all, in a highly integrated society, what action does anyone take that does not *ultimately* have an impact on "society"?

Can Mill's antagonism to paternalism serve as a basis for an ethics of public health? If Mill's doctrine is very broadly construed, does it compel justifications for public health that ultimately involve gross contortions, finding harms to others when they can only remotely be understood as such? For example, when states imposed mandatory motorcycle helmet laws, they claimed to be doing so to protect the public from the costs of accidents rather than to protect cyclists from their own risky behavior. The alternative would have been to embrace paternalism explicitly as a core value of public health. While such a strategy might be politically untenable, it would open the way to a more candid discussion of the extent to which communal well-being justifies limits on behaviors that impose harms to individuals themselves and only secondarily on others.

Part II begins with a classic selection that provides a broad foundation for thinking about the issues. Daniel Wikler compels us to consider the question of whether we have a duty to be healthy and if so why, drawing parallels with the question of whether we have an obligation to society to be maximally productive. After locating the debate over the role of the state in health protection in historical context, the next selection, by Ronald Bayer and Jonathan D. Moreno, examines three modes of policy intervention designed to modify behaviors deemed harmful to health: education, taxes, prohibition. Educational efforts are the least intrusive on the claims of individual autonomy but can pose unique questions when they begin to employ manipulative strategies. The reliance on excise taxes as a way of imposing additional costs on certain consumption patterns can serve as a deterrent but may raise questions of equity, given the regressive nature of such levies. Finally, explicit prohibitions and mandates are the most intrusive on rights and may be highly effective. But typically they raise questions about the costs, both practical and moral, of enforcement.

With this background, part II then examines two critical debates: whether currently illicit drugs should continue to be subject to a prohibitionist regime and what the appropriate public health response to tobacco should be. In both cases, sharply opposing views are paired. Robert E. Goodin, relying on utilitarian thinking, makes the case for severe restrictions on tobacco not only because of social costs but also because of the harms smokers impose on themselves. In doing so, he explicitly embraces the value of paternalism and provides the moral warrant for the neotemperance posture of the contemporary public health campaign against tobacco. Jacob Sullum, a libertarian, gives voice to Mill's perspective in opposing such restraints. In the case of currently illicit drugs, Ethan A. Nadelmann sets out to demonstrate that prohibition has been a costly disaster for individuals and society. By contrast, James Q. Wilson argues that permitting greater access to drugs would inevitably result in more widespread use and subvert the very foundations of human decency. In so doing, he parts company with other conservative thinkers, like the economist Milton Friedman, who are deeply suspicious of, indeed hostile to, government intrusions in the lives of adults.

The case studies of tobacco and illicit drugs, important in and of themselves, serve to illuminate the complex play of moral consideration in the making of public health policy regarding behaviors linked to disease and death.

Notes

1. Leichter, Howard, *Free to Be Foolish: Politics and Health Promotion in the United States and Great Britain* (Princeton, NJ: Princeton University Press, 1991).
2. Mill, John Stuart, *On Liberty* (New Haven, CT: Yale University Press, 2003).

5

Who Should Be Blamed
for Being Sick?

Daniel Wikler

Introduction

Health promotion is frequently said to proceed from the premise that *individuals are responsible for their health.*

Fine—but what does it mean? Perhaps nothing more profound than that people will usually be healthier if they try to take better care of themselves. However, if that is all it means, it is too simple an idea to serve as the philosophical foundation for a comprehensive approach to health and health care. To fulfill that latter role, it must be understood as having moral and policy implications and must involve ethical and even juridical concepts: role, obligation, and duty; perhaps fault, blame, and excuses, guilt, punishment, and compensation. Even when one who uses the slogan intends no such message, those who hear it may do so. In either case, it is important to explore the meanings and implications of the concept of personal responsibility for health before enshrining it as the motto of a new school of health promotion and education.

Concepts of Personal Responsibility
for Health

Different parties to current health policy debates have different uses for the theme of personal responsibility for health.

Advocates of self-help, and some of those devoted to holistic medicine, have encouraged individuals to eschew passive reliance on professional healers and to take the initiative in staying healthy. Some holists wax poetic, and even religious, concerning the "duty" to maintain one's physical well-being: Personal responsibility for health becomes a moral, or "spiritual" duty.[1] This moral element, however, is not inherent in their program. A toned-down holism would hold only that those who evade their "responsibility" to take care of themselves are imprudent, perhaps, or stupid, or ignorant—but not particularly evil.

Others who speak of personal responsibility for health, however, are clearly concerned with moral right and wrong.[2] People have an obligation, in this view, not only to themselves but also to their fellow citizens and taxpayers. They should keep themselves healthy so that they can avoid becoming dependent, and they must do whatever is in their power to prevent illness which could burden others with the costs of care. Accordingly, failure to accept one's responsibility for health is deemed to be grounds for penalties which would not be otherwise justified. If people fail in this responsibility and allow themselves to become sick, they may forfeit any claims to their neighbor's aid. Alternatively, they might be obligated to submit before actually becoming ill to policies which enforce this responsibility, including those which interfere with ordinary liberties through coercive health programs and prohibition of unhealthy substances and practices.

It is already clear that the term *responsibility* is being used in somewhat different senses by these groups. It follows that we cannot supply an answer to our question, "Are we responsible for our health?" unless we can achieve a more substantial and precise understanding of what is being asked. To this end, it will be worthwhile to explore the moral notions involved.

In a valuable article, Dworkin[3] has distinguished several distinct senses of "responsibility" as they occur in the context of the debate over personal responsibility for health. Three of these senses have figured in the earlier discussion. First, a person is "role-responsible" for his health because (it is said) the body in question is his own; the "role" here is the general one of being a biological organism. Neither I nor (I believe) Dworkin means to endorse the suggestion that being a biological organism carries such responsibilities, but this seems to be what some who speak of personal responsibility for health seem to have in mind. Second, one is "causally responsible" for one's health in that one's health status is determined in large part by one's own choice of behavior. Finally, a person is "liability-responsible" for one's health if, and to the extent that, one is assigned liability for the costs and other undesirable consequences of being sick.

It is useful to keep these in mind when considering the kinds of political, moral, and policy arguments in which the concept of personal responsibility for health has figured. Doing so will permit a more precise statement of, and distinction between, the lines of argument which have appeared in support of policies which either apply coercion to lifestyles or else single out those who risk their health for special treatment in health insurance and health care.

Paternalism

The first of these arguments is straightforwardly paternalistic: If we hold individuals responsible for their health, they can be required to keep better care of themselves.

They will then avoid needless suffering and expense. Our concern with their welfare justifies our intervention.

A sizable streak of paternalism runs through some of the literature on personal responsibility for health. However, paternalism is not, in this country, a respectable public rationale for coercive government policies. The paternalistic argument, then, tends to be either masked as something else or else marshalled only in support of relatively innocuous programs, such as consumer education. The retreat from motorcycle helmet laws, despite their clear health advantages, is symptomatic of the unpopularity of programs which are perceived as paternalistic.

General Utility

The second argument is addressed primarily to the general good. Illness is a terribly costly problem in a country like ours. Health care has become increasingly expensive, and containment of costs has become a national campaign. It is now a truism that actions which individuals could take on their own could be vastly more effective in combatting illness than all that doctors can do.[4] Here, then, seems to be a critically important opportunity to contain costs. Cost containment could have further consequences of moral importance. We could use the money to meet other needs, and we would have greater ease in extending health care to those who become ill but do not have the means to pay for their own care. In this view, unhealthy lifestyles are no longer affordable in this and similar societies, given the need to use our resources efficiently in meeting fundamental human needs. It may also be a part of this view that those whose lifestyle contributes to the cost problem in health care have a duty, in their role as fellow members of the community, to acquiesce in programs designed to promote healthier living.

Communitarian Rationales

There is a further rationale which is at least a cousin of the first two; whether it should be counted as a distinct argument unto itself is not wholly clear. According to the proponents of this view,[5] the public's health and safety is a special kind of good, one which is a good of the community in addition to whatever good it might be to individuals. As such, it is not simply the sum of individual goods, just as its beneficiary, the community, is not merely the sum of the individuals composing it. This collective agent may legitimately pursue its goals, such as collective health, even when doing so causes it to conflict with the private goals of some of the constituent individuals. The point is not that the community's goal always should come first, but that it constitutes a distinct interest of its own. Policies that pursue that interest do not champion some individuals over others, but rather uphold the public, community interest over that of some individuals. This remains so even when, as individuals, members of the community engage in unhealthy behavior in fulfilling their private interests.

It is easy to see how this communitarian rationale could be taken to be merely a composite of the paternalistic and utilitarian viewpoints. Either the "community" is sticking its nose into the risk takers' personal lives to benefit the risk taker (paternalism) or to benefit the group (utilitarianism), or perhaps the group as a whole simply likes the idea of everyone being healthy and is offended by risk taking. However, defenders of this rationale reject these interpretations, insisting that these fail to transcend the narrow understanding of health as necessarily a private, individual good. Their argument would be easier to make out if health could be naturally likened to those goods which are ordinarily regarded as inherently public: clean air, for example, which benefits all whether or not they pay for it, and social solidarity, which is a relational property and hence inherently collective. There are, to be sure, numerous public goods of this sort involved in public health, from highway safety to research on lung cancer. It is less clear, at least to this writer, that this supplies a "community interest" in "community health" that requires people to jog more and eat less, where this interest is taken to be something distinct from the sum of the interests of the individual and those affected by his risk taking.

Whether we count the above as two or as three rationales for assigning personal responsibility for health to the individual, they have in common a lack of dependence on any notion of liability responsibility.

Indeed, the paternalistic rationale is not at home with the notion of fault. To hold a person to be at fault for imposing costs on others through unhealthy lifestyle choices it is usually necessary to portray that individual as a free, competent agent. When we imagine forcing people, for their own good, to take better care of themselves, we may have in mind people whose behavior is not the result of free, informed choice. Thus, the compulsive eater and the addicted smoker may "need" our help. We are generally less inclined to intervene in the case of those who eat a lot because they like to and who have rationally decided to accept the risk.

Those who would attempt to influence lifestyles in order to contain costs need not take a stand on whether those who take risks are at fault. The risk takers simply present an opportunity for efforts to reduce need for health services. The policy question is whether the unhealthy choices are subject to influence and change, rather than whether they constitute fault. However, the use of penalties and other coercive measures will be more difficult to justify if fault cannot be found. Importation of a notion of civic duty may not suffice to convince those subjected to penalties that the state is being fair in leaning on them to produce the savings which the community feels it needs.

Fairness

A final rationale rests squarely on the notion of fault.[6] Those who risk illness by smoking, lack of exercise, and other unhealthy habits are unfairly burdening their neighbors. The risk takers are making choices which may have important negative consequences for others, but they are not having to take these consequences into account in their deliberations. Fairness demands, then, that these costs be imposed on those who generate them.

This view is thus based upon a certain conception of justice in the distribution of health care resources. In this view, the person who takes risks with his own health gambles with resources which belong to others. The underlying principle which seems to be assumed is that an individual's needs do not entitle him or her to social resources if these needs are created or exacerbated by his or her free decisions. Someone who would not need medical care except for his own unhealthy lifestyle is thus creating needs for medical care where none would otherwise exist. The resulting health care needs thus have a different moral status from other, "involuntary" needs.

Though the underlying principle has not been addressed by much theoretical writing on distributive justice, it is, considered in the abstract, intuitively appealing. A person who received perfectly just wages but who spends all his money on useless baubles can hardly turn around and cry poverty. The hunger resulting from a lack of cash due to such profligate spending may be just as real as hunger due to lack of a just share of dollars, but providing help at this point seems to be a matter of charity rather than of justice.

That the concept of fault is essential to this third rationale for holding individuals responsible for their health can be seen by comparing lifestyle choices to other circumstances which involve burdening on others. It costs the same to treat a person suffering from an injury caused by an earthquake or tornado as it does to treat the same kind of injury caused by refusal to wear a motorcycle helmet. All other things being equal, the costs will be the same burden on those shouldering them, be they taxpayers or co-insureds. Yet many will have a quite different attitude toward these burdens. Assuming that we hold a view of justice which includes entitlements to some measure of health care, the cost to others of the involuntary injury will be accepted as part of the burden of their fellow citizenship. To the extent that the decision not to wear the helmet is perceived as wholly informed and voluntary, the burden it imposes may be resented and ultimately rejected.

Thus, paternalists who insist that we are responsible for staying healthy will have in mind causal responsibility, perhaps conjoined with role responsibility, and the same is probably true of those whose emphasis on personal responsibility is motivated by concern for the general good. Liability responsibility, based on a finding of fault, is essential only to that approach which brands a person's unhealthy choices as positively unfair to others.

Policy Choices

Despite the vigor of the debate over personal responsibility for health, it is not entirely clear what hangs on its outcome. Many authors who press the theme of personal responsibility for health are vague on this. They may note the tragedy of preventable suffering or the seeming irrationality of spending large amounts of money on health care for diseases which could have been avoided at little or no cost. Claims to the effect that "we can no longer afford" the illnesses which result from unhealthy lifestyles are also frequent. Clearly, these authors wish that people would take better care of themselves. Our question is what they think should happen to people who do not take care of themselves.

The first policy which would follow from an emphasis on personal responsibility for health would be to increase efforts to inform people of the risks they visit upon themselves, to offer advice on how to achieve healthier lifestyles, and to attempt to induce in the public a favorable attitude toward keeping fit. The government now undertakes these tasks in any number of contexts, and few take exception to them, except on grounds of effectiveness. Some controversy might be aroused if the appeals became more strident or overtly manipulative.

Such programs lead naturally, though not inexorably, to a more active sort of encouragement. Increased taxes on cigarettes and other dangerous substances are a mild form. A stronger measure is the threat of loss of employment.[7]

Next in order of likelihood would be an attempt to change the basis on which premiums for health insurance are assessed. Those who take risks with their health would, in schemes occasionally proposed, pay more for their insurance. The higher fee for risk takers could, of course, be masked by a general increase accompanied by "incentives" for non–risk takers.

In either case, the amount of the penalty for risk taking would be fixed differently depending on the motivation for the adjustment of premiums. If the goal were that of imposing costs on those whose choices generate them, the idea might be not to deter such behavior but to "tax" it so that others are not unfairly burdened. In this case, the premiums would be decided on an actuarial basis. If, on the other hand, the motive were to discourage the behavior, whether for paternalistic reasons or out of concern for the welfare of those who might have to pay for the risk takers' care, the premium would be set after a determination of the power of various premium amounts to deter risk-taking behavior. Of course, other means, such as the requirement that motorcyclists wear safety helmets, might also be employed to deter risk taking, whichever the motivation.

More drastic policy choices following upon an emphasis on personal responsibility for health would involve the actual denial of care. If there is an actual shortage of a particular medical resource, such as transplantable organs, those whose need for the treatment was judged to be self-induced could be placed at the end of the line (all other factors being equal). The policy might be applied to entire categories of treatment. Funding for liver transplants in adults, for example, has been questioned on the grounds that most of the candidates for this very expensive treatment would be alcoholics who had created their need through their behavior. Similarly, lung cancer might be regarded as somewhat less worthy of public attention than other diseases of similar lethality because many cases are due to smoking. The government's commitment to research on the causes of and cure for AIDS has been questioned by critics who perceive a tendency to blame the disease on its victims' lifestyles.

Finally, there are more global policy choices which might be thought to follow from the assignment of responsibility for health to the individual. If people make themselves sick through their own choices, then illness is not something that "happens" to people, not a "natural" misfortune. Our tendency to feel sympathy with those who have become ill is lessened, replaced by an attitude that the sick are people who would have been fine had they not gambled and lost. In some measure, this change in attitudes undercuts some of the support which many would otherwise give for public provision of health care generally or for government's role as an insurer of last resort. Carried still further, this attitude could undermine support for the medical enterprise as a whole, except as one carried on in markets under normal business conditions, as in the trade of any ordinary commodity or service. These implications are especially powerful in combination with the present revulsion for inflation in medical costs and with the recent wave of therapeutic nihilism, in which the promise of medicine to deliver benefits in keeping with its costs is seriously questioned.

Blaming the Victim?

These claims of personal responsibility for health are sometimes answered jointly and peremptorily with one or both of a pair of rebuttals. One rebuttal is that such claims involve nothing more than "blaming the victim."[8-10] The other rebuttal is that the policy consequences of a recognition of personal responsibility for health would violate individual privacy. Each rebuttal is put forward as nearly self-evident and as sufficient reason to drop the talk of personal responsibility altogether.

A certain distaste for the whole subject is understandable. Inquiring into personal responsibility for so grave a condition as serious illness almost surely betokens an insensitivity and meanness of spirit which is unpleasant to contemplate. The focus on the individual's choices distracts us from what are, from a certain moral point of view, more important issues of health policy: access to medical care at reasonable cost; improved effectiveness of medical care; and reduction of health hazards in the environment and in the workplace. Indeed, as we have seen, emphasis on the individual undermines the ideological basis for reform. If health is mostly a function of how individuals choose to behave, then medical care is less important, and if it is less important, then it is not important enough to be made a matter of right. The same conclusion follows if the individual is assigned liability responsibility for the illness which results from his "lifestyle" rather than to the social forces which shape his behavior and thus determine that lifestyle.

Perhaps these observations show that personal responsibility for health should not be discussed at all, except to expose the ideological character of the debate. In the abortion controversy, those who pause to take the negative side of the debate over the humanity of the fetus provide the other side with partial victory; perhaps here, too, a discussion such as the present one serves to legitimize the concept even while pointing out the conceptual difficulties inherent in its application.

But it is just as likely, in this writer's view, that the lack of a debate over the merits of assigning responsibility for health to the individual will lead to the uncritical and unhesitating adoption of the associated political and moral program. What cannot be ignored is that personal responsibility for health does seem fair and fitting to much of moral common sense. If there really is some kind of conspiracy to use the concept to undermine public support for rights to health care and to protection from workplace and environmental hazards, the conspirators have chosen a popular and effective slogan. It should be discussed and evaluated lest it be accepted by default.

Questioning Assumptions

Do the rationales for assigning responsibility for health to the individual make a compelling case for seriously considering some of the policies which have been proposed? Those who sound this theme often take it for granted that they do. On closer examination, however, their arguments depend on some important assumptions on a number of fundamental matters. These assumptions, once brought to life, are anything but self-evident. The following paragraphs set some of these out. Though no attempt is made to reach firm conclusions as to their defensibility, this exposition demonstrates the difficulties involved in making a serious case for assigning responsibility for health to individuals.

"We Know What People Can Do to Stay Healthy"

There has never been a shortage of people urging others to take immediate steps to restore or maintain health.[11] We know that many of the most spirited advocates of healthful living gave useless or even dangerous advice. The ethical principle "ought implies can" itself implies that individuals cannot be responsible for staying healthy if they do not know how to do so. Those who would hold individuals responsible must insist that at last we do know what people can do for themselves; others will insist that they are mistaken.[12]

"People Who Take Risks with Their Health (Wrongly) Burden Others"

The argument from fairness proceeds from the premise that people who become ill because they do not take proper care of themselves place an unfair burden on their neighbors. Yet, the causal relationship between the risk-taking behavior and the financial status of others is often difficult to make out. In a system in which all citizens were covered by universal health insurance, and in which the decision to seek medical health through the national plan was mandatory, the relationship would be straightforward. If I take a risk with my health and become ill as a result, if I am made to see a doctor, and if you are made to pay for it, then my decision has affected your pocketbook. However, these conditions do not hold in our society. There is considerable social investment in health care institutions, and it might be true that less investment would be required if everyone took care of themselves, but this makes the relationship between an individual's taking on health risks and another's becoming financially burdened much less direct than seems to be assumed in much of the literature. If I am left to my own resources in finding a physician and paying for his or her services, then my taking on risks impoverishes myself first of all.

It is true that most Americans are members of groups of insured individuals, with the result that other members of the group may have to pay higher premiums to compensate the medical staff for treatment rendered to a person who took health risks. It does not directly follow from this fact, however, that such risk-taking behavior is an unjust burden on others. Insurance is, after all, often purchased in order to cover oneself when taking a risk. When one pools one's insurance dollars with other risk takers, then one has the comfort of knowing that if the risk turns sour, one is still not left too far behind. Of course, health insurance is probably not thought of by most who purchase it as a means of covering themselves for taking risks; it is thought, rather, to protect against medically undesirable consequences of unavoidable hazards, either those presented by nature or those imposed by the toxic environment. The risk-taking behavior in this case would simply be that of living itself. Thus, the analogy is not quite exact. A second caution is that the system of "community rating," according to which insureds are not placed in different pools according to likelihood of health need, tends to undermine the notion that health insurance is a way to cover oneself when taking risks with one's health. When the community rating requirement is imposed not really by the market but by requirement of the state, the relation between risk taking and unfair burdening becomes relatively more direct. Still, what follows from these considerations is not that my taking risks with my health counts as an unfair burden on you; we also need an argument to show that it would not be appropriate or correct to allow people to buy insurance which would cover themselves when taking health risks.

"No One Has the Right to Force Others to Pay for Their Unhealthy Behavior"

Do people whose lifestyles lead to avoidable illness make unfair demands on their more careful fellow citizens? Do the latter have cause to refuse to accept them? Or even to curb the risk-taking behavior before it results in illness?

It seems apparent to many that the correct answers to these questions are affirmative. Yet there is implicit in such answers the idea that we all can agree on which of the burdens our choices place on others is unfair, for nearly all our choices do place burdens on others. In some cases, as with freedom of speech, we have constitutional protection: We can say what we want, short of libel and slander, and the fact that harm to others may result provides no excuse for state intervention on their behalf. Our freedom of choice, regardless of consequences, extends as well to behavior which lacks explicit constitutional protection. Those who would place responsibility for health on the individual may be upset that I do not jog, but what of my failure to moonlight? If I took up a second job, then my taxes would reduce the tax burden on others and would further reduce the risk of my being admitted to the welfare rolls. Similarly, my decision to become an academic philosopher resulted in less tax dollars than I would have produced had I chosen a more lucrative career; and the decision of my rust-belt neighbors to stay put rather than to accept higher paying jobs in the Sunbelt must be put in the same category. The general point is that there are a great number of chances for becoming more of a help and less of a burden to our fellow citizens. Indeed, the opportunities to lighten our neighbor's load through maintaining our own health may be among the less important of these chances. If the reason for restricting or penalizing the person who gambles with his health lies solely in the burden placed on others thereby, then the case would seem all the stronger for some people to choose the most lucrative possible career, to live in the highest paying regions, and to reserve as little time for leisure as is practically possible. There is no apparent reason why we should restrict the scope of this principle to health.

The generalized policy just described is, of course, quite unattractive. The result would be a feed-the-meter society in which one paid for every failure to maximize contributions to the public good. Since no one endorses such a policy, we would expect those who assign responsibility of health to the individual to find a rationale for resisting the generalization of their argument. In fact, this difficulty has not been faced by advocates of personal responsibility; thus, no reply has yet been fashioned.

It seems unreasonable to suppose that the general principle would require anyone to maximize contributions to society in general or to minimize burdens, and that it is enough to contribute a decent amount and to place only moderate burdens. We are not, in this view, supposed to spend every minute of every day working for the common good, nor are we meant to investigate every conceivable opportunity to avoid needing public help. There will be, it is said, a certain threshold of initiative which will be all that the conscientious citizen needs to display to avoid being considered unfairly burdensome.

I do not want to deny that such a threshold will be a part of any reasonable conception of distributive justice, but it is fairly plain that the argument just given provides almost no guidance for use in locating it. A "live and let live" attitude might envision a perfectly just society in which people took sizable risks and passed up reasonable opportunities to help their neighbors; a puritanical attitude, at the other extreme, would condemn anyone who was less than strenuous in each of these respects. The two views differ on what should be required as the threshold for self-help and neighborliness. According to the less-stern attitude, people who take risks with their health, and thereby increase the medical expenses that must be met by others, are still "within their rights"; that is, the resulting distribution of burdens and benefits will not count as unjust. They would be seen as taking advantage of the measured amount of room for risk taking which the just society accords to each citizen. To those with the less-forgiving attitude, this room is small or nonexistent.

Thus, our question is how much one person should be permitted to burden another through choices about health, employment, and other "personal" matters. If the answer is anything other than "not at all," some rationale needs to be given for setting the threshold at one point rather than others. In the debate over personal responsibility for health, the location of the threshold is a key issue.

The problem of deciding how much risk taking to allot to each individual "for free" (i.e., before that person will be considered to have unduly and unjustly burdened his neighbors) is part of the more general debate over the limits of privacy in a closely interconnected and interdependent society, of separating "self-regarding" and "other-regarding" behavior. In popular writing, this distinction is made with apparent simplicity through the use of certain catch phrases, but the task has defied all attempts at reasoned solutions. We lack a criterion which can tell us whether unconventional hairstyles which annoy one's fellow citizens are "private," or whether the helmetless motorcyclist who, through accident, renders himself in need of publicly funded health care has engaged in other-regarding behavior because others find that their emotions do not allow them to deny health care to him.

These are actions which some reasonable persons might be perfectly happy to permit others to do if they are likewise permitted to do them; thus, they differ from murder and other actions, which are uncontroversially classified as other regarding. The claim that those whose unhealthy lifestyles are placing an unfair burden on others requires, then, a substantive theory of the public and the private, and this theory is unlikely to distinguish unhealthy lifestyles from a host of other habits and actions which we ordinarily permit people to engage in without penalty.

"People Freely Choose Their Risks"

Most who complain about having to pay for the care of people who do not take care of themselves do not express general opposition to contributing toward the care of all who become sick. The difference between, say, someone with an inherited disease and another who becomes sick because of an unhealthy lifestyle is that the latter "could have" avoided illness. However, tracing a disease back to habits of living does not make this argument work unless the habits themselves were the result of, or consisted of, free choices.

To some commentators, then, the question of free choice of lifestyles is the key to determining responsibility for health. But which choices are free, and which are not? This is a classical philosophical question regarding all behavior, but those familiar with the philosophical debates over free will know that there is no simple definition or test of freely chosen behavior. We can, it is true, distinguish certain unusual acts as unfree because of their genesis in some sort of compulsion or addiction. Once addicted, the heroin addict seems to lack the capacity to choose not to seek heroin; the compulsive hand washer is visited with overwhelming anxiety if denied access to a sink. Such behavior stands in contrast to a person who slowly, deliberately, and autonomously decides to join a mountain climbing expedition simply for the adventure. The kinds of behavior which are most commonly singled out in the debate over personal responsibility for health, such as smoking, sloth, and overweight, are, however, in a gray zone. These habits seem to be matters of personal choice, but they are notoriously difficult to give up.

Where can we look for conceptual guidance on this point? Robert Veatch, who has been the commentator most concerned with this issue,[13] has identified this debate with the general and ancient problem of free will and determinism. Veatch rehearses the classical argument briefly and notes the continuing uncertainty, but he is not content to stop short of a solution. His strategy, which ultimately brings him to the conclusion that risk-taking behavior is at least partly voluntary, is to assign the burden of proof to those who call such behavior unfree. His evaluation of available data finds that the evidence thus far put forth does not constitute such proof. In answer to the claim that the personal choices are determined by social environment, in particular one's position in the class structure, Veatch replies that the health-affecting behavior varies from individual to individual within classes. He therefore concludes that the class structure cannot by itself explain lifestyles; from this he concludes that the class structure does not determine lifestyle, and thus that the actions are at least partly free.

Veatch's empirical claim is, I think, undeniable, but it does not establish his conclusion. The fact that one single social factor—position in the class structure—does not entirely count for certain personal choices does not mean that other social factors (some thus far unidentified) do not, and those who insist that lifestyles are a product of the social environment are almost certainly assuming the existence of a broad range of social determinants. The debate between Veatch and his opponents, then, turns on the acceptance of these assumptions, together with the philosophical construal of their importance as regards to establishing voluntariness. The discussion, at this level, does indeed (as Veatch had claimed) revert to an abstract level of philosophical discourse. Clinical or experimental observations, even if amassed on great scale, will be unlikely to change any opinions.

Even so, it is unsatisfying to consign the issue to pure metaphysics. It is also out of keeping with our ordinary practice. Issues of voluntariness arise in everyday life all the time, and we do find ourselves taking stands one way or the other. In some of these arenas, such as criminal justice, arguments of a quite general character serve on occasion to turn the tide of argument or at least to blunt the force of some sorts of evidence. Clarence Darrow was able to win the acquittal of some of his clients by turning the courtroom into a philosophy class.

Ordinarily, however, the voluntariness of an action is not judged by its abstract metaphysical possibility but as an empirical matter. Those who argue that unhealthy lifestyles are the result of social determinants have not premised their view on any general hard-determinist metaphysics, but on claims of specific constraints. Some authors, it is true, simply dismiss the possibility that those with unhealthy habits had any real choice. Others, such as the influential U.S. government report *Healthy People*,[14] are relatively indulgent (". . . although socioeconomic factors are powerful determinants, individuals have limited control over them. . . . People must make personal lifestyle choices . . . in the context of a society that glamorizes many hazardous behaviors through advertising and the mass media. . . . Even when the individual knows that a habit such as eating excessive amounts of high-calorie, fatty foods is not good, available options may be limited"; pp. 17–18), but still hold open the possibility of redemption through individual choice (*Healthy People*: "Even awareness of risk factors difficult or impossible to change may prompt people to make an extra effort to reduce risks more directly under their control and thus lessen overall risk of disease and injury"; p. 18). The policy question, however, is whether it is fair to penalize them if they fail to do so.

The debate over whether such health risks as are involved in unhealthy lifestyles are freely chosen, then, may proceed at any of a number of levels of abstractness. Veatch, as mentioned, speaks of the general compatibility of free will with physical determinism. At the other pole, the argument may involve the simple question of whether the means for executing a choice existed (e.g., did the car have a seat belt in it?). The first of these approaches is not likely to be settled in the context of the debate over lifestyle than it has generally been in philosophy. The latter of these has more potential for yielding firm conclusions on freedom of choice, in that no acts will be considered free if alternative choices were physically unavailable or impossible.

This approach will not get us very far. Most of the unhealthy acts under consideration in this debate are decided upon in the presence of alternatives: No authorities stand by to stop the slothful from jogging, or command the obese to eat, or penalize anyone for not smoking. It is just as clear, however, that the mere existence of alternative courses of action will not count as proof that the unhealthy actions were free. One way of articulating the position that such choices are not fully free is by positing the presences of encumbrances on the will, that is, psychological factors which preclude or impede authentic, reasoned choice. This approach is most natural for such habits as smoking which involve a degree of physical addiction. Conditions of ghetto life might cause a general debilitation of spirit or hopelessness concerning long-term survival which could be taken as factors making reasoned, healthy choices difficult or impossible.

These kinds of explanations and defenses, however, quickly become artificial. It is one thing to explain a junkie's poor diet by his mental state and unopposable drives; it is quite another thing to blame a wide variety of lifestyle elements on a factor as undifferentiated as "ghetto life." The list of factors encumbering the will is presented as matters of psychological fact and morally neutral. Accepted as such, the interpretation of the data seems strained and seems instead to be a rationalization for a (laudable) political and moral program, that of refusing to blame the already downtrodden. In this guise, the argument is not likely to convince those who would deem the unhealthy choices free and hence find the individual responsible.

The argument that unhealthy people are not acting freely is unconvincing when it has the appearance of being covertly moral. Perhaps those who press it believe that arguing in an overtly moral way would defeat their purpose. I want, however, to briefly explore the possibility that an overtly moral argument might be defensible. The key idea here is that, in the present context at least, the judgment of whether a given choice is free is in part a judgment on whether the terms of the choice were fair. One might argue, if this proposal is correct, that the reason an unhealthy habit is unfree is not because the individual is psychologically unfit or encumbered, nor because alternative courses of action were unavailable, but because the alternatives which were available were less attractive than they should have been, morally speaking.

A recent argument regarding fairness and free choice in another context—in a discussion by Norman Daniels[15] on whether workers are overprotected by safety regulations—is instructive for our concerns. In his analysis, Daniels notes that certain occupations are not only inherently risky but are chosen because of that risk. The clearest example is that of an individual who, though holding down a decent job, tries to get rich by becoming a stunt man. Other jobs, however, involve risk but are not chosen because of the risk, but in spite of it. Coal mining is a good example. Why would an individual accept such a job when it is known to carry a risk to himself? The answer, obviously, is that alternatives might be simply unavailable. (Of course, it will remain true that a few jobs will be available in coal mining areas which do not carry such a risk, but not all miners could obtain such jobs.) Daniels concludes that since there are few real alternatives to such jobs, it would be unjust to place safety on the marketing table along with wages at the time of hiring. Protection by federal authorities is thus justified.

This suggests, albeit indirectly, a strategy for investigating the question of voluntariness as it applies to health-related behavior. We will be concerned with the availability of meaningful choices, just as Daniels was. However, it would not do to simply take over Daniels' analysis unchanged since it is untrue that smokers and nonjoggers lack suitable alternatives. Nevertheless, we might obtain what we need by means of a generalization of this strategy, considering instead the range of sets of choices available to each individual for accomplishing certain ends. The ends in question will be those for the sake of which people behave in unhealthy ways, such as stress reduction and enjoyment. The distribution of these sets of choices within society is, according to this suggestion, a matter of distributive justice. Each person is due a fair share of such choices. The strategy, then, would be to argue that although a smoker may have the option of not smoking (and thus be in a different position from the coal miner), the smoker may be one of those individuals who lacks other avenues for stress reduction and enjoyment. Suppose that this person is entitled to a minimally decent set of such avenues. It follows that this individual cannot realize his entitlement (as determined by our general scheme of distributive justice) without accepting a certain risk, that is, that risk associated with smoking. Though, like the coal miner, this individual makes a choice which results in being exposed to a certain known risk, we ought not regard such a choice as free. Its lack of voluntariness results from the fact that this person would not be given just treatment (i.e., receive the stress reduction and enjoyment he ought to have) unless the risk were taken. It must be kept in mind that this is not an argument for compensating the individual for the injury thus sustained (e.g., lung cancer); it attempts, rather, to assign a special status to what would otherwise seem to be a free choice, a status which ought to block the ascription of responsibility to the individual for accepting risk.

This argument, presented here only tentatively, suggests that the question of voluntariness cannot be decided independently of the question of responsibility. The argument given in this preliminary sketch is really a moral argument concerning who should be held responsible for accepting risk. It, like the other attempts to assign responsibility, may have to depend on strictly moral premises rather than on any morally neutral solution to the problem of determining freedom of choice.

Conclusion

The debate over personal responsibility for health, which has continued for a decade in health policy forums, is a complex phenomenon. It is also about the degree of responsibility for the health of the public which ought to be placed on nonpersons, primarily industry and government. The argument for assigning responsibility for health to the individual is often an attempt to absolve these larger institutions of blame for having caused sickness or for having failed to provide care, respectively.

Political scientists and historians are better equipped than philosophers to determine the real agendas operating in the lifestyle debate. I have been concerned here with discussion of only one component issue: whether those who indulge in unhealthy habits ought to be singled out for certain kinds of special treatment at the hands of the state. In particular, I have sought to review and to evaluate arguments which would justify attempts to prevent risk taking or to force those who become ill through unhealthy habits to pay more for their care than others (or, in extreme cases, to be denied care altogether).

These arguments come in two distinct varieties, one "right" and one "left." The approach from the right is reminiscent of the theme of the "deserving poor," which guided welfare policy. It unabashedly recognizes a category of the "undeserving sick" and wants to show them no mercy. However, the approach requires a criterion for judging when an individual has done enough to protect his health, and this is as intractable a problem as finding a threshold for adequacy in personal contribution to the nation's overall welfare. On an extreme interpretation, nothing would be enough. The "health nut" who does all he can to stay in shape could be deemed a parasite if he asked for help in paying for medical care for an "involuntary" illness (e.g., genetically based)—for could he not have worked harder and bought private insurance so as to avoid placing burdens on others?

The champions of personal responsibility for health are not always found, however, on the right. Those opposed to institutional medicine have urged individuals to take health matters into their own hands. Most of the (relatively few, thus far) calls for coercive measures to promote healthful living have come from liberal voices in public health.

If the arguments in this paper are correct, the debate over personal responsibility for health involves fundamental moral and philosophical questions whose intractability will founder attempts to achieve a reasoned solution. This pessimism will, I suspect, be congenial to political scientists and to activists, who generally lack the philosopher's interest in establishing conclusions through moral argument. All parties in this dispute, however, will need to examine the logic of the respective positions. The premises used by ideologically opposed commentators in this debate sometimes sound remarkably similar. We need to know what policy conclusions follow from what premises on causation, blame, and voluntariness if each side is to get its bearings.

References

1. Wikler D: Holistic medicine: concepts of personal responsibility for health, in D Stalker and C Glymour (eds): *Examining Holistic Medicine*. Buffalo: Prometheus Press, 1985.

2. Knowles JH: The responsibility of the individual, in H Knowles (ed): *Doing Better and Feeling Worse*. New York: Norton, 1977.

3. Dworkin G: Voluntary health risks and public policy. *Hastings Center Rep* 11(5): 26–31, 1981.

4. Lalonde M: *A New Perspective in the Health of Canadians*. Report of the Government of Canada. Ottawa, 1974.

5. Forster JL: A communitarian ethical model for public health interventions: an alternative to individual behavior change strategies. *J Public Health Policy* June 1982.

6. Knowles JH: The responsibility of the individual, in JH Knowles (ed): *Doing Better and Feeling Worse*. New York: Norton, 1977.

7. Lavine MP: Industrial screening programs for workers. *Environment* 24(5): 26–38, 1982.

8. Crawford R: Individual responsibility and health politics in the 1970's, in S Reverby and D Rosner (eds): *Health Care in America*. Philadelphia: Temple University Press, 1979, pp. 247–268.

9. Crawford R: You are dangerous to your health: the ideology and politics of victim blaming. *Int J Health Services* 7(4): 663–680, 1977.

10. Crawford R: Healthism and the medicalization of the everyday life. *Int J Health Serv* 10(3): 365–388, 1980.

11. Whorton JC: *Crusaders for Fitness: The History of American Health Reformers*. Princeton, NJ: Princeton University Press, 1982.

12. Eisenberg L: The perils of prevention: a cautionary note. *N Engl J Med* 297(22): 1230–1232, 1977.

13. Veatch RM: Voluntary risks to health. *JAMA* 243(1): 50–55, 1980.

14. *Healthy People: The Surgeon General's Report on Health Promotion and Disease Prevention.* Washington, DC: U.S. Government Printing Office, 1979.

15. Daniels N: Doth OSHA protect too much? Chap. 7 of *Just Health Care.* Cambridge: Cambridge University Press, 1985.

6

Health Promotion

Ethical and Social Dilemmas
of Government Policy

Ronald Bayer and
Jonathan D. Moreno

That health is endangered, lives are lost, and illness increased as a result of poor or destructive personal habits are by now well-established facts.[1] In the United States, as well as in other societies with advanced systems of medical care, repeated calls are made for efforts to alter or modify behavioral patterns with negative consequences for health.[2] Interest in such policies stems partly from growing doubts about the ability of therapeutic medicine to solve the problems posed by the current pattern of morbidity and mortality.[3] The interest also stems from the realization that an upper limit may have been reached in the willingness of the citizenry to shoulder the burden of an expanding health care sector that now consumes close to 11 percent of the gross national product. But whatever the sources of the interest in the modification of personal habits and behaviors that affect the health of men and women, it is clear that many now believe that something must be done.

Despite the popularity of this perspective, there is considerable doubt and confusion as to the appropriate course of action. Who has the right to modify whose behavior and under what circumstances? What should the role of government be in promoting or mandating those behaviors that presumably produce good health and in discouraging or forbidding those behaviors that presumably produce illness and lead to early death? Issues in this arena raise difficult questions about the appropriate relationship between the individual and the state. We are compelled to deal in a concrete fashion with the conflict between liberty and paternalism, between personal preference and social welfare. We must address complex issues regarding the relationships between coercion and incentives, between education and manipulation.

How may the state justify the control of personal behavior that appears, at first, to affect only the individual? To what extent do individuals have the right to behave foolishly and self-destructively? Can state action only be justified by arguing that self-destructive behavior is not truly voluntary (the product of coercive factors—either psychological or social), and that state intervention thus represents a restoration of "true" autonomy? When an individual argues that he or she has freely chosen to engage in certain behaviors despite the possibility of disease and premature death, can the state legitimately attempt to behave paternalistically?[4]

It is of course possible to argue that though the individuals who engage in hazardous behaviors suffer the primary consequences themselves, society must bear the cost of such "self-regarding" acts. Because of the tendency to place greater and greater obligations on society for the provision of health care through third-party mechanisms, the burden has increasingly become communal and not just individual. Additionally, because morbidity and mortality affect the general well-being of society in terms of its productive capacity, such behavior produces a social impact.[5] To the extent that these arguments are accepted, the realm of individual action will become harder to distinguish from that of social action. Self-regarding behavior will cease to exist, and the claims of liberty will increasingly be subordinated to those of community. To what degree should the imperatives of health be permitted to provide the justification for so fundamental a change in our deepest ethical and political commitments? Should the ideal of health provide the warrant for such a transformation when other social goods do not?

This paper sets out the ethical principles that ought to guide policymakers as they attempt to fashion government policy regarding personal behavior and health. Second, the paper examines the ethical issues that must be confronted as alternative strategies to affect personal behavior are considered and applies this set of ethical considerations to three critical cases.

Though it is clear that virtually every dimension of personal behavior can contribute to the onset of disease or to its prevention, we have chosen to limit our discussion to cigarette smoking, alcohol consumption, and vehicular behavior. Though limiting discussion of policy interventions to these activities that occur in public or which can be controlled through the regulation of commerce may appear to be a timid gesture, to include changes in the patterns of exercise, diet, and sleep along with these more public forms of behavior conjures up images of profound invasions of privacy, scarcely tolerable in a liberal society. In fact, it is the precondition for a serious discussion of whether government should seek to modify personal behaviors linked to disease and untimely death.

Personal Behavior and Health

If a single event could be pinpointed as representing the commencement of the public and official discussion of the role of government in health promotion, it would be the publication in 1975 of *A New Perspective on the Health of Canadians*. In that report Marc Lalonde, the Minister of National Health and Welfare, bluntly stated:

"Self-imposed risks and the environment are the principal or important underlying factors in each of the five major causes of death between ages 1 and 70, and one can only conclude that unless the environment is changed and the self-imposed risks are reduced, the death rates will not be significantly reduced."[6]

But even the pursuit of health had to be bounded by other considerations, especially when matters of liberty and privacy were at stake. Lalonde not only recognized the risks involved, but was alert to the nature of the opposition his challenge could well provoke: "The ultimate philosophical issue . . . is whether and to what extent government can get into the business of modifying human behavior, even if it does so to improve health."[7]

Involved were not only issues that would arise in the course of direct efforts at restriction and prohibition, but those that would surface if the government took on the function of "marketing ideas." These themes found expression 2 years later in the United States in the widely read and cited essay by John Knowles, "The Responsibility of the Individual," that appeared as part of the *Daedalus* symposium, "Doing Better and Feeling Worse: Health in the United States." Though he noted the extent to which environmental and socioeconomic factors contributed to behavior with disastrous consequences for health, it was his striking comments on personal responsibility for morbidity that were to provoke a lively and important debate. For Knowles, the social consequences of individual behavior in terms of the cost of medical intervention could no longer be tolerated: "The costs of individual irresponsibility in health have now become prohibitive. The choice is individual responsibility or social failure. Responsibility and duty must gain some degree of parity with right and freedom."[8]

The untoward social consequences of individual behavior were to become the leitmotiv of the American debate over health, lifestyles, and government responsibility. It clearly was central for Department of Health and Human Services Secretary Joseph Califano in his introduction to *Healthy People*. "Indulgence in private excess," wrote Califano, "has results that are far from private. Public expenditures for health care are only one of the results."[9] While acknowledging that there might well be controversy and debate about the appropriate role of government in urging citizens to give up their "pleasurable but harmful habits," Califano argued that "there could be no denying the public consequences of these private acts."[10]

Ethical Issues at the Threshold: Autonomy, Equity, and Community

From an ethical perspective, the determination of whether government should regulate the behavior of individuals in the name of health requires that policymakers go beyond the questions of efficiency and political acceptability. What moral warrant is there for such intervention? Does such a warrant also impose an obligation on the part of government to intercede? The demands of autonomy, equity, and community are central to any attempt to fashion an ethically sensitive public policy in this domain.

Autonomy

No issue has received more attention in the public and professional discussions of the appropriateness of government policy designed to affect personal behavior in the name of health than that of autonomy. Reflecting the profound influence of liberalism in American social thought, any attempt by the state to affect behavior that is conceived of as self-regarding is viewed with great suspicion.

The realm of privacy is held to be inviolate, except for those occasions when it can be demonstrated that what initially appears to be self-regarding is in fact behavior with demonstrable and marked consequences for others, or when it can be demonstrated that what appears to be the decision of a competent adult acting under his or her own volition is in fact the consequence of some powerful, dominating, or coercive force. Given this commitment to individual autonomy, state actions directed at individuals in the name of their own health—paternalistic actions—are difficult to justify. Though there is, in fact, a broad range of extant regulatory provisions that are demonstrably paternalistic, each contemporary effort to overcome the predilection for autonomy must show that apparently voluntary behavior is the product of misinformation or the result of an irresistible compulsion. The goal of justifiable paternalism is to protect the individual from the consequences of actions that he or she would not choose to engage in were the capacity for free choice truly present.

Though it would be theoretically possible to argue that many forms of personal behavior that produce ill health are undertaken only because the individual does not fully appreciate the ultimate consequences of such behavior, this would be a difficult proposition to defend today. Given the widespread dissemination of public health information regarding smoking, alcohol consumption, and reckless vehicular behavior, it would be necessary to argue that individuals cannot appreciate the consequences of behaviors that produce their effects in the (personally) remote future, or that the statistical risk to any individual is so small that it is not possible to make personal decisions incorporating such information.

The difficulty that attends efforts to provide the justifications of paternalism has made such arguments largely unattractive to those seeking a moral foundation for regulatory policies put forth in the name of health. As an alternative, advocates of government intervention have sought to demonstrate that the consequences of personal behavior are social burdens that warrant public action. Thus shifting the grounds of discussion obviates the necessity of putting forth arguments to demonstrate that the individual must be protected from his own ill-conceived actions. Instead, since the burden generated by personal behavior causing ill health must be assumed by others, it has been argued that an issue of equity is involved.

Equity

The discovery of the social impact of personal behavior on morbidity and mortality has provided the foundation for public discussions of the appropriate scope of governmental activity. Both the Lalonde report and *Healthy People* provide ample evidence of this fact.

Invariably such discussions are based upon economic analyses of the externalities associated with personal behavior. The cost of health care and of health insurance, the burden of social security payments to those who are disabled, the necessity of providing social supports to families deprived of primary wage earners, the toll of reduced productivity, these are typically the costs traced back to the "private" acts of those who engage in behavior that produces disease and untimely death.

What from the point of view of economics is a negative externality requiring efforts at internalization of costs, from the vantage point of ethics becomes a matter of distributive justice. What does equity demand in terms of the burdens generated by the costs of behaviorally induced ill health? Why should nonsmokers be forced to bear the burden of smokers' behavior? Why should nondrivers or drivers who do wear seat belts be required to bear the burdens of those who refuse to do so? Equity, some have argued, demands that those who choose to smoke or to drive without seat belts be forced to bear the economic consequences of their own behavior. In those instances where no mechanism exists to internalize the costs of behavior, equity might necessitate the application of disincentives, and even prohibitions of the behavior itself.

The focus on the social costs of personal behavior seems to suggest that if it were possible to avoid the problem of negative externalities by internalizing such costs, there would be little justification for social intervention, for tolerating government intrusion. But does the characterization of the problem of morbidity and mortality associated with personal behavior in terms of economic costs alone adequately capture the extent of our moral intuitions? Limiting the costs of smoking (including death from lung cancer) to smokers themselves, or limiting the cost of neurosurgery to the unbelted victims of automobile accidents, cannot be viewed as a satisfactory moral solution.

The contemporary stress upon quantifiable economic social costs of personal behavior presses upon us a conception of public concern for health that begins and ends with an accountant's ledger and which is in fact at variance with the desire to prevent untimely death, suffering, and illness as ends in themselves. A reading of court cases in this area—especially those associated with motorcycle helmet laws—reveals a strained quality in the argumentation. While data on social costs are mobilized in defense of state regulation, another set of motivations is clearly involved. The acceptable public rationale appears to be at odds with the unspoken, perhaps unspeakable, commitment to health and well-being of individuals and the community.

Community and the Public Health

Most contemporary court decisions involving cases testing the constitutionality of government efforts to regulate behavior in the name of health have focused on the state's interest in reducing the cost of negative externalities. But Dan E. Beauchamp has noted that there is an older, "radical republican" constitutional tradition in which a more robust definition of the community's interest in the well-being of its members finds expression. Thus, one late-nineteenth-century Supreme Court decision involving the state's effort to prevent the sale of alcohol held: "We cannot shut out of view the fact, within knowledge of all, that the public health, the public morals, and the public safety may be endangered by the general use of intoxicating drinks."[11]

Unlike those who have argued that the central issue raised by government intervention is that of autonomy and paternalism, Beauchamp asserts that "the individual's liberty is not being restricted to produce benefits to himself as an isolated individual, but rather to maximally protect an entire class of individuals of which he is only a small part."[12] Nor is the central issue the protection of the interests of third parties from the undue imposition of those who insist on behaving in ways that produce ill health: "Such a perspective seeks to reduce the idea of the common good to little more than the protection of the interest of others, confusing the protection of the body politic with the protection of the rights of the private citizen."

What is for Beauchamp the signal advantage of his perspective, the stress on the community's interest in health as an irreducible good, is for those fearful of an overbearing government a threatening call for the dissolution of the essential tension between the public and private realms. Nevertheless, a consideration of the community's interest in the health and well-being of its members warrants careful attention. While privacy and autonomy provide essential standards against which to judge proposed government actions, they are not the sole standards, nor ought they be permitted to overwhelm all other values. The National Research Council, in its report on public policy and alcohol, sought to strike a balance when it said: "Individual freedom is not the only premise defining the proper role of government. There are other (equally venerable) notions of politics in which the government is called on to enhance the general welfare, promote the spread of knowledge and encourage civil behavior among its citizens as well as guarantee various liberties."[13]

Ethics and Policy Choice

As policymakers confront the prospect of fashioning governmental action in the name of health, they ought to be sensitive to the ethical tensions posed by such efforts. Sensitivity to such issues will help to determine whether or not government should take steps to affect behavior that is linked to illness and early death; it will also guide decisions about how to intervene.

Education and Health Promotion Campaigns

Health communication campaigns that warn against certain activities or encourage the adoption of certain forms of behavior would at first appear to pose no ethical problems. But Ruth Faden has provided an analysis that reveals how complex the issues can be.[14] Her critical review informs the following discussion. Health communication campaigns provide needed information and thus enhance personal autonomy in the face of health risks. They seek to reduce behavior that produces health-related burdens for society. Thus, such campaigns limit the extent to which the community as a whole may be compelled to tolerate the negative externalities generated by those who engage in activities linked to morbidity and mortality. Finally, on an expressive level, they represent a public demonstration of the community's concern for the health and well-being of its members.

The challenge to health communication campaigns derives primarily from empirical studies that question their efficacy. Kenneth Warner has thus noted that the failure of the American campaign to encourage seat belt use "is echoed by experience in Canada, Great Britain, and France: in each case, major publicity campaigns either did not increase belt use at all, or at best increased use only slightly and temporarily."[15] Since such campaigns often accomplish little, their existence may, in fact, betray an unwillingness to undertake more effective interventions.

However, health education campaigns can be successful. The cumulative impact of many efforts over time is enhanced when novel messages, conveyed in a variety of media, are supplemented by more personal interventions. It is generally believed that years of antismoking campaigns have had a marked impact on cigarette consumption. But can such campaigns be too successful? Can they undermine autonomy by their efforts to reform the way in which we think about our health-related preferences?

It is a striking feature of American distrust for governmental intrusions that fear is generated by the mere prospect of a successful state-sponsored program to influence health-related behavior. For commercial advertisers to advance exaggerated claims is almost expected. Were government to engage in similar levels of exaggeration—even in the name of health—fears of manipulation would abound. This quite understandable reaction places public health education campaigns at a disadvantage. Concern about balance in governmental education efforts should not, however, provide a subterfuge for permitting gross imbalances in the marketplace. Such an outcome would produce the very results Marc Lalonde expressed concern about 10 years ago.

Public health campaigns not only seek to influence members of the community as consumers of products, but as citizens as well. They may, in fact, Faden has noted, have as their most important consequence the creation of constituencies willing to support more aggressive health promotion strategies. Antismoking campaigns, for example, were certainly instrumental in preparing the public for legislation restricting cigarette smoking in enclosed public spaces.[16] Some have expressed concern about whether such governmental influence is appropriate in a liberal society. Though it is possible to conceive of instances in which government efforts to "educate" the people would be troubling, it would be a mistake to exaggerate such threats. Government never merely mirrors public opinion. In the case of health, to do so would represent an abdication of the responsibility to enhance the general welfare.

Taxation

Given the focus of public discussion on the economic consequences of the relationship of personal behavior to morbidity and mortality, it is not surprising that considerable theoretical attention has been devoted to the role taxes might play in government health promotion efforts. Much of the concern of the past decade has centered upon negative externalities, including the cost of health care and lost productivity. Thus, it is only natural that proposals would be made to recapture those costs through excise taxes applied against products directly implicated in disease and early death.

From the point of view of economics, such taxes would correct for market imperfections that failed to pass on to consumers the true cost of their behaviors. From an ethical point of view, it would be possible to justify such efforts as critical for the more equitable distribution of the burdens associated with certain behaviors. On the other hand, since sales taxes are always regressive, it could be argued that such levies would generate inequity. The evaluation of such competing ethical claims cannot be restricted to an analysis of the incidence of taxation. As important would be a full appreciation for the ways in which such taxes would affect the social class distribution of morbidity and mortality.

The imposition of excise taxes in the name of equity would inevitably result in price increases that would create disincentives to consumption. One analysis of the elasticity of demand for cigarettes found that a 10 percent rise in the price of cigarettes would result in an equivalent reduction in teenage smoking.[17] A study of the elasticity of demand for alcohol found that an increase in federal excise taxes and hence in the price of alcohol would "reduce total consumption and in particular . . . those portions of total consumption associated with auto fatalities and liver cirrhosis."[18] How such disincentives would affect the social class pattern of consumption is an empirical matter with important implications for ethical analysis. But in any case, it is clear that without adopting either paternalistic justifications or more far-reaching arguments regarding the community's interest in the health and well-being of its members, imposing higher taxes on tobacco and alcohol would make it possible to reduce society's burden of illness and early death.

The imposition of taxes in excess of those justified by calculable negative externalities would require arguments that go beyond the claims of society in the face of such costs. Such arguments would have to demonstrate why the community's interest in health as an end in itself, or why a concern for autonomy in the face of addictive consumption, required such interventions.

What is remarkable about the theoretical discussion of the role of taxes in health promotion and disease reduction is how limited its impact has been on actual public policy. Commercial interests have succeeded in thwarting the robust application of excise taxes. In the case of alcohol, federal taxes adjusted for inflation have actually declined. Increases in federal taxes on cigarettes have been imposed primarily for purposes of revenue enhancement rather than for purposes of recapturing the costs associated with smoking.

In the presence of enormous social costs—calculated in terms of medical care, reduced productivity, suffering, and early death—an ethical analysis would find the failure to use fiscal interventions more aggressively at least as troubling as the putative risks that might attend their overly severe application.

In arguing the regressive nature of excise taxes, some have said that the poor have at least as much right to indulge in relatively minor vices as their more comfortable neighbors, especially since these activities constitute a small measure of relief from lives largely devoid of luxuries. However, the demands of equity do not require equal opportunity for access to all forms of morbidity and mortality. The demands of community may well counsel particular concern for those especially vulnerable to the damaging effects of certain lifestyles and products. Preservation of the community's commitment to the well-being of its members might dictate the use of excise taxes to discourage behavior that would create additional burdens for those already at economic disadvantage.

Restrictions, Prohibitions, and Mandatory Behavior

The creation of disincentives through the application of taxes to certain commercial products like cigarettes and alcohol would impinge upon the autonomy of those who found the added costs burdensome, perhaps prohibitively so. Nevertheless, at some price individuals would remain free to purchase cigarettes and alcohol.

There is no such ambiguity attached to public policies that would seek to bar the purchase of certain products, prohibit certain behaviors, or mandate the performance of others. Because such prohibitions or requirements would so clearly impose the government's preference on competent adults, discussion of such options tends to arouse ardent opposition.

Prohibitions evoke the specter of Big Brother and of America's "noble experiment" with alcohol. Yet on a broad range—for both paternalistic and public health reasons—governmental regulations are an accepted part of contemporary social life. Prohibitions on the sale and prescription of many intoxicating substances are challenged only by libertarians who are opposed, in principle, to any but the most limited restrictions on individual liberty. Pure food and drug laws, as well as legislation governing the use of potentially carcinogenic food additives, are not only rarely opposed but often demanded by those committed to the public health, despite their clear impingement on the liberty and autonomy of potential consumers.

It is only when government seeks to restrict the availability of a product well integrated into the social fabric, or when it attempts to mandate a form of behavior that has not been required in the past, that the ensuing controversy brings to the fore the ethical issues that undergird even the most widely accepted practices. As Stephen Teret has pointed out, the debate surrounding mandatory motorcycle helmet laws provided a unique opportunity to examine the ethical issues raised by efforts on the part of government to mandate behavior in the name of health.[19]

In June 1967, pursuant to the Highway Safety Act, the Secretary of Commerce declared that any state that did not require motorcyclists to wear helmets would lose all federal highway safety funds and 10 percent of federal highway construction funds. Teret notes in his analysis of this effort that in the next 9 years, 49 states adopted the mandated helmet requirement. Only California refused to do so. Utah limited the statutory requirement to highways on which travel exceeded 35 miles per hour.

Despite the vehement opposition to these statutes by representatives of cycling groups, compliance with the helmet requirement was nearly universal. As a consequence, deaths from motorcycle accidents registered a substantial decline. But, because motorcyclists viewed mandatory helmet laws as an unacceptable violation of their civil liberties, as an intrusion upon their autonomy, and as an example of unjustifiable paternalism, they brought suit in state after state challenging the constitutionality of these statutes. Only in Illinois did the court hold that mandatory helmet laws were unconstitutional. In one case that was pursued to the U.S. Supreme Court, the nation's highest tribunal refused to overturn a U.S. district court's holding that government could legitimately compel the use of helmets.

In their decisions, the courts tended to avoid justifications that suggested a warrant for paternalistic interventions. Rather, they sought to demonstrate that the social impact of private behavior provided ample justification for state legislative action. Typical was the language used by a U.S. district court in Massachusetts: "From the moment of injury, [society] picks the person up off the highway; delivers him to a municipal hospital and municipal doctors; provides him with unemployment compensation if, after recovery, he cannot replace his lost job, and if the injury causes permanent disability, may assume the responsibility for his and his family's continued subsistence. We do not understand the state of mind that permits the plaintiff to think that only he himself is concerned."

What the opponents of motorcycle helmet laws had failed to do in the courts they succeeded, Teret notes, at accomplishing in the Congress when the secretary of transportation was forbidden from using the power of the purse to force the states to impose protective requirements on motorcyclists.

Within 3 years of the 1976 congressional action, 27 states had repealed their laws. Helmet wearing in the repeal states declined by 40 percent. The toll in mortality began to rise, as did the cost in terms of medical expenses, lost productivity, as well as human suffering.

The dispute surrounding mandatory helmet laws raised issues of autonomy, paternalism, and general welfare, but in a sphere of behavior engaged in by a relatively small number of individuals. These same moral concerns have emerged in the course of the debate on mandatory seat belt laws that would affect tens of millions of drivers.

After years of controversy, states have just now begun to enact such requirements. Public education campaigns that sought to encourage such behavior on a voluntary basis were by all measures a failure. One 1983 study reported that less than 10 percent of Americans regularly wore seat belts.[20] Public opinion polls revealed deep opposition to such requirements from more than three-quarters of those surveyed.[21] Nevertheless, those pressing for seat belt enforcement legislation noted repeatedly the social burden generated by each individual's choice to drive unbelted and demanded government action.

Ironically, the turn toward mandatory seat belt laws, under strong federal encouragement, is the result of a concerted effort on the part of automobile manufacturers to resist imposition of a requirement that all cars be equipped with automatically inflatable air bags. Detroit opposed the enactment of an air bag requirement because it would have forced added costs upon consumers and industry. And so, ultimately, the secretary of transportation was willing to consider the substitution of a more intrusive form of government regulation—mandated seat belts—for one that would have operated through product redesign.

Though prohibitions and restrictions such as seat belt and motorcycle helmet laws are ethically defensible, this does not suggest that such intrusions ought to be a first line of defense against all behavioral causes of disease and untimely death. The political, economic, and moral costs of such intrusions dictate that they be considered with prudence as a guide. What should be underscored, however, is that an excessive focus on autonomy entails a disregard of competing moral concerns. Indeed, in some circumstances a refusal to consider prohibitions and restrictions on personal behavior would be ethically problematic.

Conclusion

In the past, discussions of the significance of personal behavior for patterns of morbidity and mortality and about the appropriate role of government in responding to such behaviors have occurred under the shadow of the charge of "victim blaming." For those concerned about the intensifying focus on individual behavior, nothing short of an ideological effort to divert attention from the social and environmental causes of disease and death seemed involved. Though some of the public discussion and literature on health promotion provided justification for such fears, many public pronouncements have stressed both environmental and personal factors.

Instead of viewing health promotion through behavioral restrictions as antagonistic to concerns about access to health care and the environmental and occupational causes of disease, they should be viewed as mutually reinforcing. A sterile debate should not be permitted to deflect attention from a course which the public health requires. The community ought to assume greater responsibility for regulating both the environmental and behavioral causes of disease.

Cigarette smoking, excessive alcohol consumption, and the failure to make use of devices that could reduce automobile fatalities ought to be the central foci of any governmental effort to reduce the pattern of behaviorally related morbidity and mortality in America. More than exhortations about such desirable goals are necessary, however. For two decades advocates of aggressive government intervention in this arena have had to bear the burden of proof. Politics, economics, and ethics have all been relied upon to provide arguments against anything but the most modest of efforts. The sheer toll in morbidity and mortality associated with such behavior provides ample justification for shifting the burden of proof. Those who oppose government health promotion efforts, including the use of fiscal measures and even carefully designed restrictions and prohibitions, ought to be compelled to provide arguments against proceeding more aggressively.

Notes

1. Victor Fuchs, *Who Shall Live?* (New York: Basic Books, 1974).

2. See, for example, Keith Reemtsma, "'Your Fault' Insurance," *New York Times* (14 October 1976), and Marc Lalonde, *A New Perspective on the Health of Canadians* (Ottawa: Government of Canada, 1975).

3. See, for example, Thomas McKeown, *The Role of Medicine: Dream, Mirage or Nemesis* (Princeton, NJ: Princeton University Press, 1979).

4. Gerald Dworkin, "Paternalism," *Monist* (January 1972): 64–84.

5. Dan E. Beauchamp, "Public Health and Individual Liberty," *Annual Review of Public Health* (1980): 121–36.

6. Lalonde, *A New Perspective,* 15.

7. Ibid., 36.

8. John Knowles, "The Responsibility of the Individual," *Daedalus* (Winter 1979): 80.

9. U.S. Department of Health, Education, and Welfare, *Healthy People: The Surgeon General's Report on Health Promotion and Disease Prevention* (Washington, DC: U.S. Government Printing Office, 1979), p. ix.

10. Ibid.

11. Cited in Dan E. Beauchamp, "The State, the Individual, and the Common Good: The Constitutional Roots of Public Health," commissioned by The Hastings Center for its project, "Health Promotion: Ethical and Social Dilemmas of Government Policy," funded by the National Center for Health Services Research, No. S04522.

12. All quotations are from Beauchamp, "The State, the Individual."

13. National Research Council, Panel on Alternative Policies Affecting the Prevention of Alcohol Abuse and Alcoholism, *Alcohol and Public Policy: Beyond the Shadow of Prohibition* (Washington, DC: National Academy Press, 1981), 55.

14. See Ruth Faden, "Ethical Issues in Public Health Campaigns," commissioned by The Hastings Center for its project, "Health Promotion: Ethical and Social Dilemmas of Government Policy," funded by the National Center for Health Services Research, No. S04522.

15. Kenneth Warner, "Bags, Buckles, and Belts: The Debate over Mandatory Personal Restraints in Automobiles," *Journal of Health Policy, Politics, and Law* (Spring 1983): 51.

16. Kenneth Warner, "The Benefits and Costs of Antismoking Policies," unpublished report to the National Center for Health Services Research, June 1983, chap. 3, 35–36.

17. Eugene Lewit and Douglas Coate, "The Potential for Using Taxes to Reduce Smoking," *Journal of Health Economics* (1982): 143.

18. Philip J. Cook, "The Effect of Liquor Taxes on Drinking, Cirrhosis, and Auto Accidents," in National Research Council, *Alcohol and Public Policy,* 284.

19. This narrative is based on Stephen Teret, "Motor Cycle Helmet Laws: Can the State Mandate Prudence?" commissioned by The Hastings Center for its project, "Health Promotion: Ethical and Social Dilemmas of Government Policy," funded by the National Center for Health Services Research, No. S04522.

20. Warner, "Bags, Buckles, and Belts," 45.

21. Ibid., 66.

7

No Smoking

The Ethical Issues

Robert E. Goodin

. . . Having made their opposition to smoking crystal clear . . . Victorian moralists would promptly go on to say that its abatement is a matter for morals rather than legislation. Smoking is a vice, to be sure. But it is a private vice, harming only smokers themselves. . . .

On the broad outlines of that analysis the great Victorian moral philosophers—John Stuart Mill,[1] Herbert Spencer,[2] and Henry Sidgwick[3]—all seem agreed. It is the place of society to stop us from doing things that will harm others; it is not the place of society to stop us from doing things that will harm no one but ourselves. In Mill's classic formulation:

> the sole end from which mankind are warranted, individually or collectively, in interfering with the liberty of action of any of their number is self-protection. . . . The only purpose for which power can be rightfully exercised over any member of a civilized community, against his will, is to prevent harm to others. His own good, either physical or moral, is not a sufficient warrant. He cannot rightfully be compelled to do or forbear because it will be better for him to do so, because it will make him happier, because, in the opinions of others, to do so would be wise or even right. These are good reasons for remonstrating with him, or reasoning with him, or persuading him, or entreating him, but not for compelling him, or visiting him with any evil in case he do otherwise. . . . The only part of the conduct of any one, for which he is amenable to society, is that which concerns others. In the part which merely concerns himself, his independence is, of right, absolute. Over himself, over his own body and mind, the individual is sovereign.[4]

As Mill goes on to say:

> What are called duties to ourselves are not socially obligatory, unless circumstances render them at the same time duties to others. . . . The distinction between the loss of consideration which a person may rightly incur by defect of prudence or of personal dignity, and the reprobation which is due to him for an offence against the rights of others, is not a merely nominal distinction. It makes a vast difference both in our feelings and in our conduct towards him, whether he displeases us in things in which we think we have a right to control him, or in things in which we know that we have not.[5]

For Mill and his philosophical fellow travelers, smoking—along with various other forms of "intemperance" and "hurtful indulgences"—clearly falls into the latter category.

. . . The lay moralists of the medical profession editorialize in the *Journal of the American Medical Association* for "tobacco for consenting adults in private only."[6] Mill could not have put it better himself.

Among professional philosophers, too, smoking has long been an area where Mill's traditional precepts have been thought largely to rule. In a classic essay on "Legal Paternalism," for example, Joel Feinberg writes:

> Many perfectly normal, rational persons voluntarily choose to run . . . a grave risk of lung cancer or heart disease . . . for whatever pleasures they find in smoking. The way the state can assure itself that such practices are truly voluntary is to confront smokers continually with the ugly medical facts so that there is no escaping the knowledge of exactly what the medical risks to health are. . . . But to prohibit [smoking] outright for everyone would be to tell voluntary risktakers that even their informed judgments of what is worthwhile are less reasonable than those of the state and that, therefore, they may not act on them. This is paternalism of the strong kind. . . . As a principle of public policy, it has an acrid moral flavor, and creates serious risks of governmental tyranny.[7]

Or, again . . . Norman Daniels maintains:

> Though most of us would agree that promoting health[y] life-styles is an important social goal, we are also justifiably hesitant about permitting too much social intrusion into individual decision-making about life-styles. . . . We resist the suggestion that there is only one acceptable conception of the good, or that self-regarding features of those conceptions must all agree on basic points, for example, in the importance placed on avoiding risks to health. . . . Only if these decisions [to endanger health] are the result of independently defined and detected failures of competency is paternalistic intervention justified. Specifically, health-threatening behaviors— smoking or not wearing seat belts—are not themselves evidence of diminished capacity for rational decision-making. Many of these behaviors, after all, are associated with natural effects—the relaxation of smoking—that are also desirable and whose payoffs individuals may weigh differently.[8]

These and various other writing in similar veins[9] serve to confirm the hold that Mill still has on professional and lay moralists alike. For all of us, the received view is apparently very much that smoking is a private-regarding vice, best treated as such.

In current controversies surrounding smoking, that conventional wisdom is being questioned in both its parts. The proposition that smoking is merely private-regarding vice, harming only smokers themselves, is challenged by evidence of the harmful effects of "passive smoking" (i.e., nonsmokers' inhaling smoke given off by others smoking around them). The proposition that smoking is best treated as we would an ordinary private-regarding vice—by informal social pressure, rather than by formal legal sanctions—is also being challenged by evidence of the addictive nature of nicotine, making it difficult for smokers to start and stop at will.

These new developments make smoking a paradigm of another kind: an issue concerning the quality of social life, requiring codes that are formal rather than informal and enforceable rather than merely hortatory. Here, morally worthy goals cannot be achieved if backed by morals alone. Legislation is not only permissible but, in some ways, morally mandated. . . .

Harm to Self

The first and most obvious reason we may have for wanting to restrict smoking is to prevent harms that would be done to smokers themselves by their smoking. . . .

Of course, Mill and his followers would query whether "his own good, either physical or moral" is ever "sufficient warrant" for coercively interfering with a person's own behavior. But they would be the first to concede that it might be, if the behavior is not fully voluntary. If it is autonomy that we are trying to protect in opposing paternalistic legislation in general, then the same values that lead us to oppose such legislation in general will lead us to welcome it in those particular cases where what we are being protected from is something that would deprive us of the capacity for autonomous choice. Evidence of the addictiveness of nicotine . . . suggests that even advocates of personal autonomy ought to favor smoking restrictions on those grounds.

Another class of broadly utilitarian moral theories would have us look instead to people's welfare, both individually and especially collectively. Although it turns out to be a slightly longer story than one might first imagine, that too would lead us to favor restrictions on smoking. . . .

Do Smokers Voluntarily Accept the Risks?

Given what we know of the health risks from smoking, we may well be tempted to "ban cigarette manufacturers from continuing to manufacture their product on the grounds that we are preventing them from causing illness to others in the same way that we prevent other manufacturers from releasing pollutants into the atmosphere, thereby causing danger to members of the community." That would be to move too quickly, though. For as Dworkin goes on to say, "The difference is . . . that in the former but not the latter case the harm is of such a nature that it could be avoided by those individuals affected, if they so chose. The incurring of the harm requires the active cooperation of the victim. It would be a mistake in theory and hypocritical in practice to assert that our interference in such cases is just like our interference in standard cases of protecting others from harm."[10]

The courts have been as sensitive to this distinction as have moral philosophers. They appeal to the venerable legal maxim, *volenti non fit injuria,* to hold that through

their voluntary assumption of the risk smokers have waived any claims against cigarette manufacturers. In perhaps one of the most dramatic cases in this area (given the
well-established synergism between smoking and asbestos inhalation in causing lung
disease), the Fifth Circuit refused to enjoin cigarette manufacturers as codefendants
in a suit against Johns-Manville, saying that "the danger is to the smoker who willing courts it."[11]

Certainly there is, morally speaking, a world of difference between the harms that
others inflict upon you and the harms that you inflict upon yourself. The question is
simply whether, in the case of smoking, the active cooperation of the smoker really
is such as to constitute voluntary acceptance of the consequent risks of illness and
death. The question is decomposable into two further ones. The first . . . concerns
the question of whether smokers know the risks. The second . . . concerns the question of whether, even if smoking in full knowledge of the risks, they could be said to
"accept" the risks in a sense that is fully voluntary.

Do Smokers Know the Risks?

Here we are involved, essentially, with a question of "informed consent." People can
be held to have consented only if they knew to what they were supposedly consenting. In the personalized context of medical encounters, this means that each and every
person being treated is told, in terms he understands, by the attending physician what
the risks of the treatment might be.[12] For largely anonymous transactions in the market,
such personalized standards are inappropriate. Instead, we are forced to infer consent from what people know or should have known (in the standard legal construct,
what a "reasonable man" should have been expected to know) about the product.
And in the anonymous world of the market, printed warnings necessarily take the
place of face-to-face admonitions. . . .

The point being made here is not that advertising bypasses consumers' capacity
to reason, and somehow renders them unfree to choose intelligently whether or not to
partake of the product. No one is saying that consumers of tobacco are brainwashed
to quite that extent. The central point here is merely that the tobacco companies in effect are giving out—and, more important, consumers are receiving—conflicting
information. . . .

Is Acceptance of the Risks Fully Voluntary?

Obviously, people cannot voluntarily accept the health risks of smoking if they do
not know what they are. Despite tobacco companies' best efforts, though, the great
majority of people—smokers included—knows, in broad outline, what health risks
smoking entails. . . .

It is worth pausing, at this point, to consider just how we should handle that recalcitrant residual of smokers who deny the evidence. Having smoked thousands of
packets containing increasingly stern warnings, and having been exposed to hundreds
of column inches of newspaper reporting and several hours of broadcasting about
smoking's hazards, they are presumably incorrigible in their false beliefs in this regard. Providing them with still more information is likely to prove pointless.[13] People

will say "if they are so bad for you as all that the government would ban cigarettes altogether." Or they will say "the government says that nearly everything is bad for you." Or they will find still some other way of rationalizing the practice.

Ordinarily it is not the business of public policy to prevent people from relying on false inferences from full information which would harm only themselves. Sometimes, however, it is. One such case comes when the false beliefs would lead to decisions that are "far-reaching, potentially dangerous, and irreversible"—as, for example, with people who believe that when they jump out of a 10th-story window they will float upward.[14]

We are particularly inclined toward intervention when false beliefs with such disastrous results are traceable to familiar, well-understood forms of cognitive defect.[15] There is something deeply offensive—morally, and perhaps legally as well—about the "intentional exploitation of a man's known weaknesses" in these ways.[16] . . .

Interfering with people's choices in such cases is paternalistic, admittedly. But there are many different layers of paternalism.[17] What is involved here is a relatively weak form of paternalism, one that works within the individual's own theory of the good and merely imposes upon him a better means of achieving what after all are only his own ends. It is one thing to stop people who want to commit suicide from doing so, but quite another to stop people who want to live from acting in a way that they falsely believe to be safe.[18] Smokers who deny the health risks fall into that latter, easier category.

The larger and harder question is how to deal with the great majority of smokers who, knowing the risks, continue smoking anyway. Of course, it might be said that they do not *really* know the risks. Although most acknowledge that smoking is "unhealthy," in some vague sense, few know exactly what chances they run of exactly what diseases. . . .

Overestimating badly the risks of dying in other more dramatic ways (such as car crashes, etc.), people badly underestimate the relative risks of dying in the more mundane ways associated with smoking. This allows them to rationalize further their smoking behavior as being "not all that dangerous," compared to other things that they are also doing. . . .

Besides all that, there is the distinction between "knowing intellectually" some statistic and "feeling in your guts" its full implications. Consent counts—morally, as well as merely legally—only if it is truly informed consent, that is to say, only if people really know what it is to which they are consenting. That, in turn, requires not only that we can state the probabilities but also that we "appreciate them in an emotionally genuine manner."[19] There is reason to believe that smokers do not.[20]

It may still be argued that, as long as people had the facts, they can and should be held responsible if they chose not to act upon them when they could have done so. It may be folly for utilitarian policymakers to rely upon people's such imperfect responses to facts for purposes of constructing social welfare functions and framing public policies around them. But there is the separate matter of who ought to be blamed when some self-inflicted harm befalls people. There, arguably, responsibility ought to be on people's own shoulders.[21] Arguably, we ought to stick to that judgment, even if people were "pressured" into smoking by the bullying of aggressive advertising or peer group pressure.[22]

What crucially transforms the "voluntary acceptance" argument is evidence of the addictive nature of cigarette smoking. Of course, saying that smoking is addictive is not to say that all smokers are hooked and none can ever give it up. Clearly, many have done so. By the same token, though, "most narcotics users . . . never progress beyond occasional use, and of those who do, approximately 30 percent spontaneously remit."[23] Surprisingly enough, studies show that more than 70 percent of American servicemen addicted to heroin in Vietnam gave it up when returning to the United States.[24] We nonetheless continue to regard heroin as an addictive drug. The test of addictiveness is not impossibility but rather difficulty of withdrawal.

There is a tendency, in discussing . . . informed consent arguments, to draw too sharp a distinction between "voluntary" and "involuntary acts" and to put the dividing line at the wrong place, at that.[25] The tendency is often to assume that any act that is the least voluntary—that is in any respect at all, to any extent at all, within the control of the agents themselves—is to be considered fully voluntary for the purposes. If we want to claim that some sort of act was involuntary, we are standardly advised to look for evidence of "somnambulism" or "automatism" or such like.[26] . . .

There is no need to make such a strong claim, though, to vitiate arguments that the conduct was "voluntary" and the harm thus self-incurred. For purposes of excusing criminal conduct, we are prepared to count forms of "duress" that stop well short of rendering all alternative actions literally impossible. It is perfectly possible for bank tellers to let a robber break their arms instead of handing over the money; but no one expects them to do so. A credible threat of serious pain, or perhaps even very gross discomfort, is ordinarily regarded as more than sufficient to constitute duress of the sort that excuses responsibility for otherwise impermissible behavior.

So, too, I would argue should be the case with addiction-induced behavior. The issue is not whether it is literally impossible, but merely whether it is unreasonably costly, for addicts to resist their compulsive desires. If that desire is so strong that even someone with "'normal and reasonable' self-control"[27] would succumb to it, we have little compunction in saying that the addict's free will was sufficiently impaired that his apparent consent counts for naught.

This is arguably the case with nicotine addiction. . . .

None of that evidence proves that it would be literally impossible for smokers to resist the impulse to smoke. Through extraordinary acts of will, they might. Nor does any of that evidence prove it is literally impossible for them to break their dependence altogether. Many have. Recall, however, that the issue is not one of impossibility but rather of how hard people should have to try before their will is said to be sufficiently impaired that their agreement does not count as genuine consent. . . .

. . . If the product is truly addictive, then we have no more reason to respect a person's voluntary choice (however well-informed) to abandon his future volition to an addiction than we have for respecting a person's voluntary choice (however well-informed) to sell himself into slavery.[28] I am unsure how far to press this argument since after all we do permit people to bind their future selves (through contracts, e.g.). But if it is the size of the stakes or the difficulty of breaking out of the bonds that makes the crucial difference, then acquiring a lethal and hard-to-break addiction is much more like a slavery contract than it is like an ordinary commercial commitment.[29]

In any case, addictiveness thus defined makes it far easier to justify interventions that on the surface appear paternalistic. In some sense, they would then not be paternalistic at all. Where people "wish to stop smoking, but do not have the requisite willpower . . . we are not imposing a good on someone who rejects it. We are simply using coercion to enable people to carry out their own goals."[30] . . .

The real force of the addiction findings, in the context of . . . informed-consent arguments, though, is to undercut the claim that there is any *continuing* consent to the risks involved in smoking. There might have been consent in the very first instance—in smoking your first cigarette. But once you were hooked, you lost the capacity to consent in any meaningful sense on a continuing basis.[31] As Hume[32] says, to consent implies the possibility of doing otherwise; and addiction substantially deprives you of the capacity to do other than continue smoking. So once you have become addicted to nicotine, your subsequent smoking cannot be taken as indicating your consent to the risks.

The most that we can now say with confidence, therefore, is that "cigarette smoking, at least initially, is a voluntary activity," in the words of a leading court case in this area.[33] If there is to be consent at all in this area, it can only be consent in the very first instance, that is, when you first begin to smoke. . . .

. . . A vast majority of smokers began smoking in their early to middle teens. Evidence suggests that "of those teenagers who smoke more than a single cigarette only 15 percent avoid becoming regular dependent smokers."[34] Studies show that, "of current smokers, about 60 percent began by the very young age of thirteen or fourteen,"[35] and the great majority—perhaps up to 95 percent—of regular adult smokers are thought to have been addicted before coming of age.[36]

The crux of the matter, then, is just this: being below the age of consent when they first began smoking, smokers were incapable of meaningfully consenting to the risks in the first instance. Being addicted by the time they reached the age of consent, they were incapable of consenting later, either.

Do the Benefits Outweigh the Costs?

In addition to Kantian-style questions about informed consent, there are also utilitarian-style questions of overall social welfare to be considered in this connection. Calculations of the social costs of smoking—both to smokers themselves and to the larger society—establish a prima facie case against smoking on such grounds. . . .

The Disutility of Smoking

Presumably it is in straightforward utilitarian terms that public health measures of all sorts are standardly justified. We do not leave it to the discretion of customers, however well-informed, whether or not to drink grossly polluted water, ingest grossly contaminated foods, or inject grossly dangerous drugs. We simply prohibit such things on grounds of public health. That appeal is justified, in turn, most standardly by recourse to utilitarian calculations of one sort or another.

Of course, we might try to dress those utilitarian arguments up as something else. To some extent, the same considerations that lead us to believe that such public health measures are justified on grounds of social utility might also give us grounds for presuming people's (at least hypothetical) consent to them, also. To some extent, we can appeal to the unfairness as well as the social disutility of external costs imposed on others in order to justify public health measures: contagious diseases and costly cures affect the community as a whole, burdening others with bills they have done nothing to incur but which the perpetrators have no (narrowly self-interested) incentive to avoid, either. While bearing those other, nonutilitarian interpretations as well, those at root seem to be most naturally seen as utilitarian considerations in favor of public health measures.

To a very large extent, though, the justification of public health measures in general must be baldly paternalistic. Their fundamental point is to promote the well-being of people who might otherwise be inclined cavalierly to court certain sorts of diseases. The ultimate ethical justification for such paternalism, in turn, must be essentially utilitarian, turning on the way that overall social utility is maximized when the utilities of all members of the society are maximized.

All of those broadly utilitarian considerations are in play in the case of smoking. Paternalistic elements have been canvassed above. There are contagion effects, too:[37] Being among smokers exerts strong social pressure upon people to start smoking and makes it difficult for people to stop; and these contagion effects are particularly pronounced among young people, whose smoking behavior is strongly affected by that of parents and peers.[38] As regards externalities, smoking is believed to cause at least half of residential fires, harming family and neighbors as well as the smokers themselves;[39] treating smoking-induced illness is costly . . . ; premature deaths cost the economy productive members and entail pain and suffering for family and friends; and so on.[40] . . .

Dealing just in those . . . human costs, smoking must surely stand indicted.

Notes

1. Mill, John Stuart. 1859. On Liberty. In *Three Essays,* ed. Richard Wollheim, pp. 1–141. Oxford: Oxford University Press, 1975, chaps. 4, 5.

2. Spencer, Herbert. 1893. *The Principles of Ethics.* London: Williams and Norgate, pt. 3, secs. 214–215.

3. Sidgwick, Henry. 1907. *The Methods of Ethics.* 7th ed. London: Macmillan, bk. 3, chap. 9, sec. 2.

4. Mill, On Liberty, p. 15.

5. Ibid., pp. 96–97.

6. Lundberg, George D., and Knoll, Elizabeth. 1986. Editorial: Tobacco for Consenting Adults in Private Only. *Journal of the American Medical Association* 255: 1051–1053.

7. Feinberg, Joel. 1971. Legal Paternalism. *Canadian Journal of Philosophy* 1: 106–124. Reprinted in Sartorius, Rolf, ed. 1983. *Paternalism.* Minneapolis: University of Minnesota Press, pp. 3–18, citing p. 11.

8. Daniels, Norman. 1985. *Just Health Care.* Cambridge: Cambridge University Press, pp. 156–158.

9. Dworkin, Gerald. 1972. Paternalism. *Monist* 56, no. 1:64–84. Reprinted in Sartorius, *Paternalism*, pp. 32–33; Wikler, Daniel. 1978. Persuasion and Coercion for Health:

Ethical Issues in Government Efforts to Change Life-Styles. *Health and Society* (now *Milbank Quarterly*) 56: 303–338. Reprinted in Sartorius, *Paternalism*, pp. 35–59; Wikler, Daniel. 1987. Personal Responsibility for Illness. In *Health Care Ethics,* ed. D. van der Veer and T. Regan, pp. 326–358. Philadelphia: Temple University Press.

10. Dworkin, Gerald. 1972. Paternalism. *Monist* 56, no. 1:64–84. Reprinted in Satorius, *Paternalism*, p. 22.

11. *Johns-Manville Sales Corp. v. International Association of Machinists, Machinists Local 1609*, 621 F.2d 756, 759 (5th Cir. 1980). See, further, Daniels, *Just Health Care*, p. 155, n. 8, cf. Anonymous, 1986.

12. Gorovitz, Samuel. 1982. *Doctors' Dilemmas*. New York: Oxford University Press, chap. 3.

13. Cf. Feinberg, Joel. 1971. Legal Paternalism. *Canadian Journal of Philosophy* 1: 106–124. Reprinted in Sartorius, *Paternalism*, p. 11.

14. Dworkin, Paternalism, reprinted in Sartorius, *Paternalism*, p. 31; see also Feinberg, Legal Paternalism, reprinted in Sartorius, *Paternalism*, p. 7.

15. Sunstein, Cass R. 1986. Legal Interference with Private Preferences. *University of Chicago Law Review* 53: 1129–1174, pp. 1161–1164.

16. White, A. A. 1972. The Intentional Exploitation of Man's Known Weaknesses. *Houston Law Review* 9: 889–927.

17. Sartorius, *Paternalism*; Feinberg, Joel. 1986. *Harm to Self.* New York: Oxford University Press.

18. Feinberg, Legal Paternalism, reprinted in Sartorius, *Paternalism*, p. 10; Dworkin, Paternalism, reprinted in Sartorius, *Paternalism*, pp. 23, 33.

19. Dworkin, Paternalism, reprinted in Sartorius, *Paternalism*, p. 30.

20. U.S. Federal Trade Commission (U.S. FTC). 1981. *Staff Report on the Cigarette Advertising Investigation*, Matthew L. Meyers, chairman. Public version. Washington, DC: FTC, p. 428a.

21. Knowles, John H. 1977. The Responsibility of the Individual. *Daedalus* 106, no. 1: 57–80; Wikler, Personal Responsibility, pp. 326–358.

22. Cf. Gewirth, Alan. 1980. Health Rights and the Prevention of Cancer. *American Philosophical Quarterly* 17: 117–125, citing pp. 124–125; Daniels, *Just Health Care*, p. 159.

23. U.S. Department of Health and Human Services (DHHS). Surgeon General. 1988. *The Health Consequences of Smoking: Nicotine Addiction.* Washington, DC: Government Printing Office, p. v.

24. Robins, L. 1973. *A Follow-up of Vietnam Drug Users.* Interim Final Report, Special Actions Office for Drug Abuse Prevention. Washington, DC: Executive Office of the President; Pollin, William. 1984. The Role of the Addictive Process as a Key Step in Causation of All Tobacco-Related Diseases. *Journal of the American Medical Association* 252: 2874; Fingarette, Herbert. 1975. Addiction and Criminal Responsibility. *Yale Law Journal* 84: 413–444, citing pp. 429–431.

25. Feinberg, *Harm to Self*, chap. 20.

26. Prevezer, S. 1958. Automatism and Involuntary Conduct. *Criminal Law Review* 1958: 361–367, 440–452; Fox, S. J. 1963. Physical Disorder, Consciousness and Criminal Liability. *Columbia Law Review* 63: 645–668.

27. Watson, Gary. 1977. Skepticism about Weakness of Will. *Philosophical Review* 86: 316–339, p. 331.

28. Mill, On Liberty, pp. 126–127.

29. Cf. Feinberg, *Harm to Self*, pp. 71–81.

30. Dworkin, Paternalism, reprinted in Sartorius, *Paternalism*, p. 32.

31. White, Intentional Exploitation.

32. Hume, David. 1760. Of the Original Contract. In *Essays, Literary, Moral and Political.* London: Millar.

33. Brown, John R. 1987. Opinion of the U.S. Court of Appeals. *Palmer v. Liggett Group, Inc.* 825 F.2d 620 (1st Cir. 1987), p. 627.

34. Russell, M. A. H. 1974. Realistic Goals for Smoking and Health. *Lancet* 7851: 254–258, citing p. 255.

35. Blasi, Vincent, and Monaghan, Henry Paul. 1986. The First Amendment and Cigarette Advertising. *Journal of the American Medical Association* 256: 502–509, citing p. 503.

36. Califano, Joseph A., Jr. 1981. *Governing America.* New York: Simon and Schuster, p. 183; Lewit, E. M., Coate, D., and Grossman, M. 1981. The Effects of Government Regulation on Teenage Smoking. *Journal of Law and Economics* 24: 545–569, citing p. 547, n. 8; Pollin, Role of the Addictive Process, p. 2874; Leventhal, Howard, Glynn, Kathleen, and Fleming, Raymond. 1987. Is the Smoking Decision an "Informed Choice"? *Journal of the American Medical Association* 257: 3373–3376, citing p. 3373; Davis, Ronald M. 1987. Current Trends in Cigarette Advertising and Marketing. *New England Journal of Medicine* 316: 725–732, citing p. 730; U.S. DHHS, p. 397.

37. Preston, M. H. 1971. Economics of Cigarette Smoking. In *Proceedings of the Second World Conference on Smoking and Health,* ed. Robert G. Richardson, pp. 100–110. London: Pittman Medical; Schelling, Thomas C. 1986. Whose Business Is Good Behavior? In *American Society: Public and Private Responsibilities,* ed. Winthrop Knowlton and Richard Zeckhauser, pp. 153–180. Cambridge, MA: Ballinger, citing pp. 161–162.

38. Leventhal, Howard, and Cleary, Paul D. 1980. The Smoking Problem: A Review of the Research and Theory in Behavioral Risk Modification. *Psychological Bulletin* 88: 370–405.

39. Schelling, Thomas C. 1986. Economics and Cigarettes. *Preventive Medicine* 15: 549–560, citing p. 550; U.S. Council of Economic Advisors (U.S. CEA). 1987. Annual Report of the Council of Economic Advisors, 1987. In *Economic Report of the President,* pp. 9–368. Washington, DC: Government Printing Office, citing p. 185; Botkin, Jeffrey R. 1988. The Fire-Safe Cigarette. *Journal of the American Medical Association* 260: 226–229.

40. Atkinson, A. B., and Meade, T. W. 1974. Methods and Preliminary Findings in Assessing the Economic and Health Services Consequences of Smoking, with Particular Reference to Lung Cancer. *Journal of the Royal Statistical Society,* ser. A., 137: 297–312; Schelling, Economics and Cigarettes; cf. Littlechild, S. C. 1986. Smoking and Market Failure. In Tollison, ed., 1986, *Smoking and Society.* Lexington Books, pp. 271–284.

8

For Your Own Good

The Anti-Smoking Crusade and the Tyranny of Public Health

Jacob Sullum

Terms of Engagement

The vigilance against deviation from the correct portrayal of smoking is accompanied by absurd rhetorical excesses, even in supposedly sober scientific journals. *JAMA*'s [*Journal of the American Medical Association*'s] vociferousness on the issue of smoking . . . may be an attempt to make up for past sins: The journal carried cigarette ads until 1953, and the AMA [American Medical Association] accepted research money from the tobacco industry in the 1960s and 1970s, during which decades activists accused the organization of inexcusable timidity on an important public health issue. Since the 1980s, however, *JAMA* has been second to none in its denunciations of tobacco. A 1986 editorial compared smoking-related deaths to Nazi genocide, calling for "a declaration of all-out war" to save "the victims of the tobaccoism holocaust."[1] A 1990 editorial, this one by a former CDC director, said tobacco executives and the advertising firms that work for them "daily make the decision to kill for money, to become 'hit men' on a colossal scale."[2] Picking up on the same theme in yet another *JAMA* editorial, then-Secretary of Health and Human Services Louis Sullivan called revenue from tobacco advertising accounts "blood money."[3]

Longtime antismoking activist Stanton Glantz, a professor at the University of California at San Francisco, has compared the tobacco companies to Timothy McVeigh, convicted of murdering 168 people in Oklahoma City. "The tobacco industry has killed 10 million Americans since 1964," he wrote in a 1997 *Los Angeles Times* op-ed piece. "No attorney general or politician even considered letting McVeigh cop a plea; the same should be true for the tobacco industry."[4] *New York Times* reporter Philip J. Hilts, who portrays himself as a moderate on smoking issues, nevertheless likens tobacco industry employees to "the guards and doctors in the Nazi death camps."[5] According to Texas Attorney General Daniel Morales, "History will record the modern-day tobacco industry alongside the worst of civilization's evil empires."[6]

Facing such an enemy, tobacco's opponents feel justified in using any weapon that comes to hand. "From my point of view," former surgeon general C. Everett Koop told the *Philadelphia Inquirer* in 1996, "anything that stops smoking is good."[7] Former AMA president Lonnie Bristow, who serves on the board of the National Center for Tobacco-Free Kids, has called the fight against smoking a "black flag" battle, explaining, "During the Civil War, when some Union troops with black soldiers went into combat against Confederate troops, both sides would wave a black flag. This meant the opposite of a white flag—a fight to the death, with no surrenders, no prisoners. Mercy was neither expected nor given. That's what it's like fighting against tobacco interests."[8]

In reality, however, the antismoking movement is not fighting "tobacco interests" so much as smokers themselves, without whom the cigarette companies would not exist. The fraction of American adults who smoke has dropped from more than two-fifths in the 1960s to about one-quarter today, but the trend has been gradual and seems to have leveled off in recent years.[9] Meanwhile, tobacco's opponents, who initially emphasized education and persuasion, have turned to increasingly coercive measures, including punitive taxes, censorship, and government-imposed smoking bans on private property. The Food and Drug Administration is poised to take charge of tobacco regulation, and the authority it claims would allow a wide range of restrictions, including a partial or complete ban on cigarettes. Prohibition would be disastrous for the tobacco companies, of course, but the results would not be very pleasant for smokers, either (or for the rest of us, given the nasty side effects of creating a black market). Even private and state-sponsored lawsuits against cigarette companies have been aimed, in part, at their customers, who would have to pay higher prices—which tobacco's opponents hope will deter smoking—to cover the cost of damage awards or settlements.

The point, in short, is to make life harder for smokers so they will stop misbehaving. The pressure works at a practical level, making smoking more expensive and less convenient, and at a symbolic level, transforming what was once a mainstream habit into a shameful addiction. Bans on smoking in public places (meaning any building other than a private residence) operate at both levels, literally and figuratively pushing smokers out into the cold—a phenomenon satirized in those Benson & Hedges ads that show smokers congregating on airplane wings and the tops of trains.

. . . The cigar boom of the 1990s can be seen as a rebellion against this attempt to redefine smoking. Sales of premium cigars (costing more than a dollar each) rose 42 percent from 1989 to 1994, and overall cigar sales, which had been declining since 1970, rose 45 percent from 1993 to 1996.[10] The demand for some premium cigars outstripped supplies, with customers waiting months for delivery. Launched in 1992, the glossy magazine *Cigar Aficionado,* fat with ads and featuring celebrity smokers on the cover, has been a big success, inspiring imitators. In increasingly smoke-free cities such as Los Angeles and New York, cigar banquets and cigar bars offer havens for smokers who can afford them. Rejecting the attempt to stigmatize smoking as low class and antisocial, the new cigar smokers see it as sophisticated and convivial. Their mood is summed up by an ad campaign for Johnnie Walker Red Label scotch that shows a man sitting in a chair with a glass in one hand and a cigar in the other. The copy reads: "Big fat cigar. Glass of Red Label. Back whether they like it or not."

The Johnnie Walker slogan calls attention to the true nature of the crusade for a smoke-free society. It is an attempt by one group of people to impose their tastes and preferences on another—a point that is often obscured by focusing on the misdeeds of the tobacco industry. As I write, Congress is considering a nationwide settlement proposal under which the tobacco companies would cough up a ton of money and swallow a mass of humiliating requirements in exchange for protection against the vicissitudes of regulation and litigation. Among other things, the companies have agreed to pay what amounts to a huge fine ($368.5 billion) for the crime of selling cigarettes; have conceded the authority of the Food and Drug Administration (FDA) over tobacco products; have accepted sweeping restrictions on advertising and promotion; have endorsed a federal ban on smoking in most nonresidential buildings; have promised to finance a $500-million-a-year national media campaign aimed at discouraging consumption of their products; and have committed themselves, under the threat of further fines, to utterly unrealistic goals for reducing smoking by teenagers. Tobacco's opponents are complaining that the agreement does not go far enough.

Whatever Congress decides, the crusade for a smoke-free society will continue because it is aimed at the behavior of individuals, not the behavior of corporations. Long before Philip Morris and R. J. Reynolds existed, the tobacco habit had plenty of detractors. . . . Initially condemned as an unsavory practice of savages, smoking quickly caught on in Europe and throughout the world, but attempts to suppress tobacco use, including cigarette bans in 19 U.S. states early in this century, have been a recurring theme. The emergence of definitive scientific evidence that smoking is hazardous . . . has given a new impetus to antitobacco forces. According to contemporary public health doctrine, the government has a right and a duty to discourage behavior that might lead to disease or injury, a principle that gives the antismoking movement a rationale for enlisting the state's assistance.

Given this country's tradition of limited government, however, most Americans are not prepared to accept "public health" as an adequate reason for joining the march toward a smoke-free society. Hence, tobacco's opponents have offered additional rationales, all designed to overcome suspicions of paternalism. They have argued that tobacco advertising is an insidious force that seduces people into acting against their interests. . . . They have said that smoking imposes costs on society that need to be recouped through special taxes. . . . They have claimed that secondhand smoke poses a grave threat to bystanders and that smoking should therefore be confined to private residences. . . . They have accused the tobacco companies of hiding the truth about smoking, thereby preventing their customers from making informed decisions. . . . They have described nicotine addiction as a compulsive and possibly contagious illness, a portrayal that fits nicely with the public health mission to control disease. . . . Often these arguments are combined with appeals to protect children, who are said to be especially vulnerable to advertising, secondhand smoke, and addiction. The best-funded antismoking group in Washington these days is the National Center for Tobacco-Free Kids, which played a key role in the negotiations that led to the nationwide settlement proposal. Former FDA commissioner David A. Kessler calls smoking a "pediatric disease," and who could be in favor of that?[11]

Since . . . none of these claims is very convincing, we are left with the argument that I understood and fervently adopted as a 10-year-old: You shouldn't smoke because it's bad for you. In the realm of public policy, the impulse behind this injunction takes the form of two complementary beliefs: that the government should suppress the use of hazardous drugs and that it should deter activities that impair "the public health." . . . the dangerous implications of these ideas extend far beyond tobacco.

. . . Because the public health field developed in response to deadly threats that spread from person to person and place to place, its practitioners are used to dictating from on high. Writing in 1879, U.S. Army surgeon John S. Billings put it this way: "All admit that the State should extend special protection to those who are incapable of judging of their own best interests, or of taking care of themselves, such as the insane, persons of feeble intellect, or children; and we have seen that in sanitary matters the public at large are thus incompetent."[12] Billings was defending traditional public health measures aimed at preventing the spread of infectious diseases and controlling hazards such as toxic fumes. It's reasonable to expect that such measures will be welcomed by the intended beneficiaries, once they understand the aim. The same cannot be said of public health's new targets. Even after the public is informed about the relevant hazards (and assuming the information is accurate), many people will continue to smoke, drink, take illegal drugs, eat fatty foods, buy guns, speed, eschew seat belts and motorcycle helmets, and otherwise behave in ways frowned upon by the public health establishment. This is not because they misunderstood; it's because, for the sake of pleasure, utility, or convenience, they are prepared to accept the risks. When public health experts assume these decisions are wrong, they are indeed treating adults like incompetent children.

One such expert, writing in the *New England Journal of Medicine* two decades ago, declared, "The real malpractice problem in this country today is not the one described on the front pages of daily newspapers but rather the malpractice that people are performing on themselves and each other—It is a crime to commit suicide quickly. However, to kill oneself slowly by means of an unhealthy life style is readily condoned and even encouraged."[13] The article prompted a response from Robert F. Meenan, a professor at the University of California School of Medicine in San Francisco, who observed: "Health professionals are trained to supply the individual with medical facts and opinions. However, they have no personal attributes, knowledge, or training that qualifies them to dictate the preferences of others. Nevertheless, doctors generally assume that the high priority that they place on health should be shared by others. They find it hard to accept that some people may opt for a brief, intense existence full of unhealthy practices. Such individuals are pejoratively labeled 'noncompliant' and pressures are applied on them to reorder their priorities."[14]

The dangers of basing government policy on this attitude are clear, especially given the broad concerns of the public health movement. According to John J. Hanlon's *Public Health Administration and Practice,* "Public health is dedicated to the common attainment of the highest levels of physical, mental, and social well-being and longevity consistent with available knowledge and resources at a given time and place."[15] The textbook *Principles of Community Health* tells us, "The most widely accepted definition of individual health is that of the World Health Organization: 'Health is a state of complete physical, mental, and social well-being and not merely the absence of disease or infirmity.'"[16] A government empowered to maximize health is a totalitarian government.

In response to such fears, the public health establishment argues that government intervention is justified because individual decisions about risk affect other people. "Motorcyclists often contend that helmet laws infringe on personal liberties," noted Surgeon General Julius Richmond's 1979 report *Healthy People,* "and opponents of mandatory [helmet] laws argue that since other people usually are not endangered, the individual motorcyclist should be allowed personal responsibility for risk. But the high cost of disabling and fatal injuries, the burden on families, and the demands on medical care resources are borne by society as a whole."[17] This line of reasoning, which is also used to justify taxes on tobacco and alcohol, implies that all resources—including not just taxpayer-funded welfare and health care but private savings, insurance coverage, and charity—are part of a common pool owned by "society as a whole" and guarded by the government.

As Meenan noted in the *New England Journal of Medicine,* "Virtually all aspects of life style could be said to have an effect on the health or well-being of society, and the decision [could then be] reached that personal health choices should be closely regulated."[18] Writing 18 years later in the same journal, Faith T. Fitzgerald, a professor at the University of California, Davis, Medical Center, observed: "Both health care providers and the commonweal now have a vested interest in certain forms of behavior, previously considered a person's private business, if the behavior impairs a person's 'health.' Certain failures of self-care have become, in a sense, crimes against society, because society has to pay for their consequences. . . . In effect, we have said that people owe it to society to stop misbehaving, and we use illness as evidence of misbehavior."[19]

Most public health practitioners would presumably recoil at the full implications of the argument that government should override individual decisions affecting health because such decisions have an impact on "society as a whole." C. Everett Koop, for his part, seems completely untroubled. "I think that the government has a perfect right to influence personal behavior to the best of its ability if it is for the welfare of the individual and the community as a whole," he writes. This is paternalistic tyranny in its purest form, arrogating to government the authority to judge "the welfare of the individual" and elevating "the community as a whole" above mere people. Ignoring the distinction between self-regarding behavior and behavior that threatens others, Koop compares efforts to discourage smoking and other risky behavior to mandatory vaccination of schoolchildren and laws against assault.[20]

While Koop may simply be confused, some defenders of the public health movement explicitly recognize that its aims are fundamentally collectivist and cannot be reconciled with the American tradition of limited government. In 1975 Dan E. Beauchamp, then an assistant professor of public health at the University of North Carolina, presented a paper at the annual meeting of the American Public Health

Association in which he argued that "the radical individualism inherent in the market model" is the biggest obstacle to improving public health. "The historic dream of public health that preventable death and disability ought to be minimized is a dream of social justice," Beauchamp said. "We are far from recognizing the principle that death and disability are collective problems and that all persons are entitled to health protection." He rejected "the ultimately arbitrary distinction between voluntary and involuntary hazards" and complained that "the primary duty to avert disease and injury still rests with the individual." Beauchamp called upon public health practitioners to challenge "the powerful sway market-justice holds over our imagination, granting fundamental freedom to all individuals to be left alone."[21]

Of all the risk factors for disease and injury, it seems, freedom is the most pernicious. And you thought it was smoking.

Notes

1. Byron J. Bailey, "Tobaccoism Is the Disease: Cancer Is the Sequela," *Journal of the American Medical Association,* 255: 14 (11 April 1986), p. 1923.

2. William H. Foege, "The Growing Brown Plague," *Journal of the American Medical Association,* 264: 12 (26 September 1990), p. 1580.

3. Louis Sullivan, "An Opportunity to Oppose: Physicians' Role in the Campaign Against Tobacco," *Journal of the American Medical Association,* 264: 12 (26 September 1990), pp. 1581–1582.

4. Stanton Glantz, "What Deal? We Got Suckered," *Los Angeles Times,* 23 June 1997, p. B5.

5. Philip J. Hilts, *Smokescreen: The Truth Behind the Tobacco Industry Cover-Up,* Reading, MA: Addison-Wesley, 1996, pp. 216–217.

6. Barnaby J. Feder, "Texas Joins Other States in Suing Tobacco Industry," *New York Times,* 29 March 1996, p. B9.

7. Shankar Vedantam, "Antismoking Campaign Often Invokes Moral Terms," *Philadelphia Inquirer,* 24 August 1996, p. A8.

8. Dennis L. Breo, "Kicking Butts," *Journal of the American Medical Association,* 270: 16 (27 October 1993), p. 1978.

9. U.S. Centers for Disease Control and Prevention, "Smoking Prevalence Among U.S. Adults," 24 April 1996. "Cigarette Smoking Among Adults—United States, 1994," *Morbidity and Mortality Weekly Report,* 12 July 1996, p. 588.

10. Susan Steinberg, "Smoke Rings," *Los Angeles Times,* 15 June 1995, p. J14. Sheryl Gay Stolberg, "Cigar Fad Reported to Be Recruiting Legions of Teen-Agers," *New York Times,* 23 May 1997, p. A24.

11. Suein L. Hwang, "FDA Seeks to Mount Attack on Smoking by Minors That Could Mean Regulation," *Wall Street Journal,* 13 July 1995, p. A1.

12. Introduction to Albert H. Buck, ed., *A Treatise on Hygiene and Public Health,* New York: Arno Press, 1977 (originally published in 1879), p. 38.

13. Leon S. White, "How to Improve the Public's Health," *New England Journal of Medicine,* 293: 15 (9 October 1975), pp. 773–774.

14. Robert F. Meenan, "Improving the Public's Health: Some Further Reflections," *New England Journal of Medicine,* 294: 1 (1 January 1976), pp. 45–46.

15. John J. Hanlon, *Public Health Administration and Practice,* St. Louis: Mosby, 1974.

16. Jack Smolensky, *Principles of Community Health*, Philadelphia: Saunders, 1977, p. 5.

17. U.S. Department of Health, Education, and Welfare, *Healthy People: The Surgeon General's Report on Health Promotion and Disease Prevention,* U.S. Public Health Service, 1979, pp. 9–20.

18. Meenan, "Improving the Public's Health," p. 45.

19. Faith T. Fitzgerald, "The Tyranny of Health," *New England Journal of Medicine,* 331: 3 (21 July 1994), pp. 196–198.

20. C. Everett Koop, "C. Everett Koop: A Surgeon General Speaks," *Priorities,* 8: 2 (1996), p. 25.

21. Dan E. Beauchamp, "Public Health as Social Justice," *Inquiry,* 13 (March 1976), pp. 3–14.

9

Drug Prohibition in the United States

Costs, Consequences, and Alternatives

Ethan A. Nadelmann

As frustrations with the drug problem and current drug policies rise daily, growing numbers of political leaders, law enforcement officials, drug abuse experts, and common citizens are insisting that a radical alternative to current policies be fairly considered: the controlled legalization (or decriminalization) of drugs.[1]

Just as "Repeal Prohibition" became a catchphrase that swept together the diverse objections to Prohibition, so "Legalize (or Decriminalize) Drugs" has become a catchphrase that means many things to many people. The policy analyst views legalization as a model for critically examining the costs and benefits of drug prohibition policies. Libertarians, both civil and economic, view it as a policy alternative that eliminates criminal sanctions on the use and sale of drugs that are costly in terms of both individual liberty and economic freedom. Others see it simply as a means to "take the crime out of the drug business." In its broadest sense, however, legalization incorporates the many arguments and growing sentiment for deemphasizing our traditional reliance on criminal justice resources to deal with drug abuse and for emphasizing instead drug abuse, prevention, treatment, and education, as well as noncriminal restrictions on the availability and use of psychoactive substances and positive inducements to abstain from drug abuse.

There is no one legalization option. At one extreme, some libertarians advocate the removal of all criminal sanctions and taxes on the production and sale of all psychoactive substances—with the possible exception of restrictions on sales to children. The alternative extremes are more varied. Some would limit legalization to one of the safest (relatively speaking) of all illicit substances: marijuana. Others prefer a "medical" oversight model similar to today's methadone maintenance programs. The middle ground combines legal availability of some or all illicit drugs with vigorous efforts to restrict consumption by means other than resort to criminal sanctions. Many supporters of this dual approach simultaneously advocate greater efforts to limit tobacco consumption and the abuse of alcohol as well as a transfer of government resources from antidrug law enforcement to drug prevention and treatment. Indeed, the best model for this view of drug legalization is precisely the tobacco control model advocated by those who want to do everything possible to discourage tobacco consumption short of criminalizing the production, sale, and use of tobacco.

Clearly, neither drug legalization nor enforcement of antidrug laws promises to "solve" the drug problem. Nor is there any question that legalization presents certain risks. Legalization would almost certainly increase the availability of drugs, decrease their price, and remove the deterrent power of the criminal sanction—all of which invite increases in drug use and abuse. There are at least three reasons, however, why these risks are worth taking. First, drug control strategies that rely primarily on criminal justice measures are significantly and inherently limited in their capacity to curtail drug abuse. Second, many law enforcement efforts are not only of limited value but also highly costly and counterproductive; indeed, many of the drug-related evils that most people identify as part and parcel of "the drug problem" are in fact the costs of drug prohibition policies. Third, the risks of legalization may well be less than most people assume, particularly if intelligent alternative measures are implemented.

The Limits of Drug Prohibition Policies

Few law enforcement officials any longer contend that their efforts can do much more than they are already doing to reduce drug abuse in the United States. This is true of international drug enforcement efforts, interdiction, and both high-level and street-level domestic drug enforcement efforts.

The United States seeks to limit the export of illicit drugs to this country by a combination of crop eradication and crop substitution programs, financial inducements to growers to abstain from the illicit business, and punitive measures against producers, traffickers, and others involved in the drug traffic. These efforts have met with scant success in the past and show few indications of succeeding in the future. The obstacles are many: marijuana and opium can be grown in a wide variety of locales, and even the coca plant "can be grown in virtually any subtropical region of the world which gets between 40 and 240 inches of rain per year, where it never freezes, and where the land is not so swampy as to be waterlogged. In South America this comes to [approximately] 2,500,000 square miles," of which less than 700 square miles are currently being used to cultivate coca.[2] Producers in many countries have reacted to crop eradication programs by engaging in "guerrilla" farming methods, cultivating their crops in relatively inaccessible hinterlands and camouflaging them with legitimate crops. Some illicit drug-producing regions are controlled not by the central government but by drug trafficking gangs or political insurgents, thereby rendering eradication efforts even more difficult and hazardous.

Even where eradication efforts prove relatively successful in an individual country, other countries will emerge as new producers, as has occurred with both the international marijuana and heroin markets during the past two decades and can be expected to follow from planned coca eradication programs. The foreign export price of illicit drugs is such a tiny fraction of the retail price in the United States [approximately 4 percent with cocaine, 1 percent with marijuana, and much less than 1 percent with heroin][3] that international drug control efforts are not even successful in raising the cost of illicit drugs to U.S. consumers.

United States efforts to control drugs overseas also confront substantial, and in some cases well-organized, political opposition in foreign countries.[4] Major drug traffickers retain the power to bribe and intimidate government officials into ignoring or even cooperating with their enterprises.[5] Particularly in many Latin American and Asian countries, the illicit drug traffic is an important source of income and employment, bringing in billions of dollars in hard currency each year and providing livable wages for many hundreds of thousands. The illicit drug business has been described—not entirely in jest—as the best means ever devised by the United States for exporting the capitalist ethic to potentially revolutionary Third World peasants. By contrast, United States-sponsored eradication efforts risk depriving those same peasants of their livelihoods, thereby stimulating support for communist insurgencies ranging from Peru's Shining Path[6] to the variety of ethnic and communist organizations active in drug-producing countries such as Colombia and Burma. Moreover, many of those involved in producing illicit drugs overseas do not perceive their moral obligation as preventing decadent gringos from consuming cocaine or heroin; rather it is to earn the best living possible for themselves and their families. In the final analysis, there is little the U.S. government can do to change this perception.

Interdiction efforts have shown little success in stemming the flow of cocaine and heroin into the United States.[7] Indeed, during the past decade, the wholesale price of a kilo of cocaine has dropped by 80 percent even as the retail purity of a gram of cocaine has quintupled from 12 to about 60 percent; the trend with heroin over the past few years has been similar if less dramatic.[8] Easily transported in a variety of large and small aircraft and sea vessels, carried across the Mexican border by legal and illegal border crossers, hidden in everything from furniture, flowers, and automobiles to private body parts and cadavers, heroin and cocaine shipments are extraordinarily difficult to detect. Despite powerful congressional support for dramatically increasing the role of the military in drug interdiction, military leaders insist that they can do little to make a difference. The Coast Guard and U.S. Customs continue to expand their efforts in this area, but they too concede that they will never seize more than a small percentage of total shipments. Because cocaine and heroin are worth more than their weight in gold, the incentives to transport these drugs to the United States are so great that we can safely assume that there will never be a shortage of those willing to take the risk.

The one success that interdiction efforts can claim concerns marijuana. Because marijuana is far bulkier per dollar of value than either cocaine or heroin, it is harder to conceal and easier to detect. Stepped-up interdiction efforts in recent years appear to have reduced the flow of marijuana into the United States and to have increased its price to the American consumer.[9] The unintended consequences of this success are twofold: The United States has emerged as one of the world's leading producers of marijuana; indeed, U.S. producers are now believed to produce among the finest strains in the world;[10] and many international drug traffickers appear to have redirected their efforts from marijuana to cocaine. The principal consequence of U.S. drug interdiction efforts, many would contend, has been a glut of increasingly potent cocaine and a shortage of comparatively benign marijuana.

Domestic law enforcement efforts have proven increasingly successful in apprehending and imprisoning rapidly growing numbers of illicit drug merchants, ranging from the most sophisticated international traffickers to the most common street-level drug dealers. The principal benefit of law enforcement efforts directed at major drug trafficking organizations is probably the rapidly rising value of drug trafficker assets forfeited to the government. There is, however, little indication that such efforts have any significant impact on the price or availability of illicit drugs. Intensive and highly costly street-level law enforcement efforts such as those mounted by many urban police departments in recent years have resulted in the arrests of thousands of low-level drug dealers and users and helped improve the quality of life in targeted neighborhoods.[11] In most large urban centers, however, these efforts have had little impact on the overall availability of illicit drugs.

The logical conclusion of the foregoing analysis is not that criminal justice efforts to stop drug trafficking do not work at all; rather, it is that even substantial fluctuations in those efforts have little effect on the price, availability, and consumption of illicit drugs. The mere existence of criminal laws combined with minimal levels of enforcement is sufficient to deter many potential users and to reduce the availability and increase the price of drugs. Law enforcement officials acknowledge that they alone cannot solve the drug problem but contend that their role is nonetheless essential to the overall effort to reduce illicit drug use and abuse. What they are less ready to acknowledge, however, is that the very criminalization of the drug market has proven highly costly and counterproductive in much the same way that the national prohibition of alcohol did 60 years ago.

[Drugs and Crime]

. . . The connection between drugs and crime is one that continues to resist coherent analysis both because cause and effect are so difficult to distinguish and because the role of the drug prohibition laws in causing and labeling "drug-related crime" is so often ignored. There are five possible connections between drugs and crime, at least three of which would be much diminished if the drug prohibition laws were repealed. First, the production, sale, purchase, and possession of marijuana, cocaine, heroin, and other strictly controlled and banned substances are crimes in and of themselves, which occur billions of times each year in the United States alone. In the absence of drug prohibition laws, these activities would largely cease to be considered crimes. Selling drugs to children would, of course, continue to be criminalized, and other evasions of government regulation of a legal market would continue to be prosecuted, but by and large the connection between drugs and crime that now accounts for all of the criminal justice costs noted above would be severed.

Second, many illicit drug users commit crimes such as robbery and burglary, as well as other vice crimes such as drug dealing, prostitution, and numbers running, to earn enough money to purchase cocaine, heroin, and other illicit drugs—drugs that cost far more than alcohol and tobacco not because they cost much more to produce but because they are illegal.[12] Because legalization would inevitably lead to a reduction in the cost of the drugs that are now illicit, it would also invite a significant reduction in this drug-crime connection. At the same time, current methadone maintenance programs represent a limited form of drug legalization that attempts to break this connection between drugs and crime by providing an addictive opiate at little or no cost to addicts who might otherwise steal to support their illicit heroin habits. Despite their many limitations, such programs have proven effective in reducing the criminal behavior and improving the lives of thousands of illicit drug addicts;[13] they need to be made more available, in part by adapting the types of outreach programs for addicts devised in the Netherlands.[14] Another alternative, the British system of prescribing not just oral methadone but also injectable heroin and methadone to addicts who take drugs intravenously, persists on a small scale even today despite continuing pressures against prescribing injectables. This, too, merits adoption in the United States, particularly if one accepts the assumption that the primary objective of drug policy should be to minimize the harms that drug abusers do to others.[15]

The third connection between drugs and crime is more coincidental than causal in nature. Although most illicit drug users do not engage in crime aside from their drug use, and although many criminals do not use or abuse illicit drugs or alcohol, substance abuse clearly is much higher among criminals than among noncriminals. A 1986 survey of state prison inmates found that 43 percent were using illegal drugs on a daily or near-daily basis in the month before they committed the crime for which they were incarcerated; it also found that roughly one-half of the inmates who had used an illicit drug did not do so until after their first arrest.[16] Perhaps many of the same factors that lead individuals into lives of crime also push them in the direction of substance abuse. It is possible that legalization would diminish this connection by removing from the criminal subculture the lucrative opportunities that now derive from the illegality of the drug market. But it is also safe to assume that the criminal milieu will continue to claim a disproportionately large share of drug abusers regardless of whether or not drugs are legalized.

The fourth link between drugs and crime is the commission of violent and other crimes by people under the influence of illicit drugs. It is this connection that seems to most infect the popular imagination. Clearly, some drugs do "cause" some people to commit crimes by reducing normal inhibitions, unleashing aggressive and other asocial tendencies, and lessening senses of responsibility. . . . No illicit drug, however, is as strongly associated with violent behavior as is alcohol. . . . The impact of drug legalization on this aspect of the drug-crime connection is the most difficult to assess, largely because changes in the overall level and nature of drug consumption are so difficult to predict.

The fifth connection is the violent, intimidating, and corrupting behavior of the drug traffickers. In many Latin American countries, most notably Colombia, this connection virtually defines the "drug problem." But even within the United States, drug trafficker violence is rapidly becoming a major concern of criminal justice officials and the public at large. The connection is not difficult to explain. Illegal markets tend to breed violence, both because they attract criminally minded and violent individuals and because participants in the market have no resort to legal institutions to resolve their disputes.[17] During Prohibition, violent struggles between bootlegging gangs and hijackings of booze-laden trucks and sea vessels were frequent and notorious occurrences. Today's equivalents are the booby traps that surround some marijuana fields, the pirates of the Caribbean looking to rob drug-laden vessels en route to the shores of the United States, the machine gun battles and executions of the more sordid drug gangs, and the generally high levels of violence that attend many illicit drug relationships; the victims include not just drug dealers but witnesses, bystanders, and law enforcement officials. Most law enforcement authorities agree that the dramatic increases in urban murder rates during the past few years can be explained almost entirely by the rise in drug dealer killings, mostly of one another.[18] At the same time, the powerful allure of illicit drug dollars is responsible for rising levels of corruptions not just in Latin America and the Caribbean but also in federal, state, and local criminal justice systems throughout the United States.[19] A drug legalization strategy would certainly deal a severe blow to this link between drugs and crime.

Perhaps the most unfortunate victims of the drug prohibition policies have been the poor and law-abiding residents of urban ghettos. Those policies have proven largely futile in deterring large numbers of ghetto dwellers from becoming drug abusers, but they do account for much of what ghetto residents identify as the drug problem. In many neighborhoods, it often seems to be the aggressive gun-toting drug dealers who upset law-abiding residents far more than the addicts nodding out in doorways.[20] Other residents, however, perceive the drug dealers as heroes and successful role models. In impoverished neighborhoods from Medellín and Rio de Janeiro to many leading U.S. cities, they often stand out as symbols of success to children who see no other options. At the same time, the increasingly harsh criminal penalties imposed on adult drug dealers have led to the widespread recruiting of juveniles by drug traffickers.[21] Where once children started dealing drugs only after they had been using them for a few years, today the sequence is often reversed. Many children start to use illegal drugs now only after they have worked for older drug dealers for a while. And the juvenile justice system offers no realistic options for dealing with this growing problem.

Perhaps the most difficult costs to evaluate are those that relate to the widespread defiance of the drug prohibition laws: the effects of labeling as criminals the tens of millions of people who use drugs illicitly, subjecting them to the risks of criminal sanction and obliging many of those same people to enter into relationships with drug dealers (who may be criminals in many more senses of the word) in order to purchase their drugs; the cynicism that such laws generate toward other laws and the law in general; and the sense of hostility and suspicion that many otherwise law-abiding individuals feel toward law enforcement officials. It was costs such as these that strongly influenced many of Prohibition's more conservative opponents.

Among the most dangerous consequences of the drug laws are the harms that stem from the unregulated nature of illicit drug production and sale.[22] Many marijuana smokers are worse off for having smoked cannabis that was grown with dangerous fertilizers, sprayed with the herbicide paraquat, or mixed with more dangerous substances. Consumers of heroin and the various synthetic substances sold on the street face even more severe consequences, including fatal overdoses and poisonings from unexpectedly potent or impure drug supplies. In short, nothing resembling an underground Food and Drug Administration has arisen to impose quality control on the illegal drug market and provide users with accurate information on the drugs they consume. More often than not, the quality of a drug addict's life depends greatly on his or her access to reliable supplies. Drug enforcement operations that succeed in temporarily disrupting supply networks are thus a double-edged sword: They encourage some addicts to seek admission into drug treatment programs, but they oblige others to seek out new and hence less reliable suppliers, with the result that more, not fewer, drug-related emergencies and deaths occur.

. . . Other costs of current drug prohibition policies include the restrictions on using the illicit drugs for legitimate medical purposes.[23] Marijuana has proven useful in alleviating pain in some victims of multiple sclerosis, is particularly effective in reducing the nausea that accompanies chemotherapy, and may well prove effective in the treatment of glaucoma[24–26]; in September 1988, the administrative law judge of the Drug Enforcement Administration accordingly recommended that marijuana be made legally available for such purposes,[27] although the agency head has yet to approve the change. Heroin has proven highly effective in helping patients to deal with severe pain; some researchers have found it more effective than morphine and other opiates in treating pain in some patients.[28] It is legally prescribed for such purposes in Britain[29] and Canada.[30] The same may be true of cocaine, which continues to be used by some doctors in the United States to treat pain despite recently imposed bans.[31] The psychedelic drugs, such as LSD (*d*-lysergic acid diethylamide), peyote, and MDMA (known as Ecstasy) have shown promise in aiding psychotherapy and in reducing tension, depression, pain, and fear of death in the terminally ill;[32] they also have demonstrated some potential, as yet unconfirmed, to aid in the treatment of alcoholism.[33,34] Current drug laws and policies, however, greatly hamper the efforts of researchers to investigate these and other potential medical uses of illegal drugs; they make it virtually impossible for any of the illegal drugs, particularly those in Schedule I, to be legally provided to those who would benefit from them; and they contribute strongly to the widely acknowledged undertreatment of pain by the medical profession in the United States.[35]

Among the strongest arguments in favor of legalization are the moral ones. On the one hand, the standard refrain regarding the immorality of drug use crumbles in the face of most Americans' tolerance for alcohol and tobacco use. Only the Mormons and a few other like-minded sects, who regard as immoral any intake of substances to alter one's state of consciousness or otherwise cause pleasure, are consistent in this respect; they eschew not just the illicit drugs but also alcohol, tobacco, caffeinated coffee and tea, and even chocolate. "Moral" condemnation by the majority of Americans of some substances and not others is little more than a transient prejudice in favor of some drugs and against others.

On the other hand, drug enforcement involves its own immoralities. Because drug law violations do not create victims with an interest in notifying the police, drug enforcement agents must rely heavily on undercover operations, electronic surveillance, and information provided by informants. . . . These techniques are certainly indispensable to effective law enforcement, but they are also among the least desirable of the tools available to police. The same is true of drug testing. It may be useful and even necessary for determining liability in accidents, but it also threatens and undermines the right of privacy to which many Americans believe they are morally and constitutionally entitled. There are good reasons for requiring that such measures be used sparingly.

Equally disturbing are the increasingly vocal calls for people to inform not just on drug dealers but on neighbors, friends, and even family members who use illicit drugs. Intolerance of illicit drug use and users is heralded not merely as an indispensable ingredient in the war against drugs but as a mark of good citizenship. Certainly every society requires citizens to assist in the enforcement of criminal laws. But societies, particularly democratic and pluralistic ones, also rely strongly on an ethic of tolerance toward those who are different but do no harm to others. Overzealous enforcement of the drug laws risks undermining that ethic and propagating in its place a society of informants. Indeed, enforcement of drug laws makes a mockery of an essential principle of a free society, that those who do no harm to others should not be harmed by others, and particularly not by the state. Most of the nearly 40 million Americans who illegally consume drugs each year do no direct harm to anyone else; indeed, most do relatively little harm even to themselves. Directing criminal and other sanctions at them, and rationalizing the justice of such sanctions, may well represent the greatest societal cost of our current drug prohibition system.

Alternatives to Drug Prohibition Policies

Repealing the drug prohibition laws clearly promises tremendous advantages. Between reduced government expenditures on enforcing drug laws and new tax revenue from legal drug production and sales, public treasuries would enjoy a net benefit of at least $10 billion per year and possibly much more; thus billions in new revenues would be available, and ideally targeted, for funding much-needed drug treatment programs as well as the types of social and educational programs that often prove most effective in creating incentives for children not to abuse drugs. The quality of urban life would rise significantly. Homicide rates would decline. So would robbery and burglary rates. Organized criminal groups, particularly the up-and-coming ones that have yet to diversify into nondrug areas, would be dealt a devastating setback. The police, prosecutors, and courts would focus their resources on combating the types of crimes that people cannot walk away from. More ghetto residents would turn their backs on criminal careers and seek out legitimate opportunities instead. And the health and quality of life of many drug users and even drug abusers would improve significantly. Internationally, U.S. foreign policymakers would get on with more important and realistic objectives, and foreign governments would reclaim the authority that they have lost to the drug traffickers.

All the benefits of legalization would be for naught, however, if millions more people were to become drug abusers . . .

The impact of legalization on the nature and level of consumption of those drugs that are currently illegal is impossible to predict with any accuracy. On the one hand, legalization implies greater availability, lower prices, and the elimination (particularly for adults) of the deterrent power of the criminal sanction—all of which would suggest higher levels of use. Indeed, some fear that the extent of drug abuse and its attendant costs would rise to those currently associated with alcohol and tobacco.[36] On the other hand, there are many reasons to doubt that a well-designed and implemented policy of controlled drug legalization would yield such costly consequences.

The logic of legalization depends in part upon two assumptions: that most illegal drugs are not as dangerous as is commonly believed; and that those types of drugs and methods of consumption that are most risky are unlikely to prove appealing to many people precisely because they are so obviously dangerous. Consider marijuana. Among the roughly 60 million Americans who have smoked marijuana, not one has died from a marijuana overdose,[37] a striking contrast with alcohol, which is involved in approximately 10,000 overdose deaths annually, half in combination with other drugs.[38] Although there are good health reasons for people not to smoke marijuana daily, and for children, pregnant women, and some others not to smoke at all, there still appears to be little evidence that occasional marijuana consumption does much harm at all. Certainly, it is not healthy to inhale marijuana smoke into one's lungs; indeed, the National Institute on Drug Abuse (NIDA) has declared that "marijuana smoke contains more cancer-causing agents than is found in tobacco smoke."[39] On the other hand, the number of "joints" smoked by all but a very small percentage of marijuana smokers is a tiny fraction of the 20 cigarettes a day smoked by the average cigarette smoker; indeed, the average may be closer to one or two joints per week than one or two per day. Note that the NIDA defines a "heavy" marijuana smoker as one who consumes at least two joints "daily." A heavy tobacco smoker, by contrast, smokes about 40 cigarettes per day.

. . . [T]his is not to say that cocaine is not a potentially dangerous drug, especially when it is injected, smoked in the form of "crack," or consumed in tandem with other powerful substances. Clearly, many tens of thousands of Americans have suffered severely from their abuse of cocaine and a tiny fraction have died. But there is also overwhelming evidence that most users of cocaine do not get into trouble with the drug. So much of the media attention has focused on the relatively small percentage of cocaine users who become addicted that the popular perception of how most people use cocaine has become badly distorted. In one survey of high school seniors' drug use, the researchers questioned those who had used cocaine recently whether they had ever tried to stop using cocaine and found that they could not stop. Only 3.8 percent responded affirmatively, in contrast to the almost 7 percent of marijuana smokers who said they had tried to stop and found they could not, and the 18 percent of cigarette smokers who answered similarly.[40] Although a survey of crack users and cocaine injectors surely would reveal a higher proportion of addicts, evidence such as this suggests that only a small percentage of people who snort cocaine end up having a problem with it. In this respect, most people differ from captive monkeys, who have demonstrated in tests that they will starve themselves to death if provided with unlimited cocaine.[41]

With respect to the hallucinogens such as LSD and psilocybic mushrooms, their potential for addiction is virtually nil. The dangers arise primarily from using them irresponsibly on individual occasions.[42] Although many of those who have used hallucinogens have experienced "bad trips," far more have reported positive experiences, and very few have suffered any long-term harm.[43] As for the great assortment of stimulants, depressants, and tranquilizers produced illegally or diverted from licit channels, each evidences varying capacities to create addiction, harm the user, or be used safely.

Until recently, no drugs were regarded with as much horror as the opiates, and in particular heroin. As with most drugs, it can be eaten, snorted, smoked, or injected. . . . There is no question that heroin is potentially highly addictive, perhaps as addictive as nicotine. But despite the popular association of heroin use with the most down-and-out inhabitants of urban ghettos, heroin causes relatively little physical harm to the human body. Consumed on an occasional or regular basis under sanitary conditions, its worst side effect, apart from the fact of being addicted, is constipation.[44] That is one reason why many doctors in early 20th-century America saw opiate addiction as preferable to alcoholism and prescribed the former as treatment for the latter where abstinence did not seem a realistic option.[45,46]

It is both insightful and important to think about the illicit drugs as we do about alcohol and tobacco. Like tobacco, some illicit substances are highly addictive but can be consumed on a regular basis for decades without any demonstrable harm. Like alcohol, many of the substances can be, and are, used by most consumers in moderation, with little in the way of harmful effects; but like alcohol they also lend themselves to abuse by a minority of users who become addicted or otherwise harm themselves or others as a consequence. And like both the legal substances, the psychoactive effects of each of the illegal drugs vary greatly from one person to another. To be sure, the pharmacology of the substance is important, as is its purity and the manner in which it is consumed. But much also depends upon not just the physiology and psychology of the consumer but his expectations regarding the drug, his social milieu, and the broader cultural environment, what Harvard University psychiatrist Norman Zinberg called the "set and setting" of the drug.[47] It is factors such as these that might change dramatically, albeit in indeterminate ways, were the illicit drugs made legally available.

It is thus impossible to predict whether or not legalization would lead to much greater levels of drug abuse. . . .

There are however, strong reasons to believe that none of the currently illicit substances would become as popular as alcohol or tobacco even if they were legalized. Alcohol has long been the principal intoxicant in most societies, including many in which other substances have been legally available. Presumably, its diverse properties account for its popularity: it quenches thirst, goes well with food, often pleases the palate, promotes appetite as well as sociability, and so on. The widespread use of tobacco probably stems not just from its powerful addictive qualities but from the fact that its psychoactive effects are sufficiently subtle that cigarettes can be integrated with most other human activities. None of the illicit substances now popular in the United States share either of these qualities to the same extent, nor is it likely that they would acquire them if they were legalized. Moreover, none of the illicit substances can compete with alcohol's special place in American culture and history, one that it retained even during Prohibition.

Much of the damage caused by illegal drugs today stems from their consumption in particularly potent and dangerous ways. There is good reason to doubt that many Americans would inject cocaine or heroin into their veins even if given the chance to do so legally. And just as the dramatic growth in the heroin-consuming population during the 1960s leveled off for reasons apparently having little to do with law enforcement, so we can expect, if it has not already occurred, a leveling off in the number of people smoking crack.

Perhaps the most reassuring reason for believing that repeal of the drug prohibition laws will not lead to tremendous increases in drug abuse levels is the fact that we have learned something from our past experiences with alcohol and tobacco abuse. We know now, for instance, that consumption taxes are an effective method for limiting consumption rates and related costs, especially among young people.[48] Substantial evidence also suggests that restrictions and bans on advertising, as well as promotion of negative advertising, can make a difference.[49] The same seems to be true of other government measures, including restrictions on time and place of sale,[50] bans on vending machines, prohibitions of consumption in public places, packaging requirements, mandated adjustments in insurance policies, crackdowns on driving while under the influence,[51] and laws holding bartenders and hosts responsible for the drinking of customers and guests. There is even some evidence that some education programs about the dangers of cigarette smoking have deterred many children from beginning to smoke.[52] At the same time, we also have come to recognize the great harms that can result when drug control policies are undermined by powerful lobbies such as those that now block efforts to lessen the harms caused by abuse of alcohol and tobacco.

Legalization thus affords far greater opportunities to control drug use and abuse than do current criminalization policies. The current strategy is one in which the type, price, purity, and potency of illicit drugs, as well as the participants in the business, are largely determined by drug dealers, the peculiar competitive dynamics of an illicit market, and the perverse interplay of drug enforcement strategies and drug trafficking tactics. During the past decade, for instance, the average retail purities of cocaine and heroin have increased dramatically, the wholesale prices have dropped greatly, the number of children involved in drug dealing has risen, and crack has become readily and cheaply available in a growing number of American cities.[53] By contrast, marijuana has become relatively scarcer and more expensive, in part because it is far more vulnerable to drug enforcement efforts than are cocaine or heroin; the result has been to induce both dealers and users away from the relatively safer marijuana and toward the relatively more dangerous cocaine.[54] Also by contrast, while the average potency of most illicit substances has increased during the 1980s, that of most legal psychoactive substances has been declining. Motivated in good part by health concerns, Americans are switching from hard liquor to beer and wine, from high tar and nicotine cigarettes to lower tar and nicotine cigarettes as well as smokeless tobaccos and nicotine chewing gums, and even from caffeinated to decaffeinated coffees, teas, and sodas. It is quite possible that these diverging trends are less a reflection of the nature of the drugs than of their legal status.

A drug control policy based predominantly on approaches other than criminal justice thus offers a number of significant advantages over the current criminal justice focus in controlling drug use and abuse. It shifts control of production, distribution, and, to a lesser extent, consumption out of the hands of criminals and into the hands of government and government licensees. It affords consumers the opportunity to make far more informed decisions about the drugs they buy than is currently the case. It dramatically lessens the likelihood that drug consumers will be harmed by impure, unexpectedly potent, or misidentified drugs. It corrects the hypocritical and dangerous message that alcohol and tobacco are somehow safer than many illicit drugs. It reduces by billions of dollars annually government expenditures on drug enforcement and simultaneously raises additional billions in tax revenues. And it allows government the opportunity to shape consumption patterns toward relatively safer psychoactive substances and modes of consumption.

Toward the end of the 1920s, when the debate over repealing Prohibition rapidly gained momentum, numerous scholars, journalists, and private and government commissions undertook thorough evaluations of Prohibition and the potential alternatives. Prominent among these were the Wickersham Commission appointed by President Herbert Hoover and the study of alcohol regulation abroad directed by the leading police scholar in the United States, Raymond Fosdick, and commissioned by John D. Rockefeller.[55] These efforts examined the successes and failings of Prohibition in the United States and evaluated the wide array of alternative regimes for controlling the distribution and use of beer, wine, and liquor. They played a major role in stimulating the public reevaluation of Prohibition and in envisioning alternatives. Precisely the same sorts of efforts are required today.

The controlled drug legalization option is not an all-or-nothing alternative to current policies. Indeed, political realities ensure that any shift toward legalization will evolve gradually, with ample opportunity to halt, reevaluate, and redirect drug policies that begin to prove too costly or counterproductive. The federal government need not play the leading role in devising alternatives; it need only clear the way to allow state and local governments the legal power to implement their own drug legalization policies. The first steps are relatively risk free: legalization of marijuana, easier availability of illegal and strictly controlled drugs for treatment of pain and other medical purposes, tougher tobacco and alcohol control policies, and a broader and more available array of drug treatment programs.

Remedying the drug-related ills of America's ghettos requires more radical steps. The risks of a more far-reaching policy of controlled drug legalization—increased availability, lower prices, and removal of the deterrent power of the criminal sanction—are relatively less in the ghettos than in most other parts of the United States in good part because drug availability is already so high, prices so low, and the criminal sanction so ineffective in deterring illicit drug use that legalization can hardly worsen the situation. On the other hand, legalization would yield its greatest benefits in the ghettos, where it would sever much of the drug-crime connection, seize the market away from criminals, deglorify involvement in the illicit drug business, help redirect the work ethic from illegitimate to legitimate employment opportunities, help stem the transmission of AIDS by IV [intravenous] drug users, and significantly improve the safety, health, and well-being of those who do use and abuse drugs. Simply stated, legalizing cocaine, heroin, and other relatively dangerous drugs may well be the only way to reverse the destructive impact of drugs and current drug policies in the ghettos.

There is no question that legalization is a risky policy, one that may indeed lead to an increase in the number of people who abuse drugs. But that risk is by no means a certainty. At the same time, current drug control policies are showing little progress, and new proposals promise only to be more costly and more repressive. We know that repealing the drug prohibition laws would eliminate or greatly reduce many of the ills that people commonly identify as part and parcel of the "drug problem." Yet that option is repeatedly and vociferously dismissed without any attempt to evaluate it openly and objectively. The past 20 years have demonstrated that a drug policy shaped by rhetoric and fear-mongering can only lead to our current disaster. Unless we are willing to honestly evaluate all our options, including various legalization strategies, there is a good chance that we will never identify the best solutions for our drug problems.

Notes

1. The terms *legalization* and *decriminalization* are used interchangeably here. Some interpret the latter term as a more limited form of legalization involving the removal of criminal sanctions against users but not against producers and sellers.

2. Statement by Senator D. P. Moynihan, citing a U.S. Department of Agriculture report, in *Congr. Rec.* 134 (no. 77), p. S7049 (27 May 1988).

3. Drug Enforcement Administration, Department of Justice, *Intell. Trends* 14 (no. 3), 1 (1987).

4. See, for example, K. Healy, *J. Interam. Stud. World Aff.* 30 (no. 2/3), 105 (summer/fall 1988).

5. E. A. Nadelmann, *J. Interam. Stud. World Aff.* 29 (no. 4), 1 (winter 1987–1988).

6. C. McClintock, *J. Interam. Stud. World Aff.* 30 (no. 2/3), 127 (summer/fall 1988); J. Kawell, *Rep. Americas* 22 (no. 6), 13 (March 1989).

7. P. Reuter, *Public Interest* (no. 92), 51 (summer 1988).

8. See the annual reports of the National Narcotics Intelligence Consumers Committee edited by the Drug Enforcement Administration, Department of Justice, Washington, DC.

9. Ibid.

10. Ibid.

11. M. R. Chaiken, Ed., *Street-Level Drug Enforcement: Examining the Issues* (National Institute of Justice, Department of Justice, Washington, DC, September 1988).

12. B. D. Johnson et al., *Taking Care of Business: The Economics of Crime by Heroin Abusers* (Lexington Books, Lexington, MA, 1985).

13. B. D. Johnson, D. Lipton, and E. Wish, *Facts about the Criminality of Heroin and Cocaine Abusers and Some New Alternatives to Incarceration* (Narcotic and Drug Research, New York, 1986), p. 30.

14. G. F. van de Wijngart, *Am. J. Drug Alcohol Abuse* 14 (no. 1), 125 (1988).

15. A controlled trial in which 96 confirmed heroin addicts requesting a heroin maintenance prescription were randomly allocated to treatment with injectable heroin or oral methadone showed that "refusal [by doctors] to prescribe heroin is . . . associated with a considerably higher abstinence rate, but at the expense of an increased arrest rate and a higher level of illicit drug involvement and criminal activity among those who did not become abstinent." R. L. Hartnoll et al., *Arch. Gen. Psychiatry* 37, 877 (1980).

16. "Drug use and crime," *Bur. Justice Stat. Spec. Rep.* (July 1988).

17. P. J. Goldstein, in *Pathways to Criminal Violence,* N. A. Weiner and M. E. Wolfgang, Eds. (Sage, Newbury Park, CA, 1989), pp. 16–48.

18. "A tide of drug killing," *Newsweek,* 16 January 1989, p. 44.

19. P. Shenon, *New York Times,* 11 April 1988, p. A1.

20. W. Nobles, L. Goddard, W. Cavil, and P. George, *The Culture of Drugs in the Black Community* (Institute for the Advanced Study of Black Family Life and Culture, Oakland, CA, 1987).

21. T. Mieczowski, *Criminology* 24, 645 (1986).

22. C. L. Renfroe and T. A. Messinger, *Semin. Adolesc. Med.* 1 (no. 4), 247 (1985).

23. See, for example, P. Fitzgerald, *St. Louis Univ. Public Law Rev.* 6, 371 (1987).

24. L. Grinspoon and J. B. Bakalar, in *Dealing with Drugs: Consequences of Government Control,* R. Hamowy, Ed. (Lexington Books, Lexington, MA, 1987), pp. 183–219.

25. T. H. Mikuriya, Ed., *Marijuana: Medical Papers, 1839–1972* (Medi-Comp Press, Oakland, CA, 1973).

26. *In the Matter of Marijuana Rescheduling Petition,* Docket No. 86–22, 6 September 1988, Drug Enforcement Administration, Department of Justice.

27. Ibid.

28. A. S. Trebach, *The Heroin Solution* (Yale Univ. Press, New Haven, CT, 1982), pp. 59–84.

29. Ibid.

30. L. Appleby, *Saturday Night* (November 1985), p. 13.

31. F. R. Lee, *New York Times,* 10 February 1989, p. B3; F. Barre, *Headache* 22, 69 (1982).

32. L. Grinspoon and J. B. Bakalar, *Psychedelic Drugs Reconsidered* (Basic Books, New York, 1979).

33. Grinspoon and Bakalar, in *Dealing with Drugs.*

34. L. Grinspoon and J. B. Bakalar, *Psychedelic Drugs Reconsidered.*

35. M. Donovan, P. Dillon, and L. McGuire, *Pain* 30, 69 (1987); D. E. Weissman, *Narc Officer* 5 (no. 1), 47 (January 1989); D. Goleman, *New York Times,* 31 December 1987, p. B5. The Controlled Substances Act, 21 U.S.C. §801, et seq., defines a Schedule I drug as one that: (i) has a high potential for abuse; (ii) has no currently accepted medical use in treatment in the United States; and (iii) for which there is a lack of accepted safety for use under medical supervision. It is contrary to federal law for physicians to prescribe Schedule I drugs to patients for therapeutic purposes.

36. M. M. Kondracke, *New Repub.* 198 (no. 26), 16 (27 June 1988).

37. *In the Matter of Marijuana.*

38. D. R. Gerstein, in *Alcohol and Public Policy: Beyond the Shadow of Prohibition,* M. H. Moore and D. R. Gerstein, Eds. (National Academy Press, Washington, DC, 1981), pp. 182–224.

39. *Marijuana* (National Institute on Drug Abuse, Washington, DC, 1983).

40. P. M. O'Malley, L. D. Johnston, and J. G. Bachman, *NIDA Monogr. Ser. 61* (1985), pp. 50–75.

41. T. G. Aigner and R. L. Balster, *Science* 201, 534 (1978); C. E. Johnson, *NIDA Monogr. Ser. 50* (1984), pp. 54–71.

42. Grinspoon and Bakalar, *Psychedelic Drugs Reconsidered.*

43. Ibid.

44. J. Kaplan, *The Hardest Drug: Heroin and Public Policy* (University of Chicago Press, Chicago, 1983), p. 127.

45. S. Siegel, *Res. Adv. Alcohol Drug Probl.* 9, 279 (1986).

46. J. A. O'Donnell, *Narcotics Addicts in Kentucky* (Public Health Service Pub. 1881, National Institute of Mental Health, Chevy Chase, MD, 1969), discussed in *Licit and Illicit Drugs* [E. M. Brecher and the Editors of *Consumer Reports* (Little, Brown, Boston, 1972), pp. 8–10].

47. See N. Zinberg, *Drug, Set and Setting: The Basis for Controlled Intoxicant Use* (Yale University Press, New Haven, CT, 1984).

48. See P. J. Cook, in *Alcohol and Public Policy: Beyond the Shadow of Prohibition,* M. H. Moore and D. R. Gerstein, Eds. (National Academy Press, Washington, DC, 1981), pp. 255–285; D. Coate and M. Grossman, *J. Law Econ.* 31, 145 (1988); also see K. E. Warner, in *The Cigarette Excise Tax* (Harvard University Institute for the Study of Smoking Behavior and Policy, Cambridge, MA, 1985), pp. 88–105.

49. J. B. Tye, K. E. Warner, and S. A. Glantz, *J. Public Health Policy* 8, 492 (1987).

50. O. Olsson and P.-O.H. Wikstrom, *Contemp. Drug Probl.* 11, 325 (fall 1982); M. Terris, *Am. J. Public Health* 57, 2085 (1967).

51. M. D. Laurence, J. R. Snortum, and F. E. Zimring, Eds., *Social Control of the Drinking Driver* (University of Chicago Press, Chicago, 1988).

52. J. M. Polich, P. L. Ellickson, P. Reuter, and J. P. Kahan, *Strategies for Controlling Adolescent Drug Use* (RAND, Santa Monica, CA, 1984), pp. 145–152.

53. National Narcotics Intelligence Consumers Committee annual reports.

54. Ibid.

55. R. B. Fosdick and A. L. Scott, *Toward Liquor Control* (Harper, New York, 1933).

10

Against the Legalization of Drugs

James Q. Wilson

In 1972, the president appointed me chairman of the National Advisory Council for Drug Abuse Prevention. Created by Congress, the council was charged with providing guidance on how best to coordinate the national war on drugs. (Yes, we called it a war then, too.) In those days, the drug we were chiefly concerned with was heroin. When I took office, heroin use had been increasing dramatically. Everybody was worried that this increase would continue. Such phrases as "heroin epidemic" were commonplace.

That same year, the eminent economist Milton Friedman published an essay in *Newsweek* in which he called for legalizing heroin. His argument was on two grounds: As a matter of ethics, the government has no right to tell people not to use heroin (or to drink or to commit suicide); as a matter of economics, the prohibition of drug use imposes costs on society that far exceed the benefits. Others, such as the psychoanalyst Thomas Szasz, made the same argument.

We did not take Friedman's advice. (Government commissions rarely do.) I do not recall that we even discussed legalizing heroin, though we did discuss (but did not take action on) legalizing a drug, cocaine, that many people then argued was benign. Our marching orders were to figure out how to win the war on heroin, not to run up the white flag of surrender.

That was 1972. Today, we have the same number of heroin addicts that we had then—half a million, give or take a few thousand. Having that many heroin addicts is no trivial matter; these people deserve our attention. But not having had an increase in that number for over 15 years is also something that deserves our attention. What happened to the "heroin epidemic" that many people once thought would overwhelm us?

The facts are clear: a more or less stable pool of heroin addicts has been getting older, with relatively few new recruits. In 1976 the average age of heroin users who appeared in hospital emergency rooms was about 27; 10 years later it was 32. More than two-thirds of all heroin users appearing in emergency rooms are now over the age of 30. Back in the early 1970s, when heroin got onto the national political agenda, the typical heroin addict was much younger, often a teenager. Household surveys show the same thing—the rate of opiate use (which includes heroin) has been flat for the better part of two decades. More fine-grained studies of inner-city neighborhoods confirm this. John Boyle and Ann Brunswick found that the percentage of young blacks in Harlem who used heroin fell from 8 percent in 1970–1971 to about 3 percent in 1975–1976.

Why did heroin lose its appeal for young people? When the young blacks in Harlem were asked why they stopped, more than half mentioned "trouble with the law" or "high cost" (and high cost is, of course, directly the result of law enforcement). Two-thirds said that heroin hurt their health; nearly all said they had had a bad experience with it. We need not rely, however, simply on what they said. In New York City in 1973–1975, the street price of heroin rose dramatically, and its purity sharply declined, probably as a result of the heroin shortage caused by the success of the Turkish government in reducing the supply of opium base and of the French government in closing down heroin-processing laboratories located in and around Marseilles. These were short-lived gains for, just as Friedman predicted, alternative sources of supply—mostly in Mexico—quickly emerged. But the 3-year heroin shortage interrupted the easy recruitment of new users.

Health and related problems were no doubt part of the reason for the reduced flow of recruits. Over the preceding years, Harlem youth had watched as more and more heroin users died of overdoses, were poisoned by adulterated doses, or acquired hepatitis from dirty needles. The word got around: Heroin can kill you. By 1974 new hepatitis cases and drug-overdose deaths had dropped to a fraction of what they had been in 1970.

Alas, treatment did not seem to explain much of the cessation in drug use. Treatment programs can and do help heroin addicts, but treatment did not explain the drop in the number of *new* users (who by definition had never been in treatment) nor even much of the reduction in the number of experienced users.

No one knows how much of the decline to attribute to personal observation as opposed to high prices or reduced supply. But other evidence suggests strongly that price and supply played a large role. In 1972 the National Advisory Council was especially worried by the prospect that U.S. servicemen returning to this country from Vietnam would bring their heroin habits with them. Fortunately, a brilliant study by Lee Robins of Washington University in St. Louis put that fear to rest. She measured drug use of Vietnam veterans shortly after they had returned home. Though many had used heroin regularly while in Southeast Asia, most gave up the habit when back in the United States. The reason: Here, heroin was less available, and sanctions on its use were more pronounced. Of course, if a veteran had been willing to pay enough—which might have meant traveling to another city and would certainly have meant making an illegal contact with a disreputable dealer in a threatening neighborhood in order to acquire a (possibly) dangerous dose—he could have sustained his drug habit. Most veterans were unwilling to pay this price, and so their drug use declined or disappeared.

Reliving the Past

Suppose we had taken Friedman's advice in 1972. What would have happened? We cannot be entirely certain, but at a minimum we would have placed the young heroin addicts (and, above all, the prospective addicts) in a very different position from the one in which they actually found themselves. Heroin would have been legal. Its price would have been reduced by 95 percent (minus whatever we chose to recover in taxes). Now that it could be sold by the same people who make aspirin, its quality would have been assured—no poisons, no adulterants. Sterile hypodermic needles would have been readily available at the neighborhood drugstore, probably at the same counter where the heroin was sold. No need to travel to big cities or unfamiliar neighborhoods—heroin could have been purchased anywhere, perhaps by mail order.

There would no longer have been any financial or medical reason to avoid heroin use. Anybody could have afforded it. We might have tried to prevent children from buying it, but as we have learned from our efforts to prevent minors from buying alcohol and tobacco, young people have a way of penetrating markets theoretically reserved for adults. Returning Vietnam veterans would have discovered that Omaha and Raleigh had been converted into the pharmaceutical equivalent of Saigon.

Under these circumstances, can we doubt for a moment that heroin use would have grown exponentially? Or that a vastly larger supply of new users would have been recruited? Professor Friedman is a Nobel Prize–winning economist whose understanding of market forces is profound. What did he think would happen to consumption under his legalized regime? Here are his words: "Legalizing drugs might increase the number of addicts, but it is not clear that it would. Forbidden fruit is attractive, particularly to the young."

Really? I suppose that we should expect no increase in Porsche sales if we cut the price by 95 percent, no increase in whiskey sales if we cut the price by a comparable amount—because young people only want fast cars and strong liquor when they are "forbidden." Perhaps Friedman's uncharacteristic lapse from the obvious implications of price theory can be explained by a misunderstanding of how drug users are recruited. In his 1972 essay he said that "drug addicts are deliberately made by pushers, who give likely prospects their first few doses free." If drugs were legal it would not pay anybody to produce addicts because everybody would buy from the cheapest source. But as every drug expert knows, pushers do not produce addicts. Friends or acquaintances do. In fact, pushers are usually reluctant to deal with nonusers because a nonuser could be an undercover cop. Drug use spreads in the same way any fad or fashion spreads: somebody who is already a user urges his friends to try, or simply shows already-eager friends how to do it.

But we need not rely on speculation, however plausible, that lowered prices and more abundant supplies would have increased heroin usage. Great Britain once followed such a policy and with almost exactly those results. Until the mid-1960s, British physicians were allowed to prescribe heroin to certain classes of addicts. (Possessing these drugs without a doctor's prescription remained a criminal offense.) For many years this policy worked well enough because the addict patients were typically middle-class people who had become dependent on opiate painkillers while undergoing hospital treatment. There was no drug culture. The British system worked for many years, not because it prevented drug abuse, but because there was no problem of drug abuse that would test the system.

All that changed in the 1960s. A few unscrupulous doctors began passing out heroin in wholesale amounts. One doctor prescribed almost 600,000 heroin tablets—that is, over 13 pounds—in just one year. A youthful drug culture emerged with a demand for drugs far different from that of the older addicts. As a result, the British government required doctors to refer users to government-run clinics to receive their heroin.

But the shift to clinics did not curtail the growth in heroin use. Throughout the 1960s the number of addicts increased—the late John Kaplan of Stanford estimated by fivefold—in part as a result of the diversion of heroin from clinic patients to new users on the streets. An addict would bargain with the clinic doctor over how big a dose he would receive. The patient wanted as much as he could get; the doctor wanted to give as little as was needed. The patient had an advantage in this conflict because the doctor could not be certain how much was really needed. Many patients would use some of their "maintenance" dose and sell the remaining part to friends, thereby recruiting new addicts. As the clinics learned of this, they began to shift their treatment away from heroin and toward methadone, an addictive drug that, when taken orally, does not produce a "high" but will block the withdrawal pains associated with heroin abstinence.

Whether what happened in England in the 1960s was a miniepidemic or an epidemic depends on whether one looks at numbers or at rates of change. Compared to the United States, the numbers were small. In 1960 there were 68 heroin addicts known to the British government; by 1968 there were 2,000 in treatment and many more who refused treatment. (They would refuse in part because they did not want to get methadone at a clinic if they could get heroin on the street.) Richard Hartnoll estimates that the actual number of addicts in England is five times the number officially registered. At a minimum, the number of British addicts increased by 30-fold in 10 years; the actual increase may have been much larger.

In the early 1980s the numbers began to rise again, and this time nobody doubted that a real epidemic was at hand. The increase was estimated to be 40 percent a year. By 1982 there were thought to be 20,000 heroin users in London alone. Geoffrey Pearson reports that many cities—Glasgow, Liverpool, Manchester, and Sheffield among them—were now experiencing a drug problem that once had been largely confined to London. The problem, again, was supply. The country was being flooded with cheap, high-quality heroin, first from Iran and then from Southeast Asia.

The United States began the 1960s with a much larger number of heroin addicts and probably a bigger at-risk population than was the case in Great Britain. Even though it would be foolhardy to suppose that the British system, if installed here, would have worked the same way or with the same results, it would be equally foolhardy to suppose that a combination of heroin available from leaky clinics and from street dealers who faced only minimal law-enforcement risks would not have produced a much greater increase in heroin use than we actually experienced. My guess is that if we had allowed either doctors or clinics to prescribe heroin, we would have had far worse results than were produced in Britain, if for no other reason than the vastly larger number of addicts with which we began. We would have had to find some way to police thousands (not scores) of physicians and hundreds (not dozens) of clinics. If the British civil service found it difficult to keep heroin in the hands of addicts and out of the hands of recruits when it was dealing with a few hundred people, how well would the American civil service have accomplished the same tasks when dealing with tens of thousands of people?

Back to the Future

Now cocaine, especially in its potent form, crack, is the focus of attention. Now as in 1972 the government is trying to reduce its use. Now as then some people are advocating legalization. Is there any more reason to yield to those arguments today than there was almost two decades ago?

I think not. If we had yielded in 1972 we almost certainly would have had today a permanent population of several million, not several hundred thousand, heroin addicts. If we yield now we will have a far more serious problem with cocaine.

Crack is worse than heroin by almost any measure. Heroin produces a pleasant drowsiness and, if hygienically administered, has only the physical side effects of constipation and sexual impotence. Regular heroin use incapacitates many users, especially poor ones, for any productive work or social responsibility. They will sit nodding on a street corner, helpless but at least harmless. By contrast, regular cocaine use leaves the user neither helpless nor harmless. When smoked (as with crack) or injected, cocaine produces instant, intense, and short-lived euphoria. The experience generates a powerful desire to repeat it. If the drug is readily available, repeat use will occur. Those people who progress to "bingeing" on cocaine become devoted to the drug and its effects to the exclusion of almost all other considerations—job, family, children, sleep, food, even sex. Dr. Frank Gawin at Yale and Dr. Everett Ellinwood at Duke report that a substantial percentage of all high-dose, binge users become uninhibited, impulsive, hypersexual, compulsive, irritable, and hyperactive. Their moods vacillate dramatically, leading at times to violence and homicide.

Women are much more likely to use crack than heroin, and if they are pregnant, the effects on their babies are tragic. Douglas Besharov, who has been following the effects of drugs on infants for 20 years, writes that nothing he learned about heroin prepared him for the devastation of cocaine. Cocaine harms the fetus and can lead to physical deformities or neurological damage. Some crack babies have for all practical purposes suffered a disabling stroke while still in the womb. The long-term consequences of this brain damage are lowered cognitive ability and the onset of mood disorders. Besharov estimates that about 30,000 to 50,000 such babies are born every year, about 7,000 in New York City alone. There may be ways to treat such infants, but from everything we now know the treatment will be long, difficult, and expensive. Worse, the mothers who are most likely to produce crack babies are precisely the ones who, because of poverty or temperament, are least able and willing to obtain such treatment. In fact, anecdotal evidence suggests that crack mothers are likely to abuse their infants.

The notion that abusing drugs such as cocaine is a "victimless crime" is not only absurd but dangerous. Even ignoring the fetal drug syndrome, crack-dependent people are, like heroin addicts, individuals who regularly victimize their children by neglect, their spouses by improvidence, their employers by lethargy, and their coworkers by carelessness. Society is not and could never be a collection of autonomous individuals. We all have a stake in ensuring that each of us displays a minimal level of dignity, responsibility, and empathy. We cannot, of course, coerce people into goodness, but we can and should insist that some standards must be met if society itself—on which the very existence of the human personality depends—is to persist. Drawing the line that defines those standards is difficult and contentious, but if crack and heroin use do not fall below it, what does?

The advocates of legalization will respond by suggesting that my picture is overdrawn. Ethan Nadelmann of Princeton argues that the risk of legalization is less than most people suppose. Over 20 million Americans between the ages of 18 and 25 have tried cocaine (according to a government survey), but only a quarter million use it daily. From this Nadelmann concludes that at most 3 percent of all young people who try cocaine develop a problem with it. The implication is clear: Make the drug legal and we only have to worry about 3 percent of our youth.

The implication rests on a logical fallacy and a factual error. The fallacy is this: The percentage of occasional cocaine users who become binge users *when the drug is illegal* (and thus expensive and hard to find) tells us nothing about the percentage who will become dependent when the drug is legal (and thus cheap and abundant). Drs. Gawin and Ellinwood report, in common with several other researchers, that controlled or occasional use of cocaine changes to compulsive and frequent use "when access to the drug increases" or when the user switches from snorting to smoking. More cocaine more potently administered alters, perhaps sharply, the proportion of "controlled" users who become heavy users.

The factual error is this: The federal survey Nadelmann quotes was done in 1985, *before* crack had become common. Thus the probability of becoming dependent on cocaine was derived from the responses of users who snorted the drug. The speed and potency of cocaine's action increases dramatically when it is smoked. We do not yet know how greatly the advent of crack increases the risk of dependency, but all the clinical evidence suggests that the increase is likely to be large.

It is possible that some people will not become heavy users even when the drug is readily available in its most potent form. So far there are no scientific grounds for predicting who will and who will not become dependent. Neither socioeconomic background nor personality traits differentiate between casual and intensive users. Thus, the only way to settle the question of who is correct about the effect of easy availability on drug use, Nadelmann or Gawin and Ellinwood, is to try it and see. But that social experiment is so risky as to be no experiment at all, for if cocaine is legalized and if the rate of its abusive use increases dramatically, there is no way to put the genie back in the bottle, and it is not a kindly genie.

Have We Lost?

Many people who agree that there are risks in legalizing cocaine or heroin still favor it because, they think, we have lost the war on drugs. "Nothing we have done has worked" and the current federal policy is just "more of the same." Whatever the costs of greater drug use, surely they would be less than the costs of our present, failed efforts.

That is exactly what I was told in 1972—and heroin is not quite as bad a drug as cocaine. We did not surrender, and we did not lose. We did not win, either. What the nation accomplished then was what most efforts to save people from themselves accomplish: The problem was contained and the number of victims minimized, all at a considerable cost in law enforcement and increased crime. Was the cost worth it? I think so, but others may disagree. What are the lives of would-be addicts worth? I recall some people saying to me then, "Let them kill themselves." I was appalled. Happily, such views did not prevail.

Have we lost today? Not at all. High-rate cocaine use is not commonplace. The National Institute of Drug Abuse (NIDA) reports that less than 5 percent of high-school seniors used cocaine within the last 30 days. Of course this survey misses young people who have dropped out of school and miscounts those who lie on the questionnaire, but even if we inflate the NIDA estimate by some plausible percentage, it is still not much above 5 percent. Medical examiners reported in 1987 that about 1,500 died from cocaine use; hospital emergency rooms reported about 30,000 admissions related to cocaine abuse.

These are not small numbers, but neither are they evidence of a nationwide plague that threatens to engulf us all. Moreover, cities vary greatly in the proportion of people who are involved with cocaine. To get city-level data we need to turn to drug tests carried out on arrested persons, who obviously are more likely to be drug users than the average citizen. The National Institute of Justice, through its Drug Use Forecasting (DUF) project, collects urinalysis data on arrestees in 22 cities. As we have already seen, opiate (chiefly heroin) use has been flat or declining in most of these cities over the last decade. Cocaine use has gone up sharply, but with great variation among cities. New York, Philadelphia, and Washington, D.C., all report that two-thirds or more of their arrestees tested positive for cocaine, but in Portland, San Antonio, and Indianapolis the percentage was one-third or less.

In some neighborhoods, of course, matters have reached crisis proportions. Gangs control the streets, shootings terrorize residents, and drug-dealing occurs in plain view. The police seem barely able to contain matters. But in these neighborhoods—unlike at Palo Alto cocktail parties—the people are not calling for legalization, they are calling for help. And often not much help has come. Many cities are willing to do almost anything about the drug problem except spend more money on it. The federal government cannot change that; only local voters and politicians can. It is not clear that they will.

It took about 10 years to contain heroin. We have had experience with crack for only about 3 or 4 years. Each year we spend perhaps $11 billion on law enforcement (and some of that goes to deal with marijuana) and perhaps $2 billion on treatment.

Large sums, but not sums that should lead anyone to say, "We just can't afford this any more."

The illegality of drugs increases crime, partly because some users turn to crime to pay for their habits, partly because some users are stimulated by certain drugs (such as crack or PCP [phencyclidine]) to act more violently or ruthlessly than they otherwise would, and partly because criminal organizations seeking to control drug supplies use force to manage their markets. These also are serious costs, but no one knows how much they would be reduced if drugs were legalized. Addicts would no longer steal to pay black-market prices for drugs, a real gain. But some, perhaps a great deal, of that gain would be offset by the great increase in the number of addicts. These people, nodding on heroin or living in the delusion-ridden high of cocaine, would hardly be ideal employees. Many would steal simply to support themselves, since snatch-and-grab, opportunistic crime can be managed even by people unable to hold a regular job or plan an elaborate crime. Those British addicts who get their supplies from government clinics are not models of law-abiding decency. Most are in crime, and though their per-capita rate of criminality may be lower thanks to the cheapness of their drugs, the total volume of crime they produce may be quite large. Of course, society could decide to support all unemployable addicts on welfare, but that would mean that gains from lowered rates of crime would have to be offset by large increases in welfare budgets.

Proponents of legalization claim that the costs of having more addicts around would be largely if not entirely offset by having more money available with which to treat and care for them. The money would come from taxes levied on the sale of heroin and cocaine.

To obtain this fiscal dividend, however, legalization's supporters must first solve an economic dilemma. If they want to raise a lot of money to pay for welfare and treatment, the tax rate on the drugs will have to be quite high. Even if they themselves do not want a high rate, the politicians' love of "sin taxes" would probably guarantee that it would be high anyway. But the higher the tax, the higher the price of the drug, and the higher the price the greater the likelihood that addicts will turn to crime to find the money for it and that criminal organizations will be formed to sell tax-free drugs at below-market rates. If we managed to keep taxes (and thus prices) low, we would get that much less money to pay for welfare and treatment and more people could afford to become addicts. There may be an optimal tax rate for drugs that maximizes revenue while minimizing crime, bootlegging, and the recruitment of new addicts, but our experience with alcohol does not suggest that we know how to find it.

The Benefits of Illegality

The advocates of legalization find nothing to be said in favor of the current system except, possibly, that it keeps the number of addicts smaller than it would otherwise be. In fact, the benefits are more substantial than that.

First, treatment. All the talk about providing "treatment on demand" implies that there is a demand for treatment. That is not quite right. There are some drug-dependent people who genuinely want treatment and will remain in it if offered; they should receive it. But there are far more who want only short-term help after a bad crash; once stabilized and bathed, they are back on the street again, hustling. And even many of the addicts who enroll in a program honestly wanting help drop out after a short while when they discover that help takes time and commitment. Drug-dependent people have very short time horizons and a weak capacity for commitment. These two groups—those looking for a quick fix and those unable to stick with a long-term fix—are not easily helped. Even if we increase the number of treatment slots—as we should—we would have to do something to make treatment more effective.

One thing that can often make it more effective is compulsion. Douglas Anglin of UCLA [the University of California at Los Angeles], in common with many other researchers, has found that the longer one stays in a treatment program, the better the chances of a reduction in drug dependency. But he, again like most other researchers, has found that dropout rates are high. He has also found, however, that patients who enter treatment under legal compulsion stay in the program longer than those not subject to such pressure. His research on the California civil-commitment program, for example, found that heroin users involved with its required drug-testing program had over the long term a lower rate of heroin use than similar addicts who were free of such constraints. If for many addicts compulsion is a useful component of treatment, it is not clear how compulsion could be achieved in a society in which purchasing, possessing, and using the drug were legal. It could be managed, I suppose, but I would not want to have to answer the challenge from the American Civil Liberties Union that it is wrong to compel a person to undergo treatment for consuming a legal commodity.

Next, education. We are now investing substantially in drug-education programs in the schools. Though we do not yet know for certain what will work, there are some promising leads. But I wonder how credible such programs would be if they were aimed at dissuading children from doing something perfectly legal. We could, of course, treat drug education like smoking education: inhaling crack and inhaling tobacco are both legal, but you should not do it because it is bad for you. That tobacco is bad for you is easily shown; the surgeon general has seen to that. But what do we say about crack? It is pleasurable, but devoting yourself to so much pleasure is not a good idea (though perfectly legal)? Unlike tobacco, cocaine will not give you cancer or emphysema, but it will lead you to neglect your duties to family, job, and neighborhood? Everybody is doing cocaine, but you should not?

Again, it might be possible under a legalized regime to have effective drug-prevention programs, but their effectiveness would depend heavily, I think, on first having decided that cocaine use, like tobacco use, is purely a matter of practical consequences; no fundamental moral significance attaches to either. But if we believe— as I do—that dependency on certain mind-altering drugs *is* a moral issue and that their illegality rests in part on their immorality, then legalizing them undercuts, if it does not eliminate altogether, the moral message.

That message is at the root of the distinction we now make between nicotine and cocaine. Both are highly addictive; both have harmful physical effects. But we treat the two drugs differently, not simply because nicotine is so widely used as to be beyond the reach of effective prohibition, but because its use does not destroy the user's essential humanity. Tobacco shortens one's life, cocaine debases it. Nicotine alters one's habits, cocaine alters one's soul. The heavy use of crack, unlike the heavy use of tobacco, corrodes those natural sentiments of sympathy and duty that constitute our human nature and make possible our social life. To say, as does Nadelmann, that distinguishing morally between tobacco and cocaine is "little more than a transient prejudice" is close to saying that morality itself is but a prejudice.

The Alcohol Problem

Now we have arrived where many arguments about legalizing drugs begin: Is there any reason to treat heroin and cocaine differently from the way we treat alcohol?

There is no easy answer to that question because, as with so many human problems, one cannot decide simply on the basis either of moral principles or of individual consequences; one has to temper any policy by a common-sense judgment of what is possible. Alcohol, like heroin, cocaine, PCP, and marijuana, is a drug—that is, a mood-altering substance—and consumed to excess it certainly has harmful consequences: auto accidents, barroom fights, bedroom shootings. It is also, for some people, addictive. We cannot confidently compare the addictive powers of these drugs, but the best evidence suggests that crack and heroin are much more addictive than alcohol.

Many people, Nadelmann included, argue that since the health and financial costs of alcohol abuse are so much higher than those of cocaine or heroin abuse, it is hypocritical folly to devote our efforts to preventing cocaine or drug use. But as Mark Kleiman of Harvard has pointed out, this comparison is quite misleading. What Nadelmann is doing is showing that a *legalized* drug (alcohol) produces greater social harm than *illegal* ones (cocaine and heroin). But of course. Suppose that in the 1920s we had made heroin and cocaine legal and alcohol illegal. Can anyone doubt that Nadelmann would now be writing that it is folly to continue our ban on alcohol because cocaine and heroin are so much more harmful?

And let there be no doubt about it—widespread heroin and cocaine use are associated with all manner of ills. Thomas Bewley found that the mortality rate of British heroin addicts in 1968 was 28 times as high as the death rate of the same age group of nonaddicts, even though in England at the time an addict could obtain free or low-cost heroin and clean needles from British clinics. Perform the following mental experiment: Suppose we legalized heroin and cocaine in this country. In what proportion of auto fatalities would the state police report that the driver was nodding off on heroin or recklessly driving on a coke high? In what proportion of spouse-assault and child-abuse cases would the local police report that crack was involved? In what proportion of industrial accidents would safety investigators report that the forklift or drill-press operator was in a drug-induced stupor or frenzy? We do not know exactly what the proportion would be, but anyone who asserts that it would not be much higher than it is now would have to believe that these drugs have little appeal except when they are illegal. And that is nonsense.

An advocate of legalization might concede that social harm—perhaps harm equivalent to that already produced by alcohol—would follow from making cocaine and heroin generally available. But at least, he might add, we would have the problem "out in the open" where it could be treated as a matter of "public health." That is well and good, *if* we knew how to treat—that is, cure—heroin and cocaine abuse. But we do not know how to do it for all the people who would need such help. We are having only limited success in coping with chronic alcoholics. Addictive behavior is immensely difficult to change, and the best methods for changing it—living in drug-free therapeutic communities, becoming faithful members of Alcoholics Anonymous or Narcotics Anonymous—require great personal commitment, a quality that is, alas, in short supply among the very persons—young people, disadvantaged people—who are often most at risk for addiction.

Suppose that today we had, not 15 million alcohol abusers, but half a million. Suppose that we already knew what we have learned from our long experience with the widespread use of alcohol. Would we make whiskey legal? I do not know, but I suspect there would be a lively debate. The surgeon general would remind us of the risks alcohol poses to pregnant women. The National Highway Traffic Safety Administration would point to the likelihood of more highway fatalities caused by drunk drivers. The Food and Drug Administration might find that there is a nontrivial increase in cancer associated with alcohol consumption. At the same time the police would report great difficulty in keeping illegal whiskey out of our cities, officers being corrupted by bootleggers, and alcohol addicts often resorting to crime to feed their habit. Libertarians, for their part, would argue that every citizen has a right to drink anything he wishes and that drinking is, in any event, a "victimless crime."

However the debate might turn out, the central fact would be that the problem was still, at that point, a small one. The government cannot legislate away the addictive tendencies in all of us, nor can it remove completely even the most dangerous addictive substances. But it can cope with harms when the harms are still manageable.

Science and Addiction

One advantage of containing a problem while it is still containable is that it buys time for science to learn more about it and perhaps to discover a cure. Almost unnoticed in the current debate over legalizing drugs is that basic science has made rapid strides in identifying the underlying neurological processes involved in some forms of addiction. Stimulants such as cocaine and amphetamines alter the way certain brain cells communicate with one another. That alteration is complex and not entirely understood, but in simplified form it involves modifying the way in which a neurotransmitter called dopamine sends signals from one cell to another.

When dopamine crosses the synapse between two cells, it is in effect carrying a message from the first cell to activate the second one. In certain parts of the brain that message is experienced as pleasure. After the message is delivered, the dopamine returns to the first cell. Cocaine apparently blocks this return, or "reuptake," so that the excited cell and others nearby continue to send pleasure messages. When the exaggerated high produced by cocaine-influenced dopamine finally ends, the brain cells may (in ways that are still a matter of dispute) suffer from an extreme lack of dopamine, thereby making the individual unable to experience any pleasure at all. This would explain why cocaine users often feel so depressed after enjoying the drug. Stimulants may also affect the way in which other neurotransmitters, such as serotonin and noradrenaline, operate.

Whatever the exact mechanism may be, once it is identified it becomes possible to use drugs to block either the effect of cocaine or its tendency to produce dependency. There have already been experiments using desipramine, imipramine, bromocriptine, carbamazepine, and other chemicals. There are some promising results.

Tragically, we spend very little on such research, and the agencies funding it have not in the past occupied very influential or visible posts in the federal bureaucracy. If there is one aspect of the "war on drugs" metaphor that I dislike, it is its tendency to focus attention almost exclusively on the troops in the trenches, whether engaged in enforcement or treatment, and away from the research-and-development efforts back on the home front where the war may ultimately be decided.

I believe that the prospects of scientists in controlling addiction will be strongly influenced by the size and character of the problem they face. If the problem is a few hundred thousand chronic, high-dose users of an illegal product, the chances of making a difference at a reasonable cost will be much greater than if the problem is a few million chronic users of legal substances. Once a drug is legal, not only will its use increase but many of those who then use it will prefer the drug to the treatment: They will want the pleasure, whatever the cost to themselves or their families, and they will resist—probably successfully—any effort to wean them away from experiencing the high that comes from inhaling a legal substance.

If I Am Wrong . . .

No one can know what our society would be like if we changed the law to make access to cocaine, heroin, and PCP easier. I believe, for reasons given, that the result would be a sharp increase in use, a more widespread degradation of the human personality, and a greater rate of accidents and violence.

I may be wrong. If I am, then we will needlessly have incurred heavy costs in law enforcement and some forms of criminality. But if I am right, and the legalizers prevail anyway, then we will have consigned millions of people, hundreds of thousands of infants, and hundreds of neighborhoods to a life of oblivion and disease. To the lives and families destroyed by alcohol we will have added countless more destroyed by cocaine, heroin, PCP, and whatever else a basement scientist can invent.

Human character is formed by society; indeed, human character is inconceivable without society, and good character is less likely in a bad society. Will we, in the name of an abstract doctrine of radical individualism, and with the false comfort of suspect predictions, decide to take the chance that somehow individual decency can survive amid a more general level of degradation?

I think not. The American people are too wise for that, whatever the academic essayists and cocktail-party pundits may say. But if Americans today are less wise than I suppose, then Americans at some future time will look back on us now and wonder, what kind of people were they that they could have done such a thing?

Further Reading

Bayer, Ronald, and James Colgrove, "Science, Politics, and Ideology in the Campaign Against Environmental Tobacco Smoke," *American Journal of Public Health* 92(6): June 2002, 949–954.

Buchanan, David R., *An Ethic for Health Promotion: Rethinking the Sources of Human Well-Being* (New York: Oxford University Press, 2000).

Crawford, Rob, "You Are Dangerous to Your Health: The Ideology and Politics of Victim Blaming," *International Journal of Health Services* 7(4): 1977, 663–680.

Dworkin, Gerald, "Voluntary Health Risks and Public Policy," *Hastings Center Report* 11(5): October 1981, 26–31.

Epstein, Richard A., "Let the Shoemaker Stick to His Last: A Defense of the 'Old' Public Health," *Perspectives in Biology and Medicine* 46(3) Suppl.: Summer 2003, S138–S159.

Gostin, Lawrence O., and M. Gregg Bloche, "The Politics of Public Health: A Reply to Richard Epstein," *Perspectives in Biology and Medicine* 46(3) Suppl.: Summer 2003, S160–S175.

Satel, Sally L., *PC, M.D.: How Political Correctness Is Corrupting Medicine* (New York: Basic Books, 2000).

Weale, Albert, "Invisible Hand or Fatherly Hand? Problems of Paternalism in the New Perspective on Health," *Journal of Public Health Politics, Policy & Law* 7(4): Winter 1983, 784–807.

PART III

JUSTICE AND HEALTH

Introduction

Insofar as public health deals with questions of justice, it deals with the question of what people ought to have as a matter of fairness, necessity, and human rights. When public health addresses questions of social stratification and the inequalities of power and wealth in a given society, there, too, issues of justice pertain. Finally, ethical questions of justice are central to the design and workings of various institutions and programs (whether involving service delivery, education, or access to resources), and these are often the key objectives of policy analysis and implementation in public health.

Inequality in patterns of morbidity and mortality are clearly tied, although for reasons not yet fully understood, to inequalities in other dimensions of human social life. One of the central tenets and findings of epidemiological research during the past 200 years has been the discovery of the so-called social gradient, which refers to the fact that inequalities of wealth, power, and social status correspond to inequalities of health, illness, and risk. This pattern is remarkably robust and resilient across societies and across time: In virtually any society at any time, those who are rich and powerful will also be healthier than those who are not. Of course, the compromised health status of the poor may be due to their exposure to pollution, lack of sanitation, poor diet, and the like. At yet, the social gradient of inequality seems to go beyond economic inequality and to be related as well to hierarchical social relations of many kinds; in other words, health disparities are also connected with inequalities of power and status.

The first selection of part III, by Angus Deaton, examines the gradient of health and wealth. The selection from Richard G. Wilkinson carries the discussion further, providing a brief overview of recent research and debates concerning the social determinants of health and the policy significance of the social gradient. Deaton urges caution in drawing conclusions from these findings; Wilkinson offers a provocative interpretation of some of the implications that the perspective of the new public health has to offer and the potentially radical political consequences to taking this perspective seriously. To be sure, the epidemiological jury is still out on a number of these suggestive findings and on the most appropriate interpretation of data.

An even more explicit exploration of the ethical perspective and implications of public health perspectives on health disparities is provided in the selection by a team of noted philosophers and public health researchers, Norman Daniels, Bruce P. Kennedy, and Ichiro Kawachi. Their work, which has been the subject of sharp criticism, is the most explicit attempt to put together the philosophical question of what pattern of health status would fit the requirements of justice with the policy question of how complex types of inequality—economic, social-cultural, and political—can be mitigated if not overcome. Daniels was trying to enlist the moral and intellectual force of careful thinking about the requirements of justice in the cause of universal health insurance and access to acute care a decade ago; today he and his collaborators are bringing careful arguments to bear against even bigger game: health status and outcomes (not just access to the means to health) themselves.

But thinking about the ethical challenges of access to care still remains important. The American health care system is by far the wealthiest, most expensive, most resource intensive, and—after many failed attempts to achieve universal access—the most willfully inegalitarian health care system in the democratic world. How might various conceptions of social and distributive justice shed light on this issue?

Almost 30 years ago, the President's Commission on Ethical Issues in Medicine and in Biomedical and Behavioral Science issued a stinging indictment of the inequality and the injustice of the American health care system entitled *Securing Access to Health Care* (1983). At that time, the largely private, employer-based health insurance system left nearly 30 million working Americans and their families without adequate coverage for all or part of the year. At the same time, health care costs consumed around 8 percent of the country's gross domestic product (GDP; the total value of all the goods and services produced in the United States in a given year). Today, the figure is closer to 48 million uninsured and 15 percent of GDP. After a brief hiatus when the rate of annual increase slowed, the cost of health care is again increasing at a rate of over 10 percent per year.

Two decades earlier, the architects of Medicare and Medicaid (health insurance coverage for the elderly and the very poor) during the Great Society period of the 1960s had thought that their programs would quickly pave the way to universal health insurance, and in this respect the United States would join all the other developed nations in the world. That did not occur.

In the early 1990s, the Clinton administration offered the most sweeping and ambitious health reform effort in American history. That plan would have provided both universal health insurance coverage for at least a basic level of services and would have, through government regulation and market competition, tried to stem the rising tide of health care costs. In the end, the Clinton plan failed. It was widely attacked for its complexity and cost.

We have now had a decade or more of the American experiment of private, largely for-profit managed care. Like a message that bears endless repetition, in 2004 the Institute of Medicine issued the latest comprehensive study of access to acute care and to health insurance coverage. In that report, this troubling story is brought up to date, and we find evidence of a situation grown markedly worse, not better, over the years.

In the final section of this chapter, Bruce Jennings, writing at a time in the early 1990s when the best prospects for health policy reform seemed to be coming from the top down, addresses the question of how democratic values and processes can inform health policy reform. Implicit in his argument is the suspicion that health reform ethics and health reform politics have been on a collision course for many years, and that part the failure of the Clinton plan was its reliance on the expertise, both ethical and practical, of intellectual elites. Their recommendations did not enjoy the support that might have emerged from deliberations and experiences of ordinary citizens at the grassroots level. The problem was at least partly due to the failure to provide the necessary time and space for such deliberation to work through the ethical aspects of health policy reform. The false and incendiary rhetoric of attack advertisements was substituted for such engagement and deliberation. Ordinary citizens became (increasingly restless and dissatisfied) spectators on the sidelines of a power struggle between wealthy and entrenched special interest groups.

What, Jennings asks, would happen if we experimented with a more robust and concerted effort at bringing democratic deliberation to bear on issues of justice, equality, and health policy reform? Would the well-off find reason to identify and connect their own interests with the interests of the excluded and the underserved? Would they find a universal system more threatening than the current arrangements simply because government would play a larger role than before in the health insurance field? Would democratic deliberation ultimately take up those multiple social, political, and environmental determinants of health status that public health so assiduously studies but that, until now, have had but little traction in health policy circles? Might such a conversation ultimately confront the core question about how to make individuals healthier by making the communities in which they live healthier?

11

Policy Implications of the Gradient of Health and Wealth

Angus Deaton

Poorer people die younger and are sicker than richer people; indeed, mortality and morbidity rates are inversely related to many correlates of socioeconomic status such as income, wealth, education, or social class. That economic deprivation is strongly related to ill health was perhaps first scientifically documented by René Villermé, who compared mortality rates and poverty across the arrondissements of Paris in the 1820s, although references to the relationship can be found in ancient Greek and Chinese texts.[1] A gradient of health with social class (defined through occupation) has been documented in the United Kingdom since the first census in 1851. In the United States, the landmark study by Evelyn Kitagawa and Philip Hauser merged census and death records to document the relationship between mortality on the one hand and education, income, occupation, race, and place of residence on the other.[2] The gradient persists in recent data. The National Longitudinal Mortality Study (NLMS) merged data from death records with responses from household surveys around 1980. People whose reported family incomes in 1980 were less than $5,000 in 1980 prices are estimated to have a life expectancy around 25 percent lower than those whose family incomes were above $50,000.[3]

What Is the Gradient?

The relationship between health and income is referred to as a "gradient" to emphasize the gradual relationship between the two; health improves with income throughout the income distribution, and poverty has more than a "threshold" effect on health. In the NLMS data the proportional relationship between income and mortality is the same at all income levels, which implies that the absolute reduction in mortality for each dollar of income is much larger at the bottom of the income distribution than at the top. The gradient is often assessed in terms of other variables; mortality declines with wealth, with rank, and with social status. One of the most famous of the current studies links ill health and mortality to occupational grade among Whitehall civil servants (in the United Kingdom); that none of them are poor further illustrates that the gradient is more than an effect of poverty.[4]

Nonincome Differences in Health

There are also marked differences in life expectancy by race and by geography. In the United States there is a 20-year gap in life expectancy between white men in the healthiest counties and black men in the unhealthiest counties.[5] These nonincome differences in health are frequently referred to, alongside differences by income group or social class, as "inequalities in health." Indeed, the most frequently cited correlate of mortality is simply "socioeconomic status" (SES). While this term is sometimes convenient, it is unhelpful for policy discussions. Quite different policies are called for to deal with health in relation to income, education, or social class.

Addressing Health Inequalities

Many people find it unjust that people should not only be unequal in the amount of goods and services they receive but also in the length and quality of their lives. They believe that addressing these income-related inequalities in health is an urgent task of health policy. The current British government sees the reduction of health inequalities as its primary health-related goal. Other commentators go further and see the economic and social structure of society—especially low income, income inequality, discrimination, and social exclusion—as the ultimate determinants, the "causes of causes," of disease and death. From this perspective, a thoroughgoing redistribution of income and wealth is the key to improving population health. Focusing on "downstream" causes such as the control of health-related behavior or health delivery systems is likely to be futile if the "upstream" causes in the underlying socioeconomic structure remain unreformed. Britain's Acheson report on health inequalities, commissioned by the first Blair government, is the leading example of a set of redistributive policy prescriptions for addressing health inequalities through primarily "upstream" policies.[6] It subsequently formed the basis for a set of government proposals, including general income-support policies such as family and child tax credits, and increases in the minimum wage, which are justified on health grounds.

In this paper I review some of the evidence on the gradient, as well as its theoretical interpretations, and ask whether it makes sense to design policy to address health inequalities. I am particularly concerned with whether redistributing income will improve population health, something that is frequently taken as obvious in the public health literature. In the final section, which discusses policy prescriptions, I argue that the evidence on the gradient strengthens the case for redistribution toward the poor. When low income and poor health go together, the poor are doubly deprived and thus have a greater claim on our attention than is warranted from their incomes alone. But I also argue that the reduction of the gradient, or of health inequalities more generally, is an inappropriate target for health policy.

What Causes the Gradient If Not Income?

Policy cannot be intelligently conducted without an understanding of mechanisms; correlations are not enough. Income might cause health, health might cause income, or both might be correlated with other factors; indeed, all three possibilities might be operating simultaneously. The relative importance of each story is almost certainly different at different times, for different causes of illness, and at different points in life. Unfortunately, there is no general agreement about causes. Worse still, what apparent agreement there is is sometimes better supported by repeated assertion than by solid evidence. I begin with a brief discussion of the most important mechanisms other than a direct causal effect of income on health: two-way causality between health and income, differential access to health care, and health-related behavior. The argument here is that the three nonincome stories, although important, do not provide a complete explanation of the gradient.

Effects of Health on Income

Part of the gradient comes from the effects of health on income. The main mechanism works through the ability to work and its effects on earnings; the effect of health on wealth through out-of-pocket costs of medical care is important for some people but is of relatively small importance overall.[7] If the effect of health on earnings were the major part of the story, the appropriate policy would be to address health directly using health-specific interventions. In addition, when calculating the returns to such interventions, we should also allow for the additional benefits on productivity. It is unfortunate and divisive that much of the public health literature on the gradient takes the position that the effects of health on socioeconomic status—known in this literature as reverse causality, "selection," or "drift"—are negligible. Yet economists and others have documented the effects of health on earnings in many contexts, perhaps most notably as a proximate cause of retirement.[8] Indeed, the relationship between income and health is much muted among retirees, among whom the effect of health on earnings has been removed. As recognized by insurance programs around the world, disability is a major cause of low income and poverty.

Some of the interactions between health and economic success operate over very long periods. Mother's cigarette smoking during pregnancy predicts teenage educational achievements; height at age 7 predicts subsequent unemployment; ill health, even poor prenatal nutrition, decreases the probability of ever being married, itself an aspect of socioeconomic status that is associated with good health; and prenatal nutrition affects cardiovascular disease and type 2 diabetes in late middle age, exactly the sort of conditions that predict early retirement.[9]

Effects of Income on Health

That there are influences from health to wealth does not deny the reverse. The risk of becoming disabled is much higher among people who are poorer, less educated, and of lower social status. The illnesses that provoke early retirement are less likely among the rich and well educated, and the nutrition and risk behavior of pregnant women is conditioned by their socioeconomic status. One of the clearest messages from the literature is that health and wealth are mutually determined.

That the effects of health on earnings and education do not account for all of the gradient is supported by direct evidence from both human and animal studies that the manipulation of socioeconomic status affects disease. In addition, there is a series of nonexperimental long-term longitudinal studies, especially those from the British birth cohorts, in which the sequence of health and economic events can be studied, as well as the longitudinal evidence in the two Whitehall studies.[10]

Several studies find that socioeconomic status predicts health and mortality, not only contemporaneously, but many years after status is measured. The contemporaneous cross-sectional correlation is magnified by the low earnings of those who are sick or about to die, and this source of correlation is reduced by waiting until those people either recover or die. Using the NLMS data, and controlling for years of schooling, doubling income reduced the probability of death by 27 percent during the first year of follow-up for those ages 25–59; the comparable effects for mortality in years 1–2, 2–5, and 5–9 after follow-up are 25 percent, 23 percent, and 17 percent, respectively.[11] While such calculations do nothing to remove the long-standing effects of health on earnings—for example, from damage in early childhood—the fact that the predictive effect of income is reduced by so little testifies to the importance either of very long-standing effects or of a causal influence running from income to mortality.

The Access Argument

If better-educated, richer, or lighter-skinned people have better access to health care, and if health care has a major effect on mortality and morbidity, then education, wealth, or race will predict health outcomes. If access to care is the major cause of the gradient, the appropriate policy is to address the structure of the health care industry, including not only the provision of insurance but also the ways in which different groups of people are treated differently within the system. Once again, much of the public health literature tends to take a strong negative view of this argument, although there is an active and contested literature in the United States on racial discrimination in treatment.

Much of the public health literature on the gradient is deeply skeptical of the value of medical care, a view that traces back to Thomas McKeown's work on the determinants of mortality in nineteenth- and early twentieth-century Britain.[12] McKeown, whose work has been an important theme underlying much of the modern work on health inequalities, found that the decline of each of the major causes of death preceded the discovery of an effective preventive measure. He also argued (although on much weaker grounds) that the "sanitary" revolution in public health had little effect and, largely by elimination rather than any positive evidence, concluded that rising living standards, especially better nutrition and housing, were primarily responsible for improvement in life expectancy. Based on direct arguments about the availability of food, Robert Fogel has made complementary arguments about the primacy of nutrition in the process of economic development and growth.[13] So, if medical care has little effect on mortality—although perhaps more on morbidity—then differences in health cannot be explained by differences in access to it.

Even among those who accept a more positive role for health services and technologies, there is a good deal of skepticism about the role of health care in explaining the gradient. If medical care does play an important role in driving the increase in life expectancy over time, it is possible that important new technologies are quickly disseminated through the health care system without ever generating a gradient. Moreover, the gradient exists, and takes much the same form, in countries with and without health care that is free at the point of service. Indeed, the failure of the mortality gradient to vanish after the introduction of Britain's National Health Service was an important stimulus to the recent literature.

Effect of Life-Saving Technology

Yet none of these arguments is entirely convincing. It is easy to imagine that the same health care system, whether public or private, could provide very different care for patients whose educational background enables them to "work the system," by calling on highly placed friends in the profession or by being both more compliant and more questioning patients. (It should be noted, however, that Whitehall II found a gradient in cardiovascular disease prior to hospitalization.) Furthermore, the gradient is steeper and the correlation stronger for cardiovascular disease than for cancer. For example, the Whitehall studies show little gradient in cancer other than in lung cancer, which is entirely attributable to differential smoking behavior across the occupational grades. There is also a marked similarity between the pattern in the gradients, substantial for heart disease and negligible for cancer, and the pattern in technical progress, with substantial gains in technique and associated lives saved since about 1970 in the treatment of heart disease and none at all in cancer. We know from previous work that new techniques and knowledge can generate a gradient, even when none previously existed. So while the public health literature contains sound arguments that differential access to medical care is not the root of the gradient, the literature probably assigns too little weight to the effectiveness of medical care itself and, beyond that, to the possibility that widening gradients are related to life-saving bursts of technical progress.

Role of Health-Related Behavior

Health-related behavior involving the use of tobacco, alcohol, and drugs; obesity; and sex play an important part in determining the gradient. Poor people who are ill find it more difficult to conform to complicated and time-intensive treatment regimens, such as for diabetes, HIV, or multidrug-resistant tuberculosis.[14] Harmful behavior of this kind is negatively associated with income and education, at least in rich countries, and so helps to induce and maintain the gradient. However, such behavior explains only a part of the relationship and, to the extent that it does, it does not necessarily follow that the policy implication is to alter the behavior, rather than to focus on income, wealth, or education, or even on remedial health care.

The Whitehall studies again provide good evidence that the gradient persists when health-related behavior is controlled for. The gradient in cardiovascular disease across five Whitehall ranks is reduced from fivefold to fourfold if the calculations are confined to nonsmokers.[15] Controls for a wide range of risk factors, observed by physician examination, explain only a small fraction of the relationship between rank and health. More generally, if somewhat less convincingly, if we multiply the effect of smoking on the risk of death by the effect of income on the risk of smoking, the result is too small to explain the direct effect of income on the risk of death.

However, all of this health-related behavior is subject to measurement problems in self-reported survey data. Given our ignorance of the biological mechanisms, these are not resolved by clinical measurement of risk factors, which, although accurate in themselves, do not deliver precise estimates of the true underlying risk. The measurement error will generally bias downward the estimates of the effects of behavior on health and, in the current context, understate the contribution of the behaviors to the gradient.[16] That said, there also may be biases in the other direction—for example, if better-off people overreport the healthy behavior that is expected of them, or if the biological effects of risky behavior interact with income or social status.

Even so, if there were less risky behavior, the population would be healthier, and, given the distribution of the behavior by socioeconomic status, inequalities in health would be less. Yet arguments for not thinking about behavior as a fundamental cause of health inequalities exist in two very different literatures. In sociology and public health, especially among those taking the view that health is socially produced, it is argued that risky behavior is only a proximate cause of poor health and is itself a consequence of low income, education, powerlessness, discrimination, and social exclusion.[17] Directing policy toward behavior will only change the behavior without changing the fact that the poor are less healthy than the rich. Some evidence for these claims comes from historical changes in the patterns of disease. Heart disease and lung cancer used to be diseases of the rich but are now diseases of the poor. More recently, HIV infection in wealthy countries has moved from being a disease of the rich to a disease of the poor and is moving in a similar direction in poor countries. The gradient across social classes in Britain in 1851 was markedly similar to that of a century and a half later, in spite of dramatic changes in the pattern of disease, so that even if policy is effective against particular diseases, it may have little effect on the gradient.

Another argument against focusing on risky behavior comes from the economics literature, which emphasizes that given the constraints that poor people face, in terms of both money and time, risky behavior may be neither irresponsible nor irrational. Relative to everyone else, poor people have little human (educational) or financial capital and relatively more health capital, if only because everyone is born with one body and a single life to lead, and not everyone gets an inheritance or a fine education. While better-off people use their wealth and education as sources of income and consumption, poor people must make relatively heavy use of their bodies for both production and consumption, working in manual occupations and taking what pleasures they can in cheap but health-compromising activities, of which cigarette smoking is perhaps the leading example.[18]

A Direct Link from Income to Health?

Suppose, finally, that there is a direct causal link to health from some aspect or correlate of socioeconomic status. There is good evidence that this is part of the story. In poor countries, income provides nutrition, housing, clean water, and sanitation and thus protects both adults and children from hunger and infectious disease. Although once again the causality runs in both directions, the nutrition from additional income will have little effect on nutritional status in the presence of disease, and susceptibility to disease is higher among those with poor nutritional status.[19] In rich countries, where chronic disease has largely replaced infectious disease as the main cause of morbidity and mortality, similar effects exist, albeit through different biological mechanisms. It has long been argued that stress increases susceptibility to disease, and a great deal of modern work has been directed at establishing the pathways through which repeated exposure to stress compromises the immune system.[20] Laboratory work with animals allows the experimental manipulation of health or status or both, and such experiments show how social rank within a monkey group acts to differentially protect individuals against experimentally induced infection. When the same monkey experiences a different rank, when the monkey groups are shuffled, the monkey's rank, not its identity, predicts the protection it receives; these experiments have been partially replicated among humans.[21]

So we have a correlation between socioeconomic status and health and evidence that the correlation is causal, at least in part. We have come a long way toward the "upstream" policy stance of (for example) the Acheson report, that population health is best addressed by income-support schemes for the poor, supported (presumably, although the sources of finance are never clearly stated) by increased taxation of the better-off. But the connection is much less clear than may at first appear. In particular, it depends on what we mean by "socioeconomic status," a term that is convenient as a shorthand for a wide range of possibilities, including income, education, rank, or social class, but that is useless for thinking about policy in the absence of an instrument that acts on them all. Redistribution of income will be effective only if health is determined by income or by something determined by income. Whether or not this is true is something on which the evidence is decidedly mixed.

Importance of Education

One line of thought is that education, not income, matters for health, so that the correlation with income is induced by the effects of education on income. In many economic models of health, education is seen as enhancing a person's efficiency as a producer of health—a suggestive phrase, but not one that is very explicit about the mechanisms involved.[22] The empirical evidence shows that education is protective of health; evidence from a range of rich countries shows that an additional year of education reduces mortality rates (at all ages) by around 8 percent.[23] Since a year of education also increases earnings by about 8 percent on average, and since income reduces mortality independently of education in the NLMS, education reduces mortality twice over, once directly and once through additional earnings.[24]

It is possible that education is standing as a proxy for something else: In particular, people who are more patient, more forward looking, and have more ability to delay gratification, are likely to be both better educated and healthier, even if the education itself plays no direct role, and there is some evidence for this position.[25] Yet there is also evidence that education is directly protective; those who were forced to go to school by U.S. schooling laws in the early twentieth century lived longer than those who did not receive the additional schooling.[26] One obvious possibility is that educated people have more information about health, and this is almost certainly the case during some episodes, such as immediately after the U.S. surgeon general's report on smoking. But the news percolated to everyone over time, and yet the negative correlation between education and smoking remains. Indeed, survey evidence frequently shows that less-educated people understand the dangers, and that the effects of education on smoking remain after controlling for that knowledge.[27]

Income versus Education

It remains controversial whether income is protective of health over and above the effects of education. The best evidence in the United States again comes from the NLMS, where both income and education are separately protective. Yet there are studies in which income drives out education and studies in which education drives out income. Yet again, studies that work with aggregate data, either over time or at the state or city level, find no effect or even find a perverse effect of aggregate income on aggregate health. Over time, in the United States and Britain, there is no stable relationship between the growth of income and the decline in mortality rates. Indeed, the productivity slowdown in the United States after 1972 and the associated slowing in the rate of growth of real family incomes coincide with an acceleration in decline of mortality rates for all but young adults. Although Britain's pattern of income growth differs from that of the United States, the two countries' age-specific mortality patterns from 1950 to 2000 are similar. These patterns can readily be explained by technological changes, particularly in the treatment of heart disease and low birth weight infants, but not at all by patterns of income growth.[28]

Theory of Relativity

This conflict between the individual-level and aggregate studies remains unresolved, but it is consistent with the view that it is not income itself that matters, but relative income, or rank. Indeed, the animal experiments do not involve income, but social status or rank relative to those of others in the relevant reference group. Raising income is not the same thing as raising relative income or rank, although raising any one person's income might be so. For example, suppose that the government, in an attempt to improve public health according to Acheson, increases the marginal rate of tax on everyone and uses the proceeds to pay everyone a fixed monthly benefit. Because the poor have low incomes, they pay little tax, and because everyone gets the same benefit, such a scheme redistributes income from the rich to the poor. But it is clear that the scheme has no effect on anyone's rank in the income distribution. Although income is more equally distributed than before, the poorest person is still the poorest, the second poorest the second poorest, and so on. This is not just hypothetical; rank is more likely than income to be the determinant of the "sense of control" that is a crucial predictor in the Whitehall studies, and rank is likely to be the aspect of income that is protective if what is harmful to health is the psychosocial stress associated with low status.[29]

Yet the matter is far from closed. Absolute income, not rank, is important for buying things that matter for health, such as health care or nutrition, and for relieving the stress that comes from the struggle to make ends meet. Also, those who argue for the importance of relative income or rank need to explain why people who find their low rank oppressive do not move on to some other group where they can do better.

Redistributing the Wealth

Suppose then that it is indeed income or wealth that matters. In this spirit, Vicente Navarro has recently argued that "the intervention that would add the most years of life to the population of Spain or the United States (or for that matter any other country) would be one that would lead to all social classes having the same mortality as those at the top. From this premise we can deduce that the most effective means of reducing mortality would be to eliminate social inequalities by redistribution of wealth."[30] It is important to understand that the second sentence does not follow from the first. Redistribution of wealth increases the wealth of the poor but reduces the wealth of the rich so that if, as is often argued, the gradient is much the same among the rich as among the poor, the loss of health among the rich must be offset against the gains among the poor. If income is what matters for health, then its redistribution will only improve population health if additional income has a lesser effect on health among the rich than among the poor. While this proposition is plausible and is supported by evidence from the NLMS, it is far from being established. But even more is needed. As economists like to point out, redistribution through the tax system typically means that the rich lose more than $1 for each dollar redistributed to the poor. This effect, known as "deadweight loss," further raises the bar for any policy of improving population health through income redistribution.

Another important plank in the platform for redistribution comes from the argument that at least in rich countries it is not income that affects health, but income inequality.[31] In this context, income inequality means not differences in income across people, as when we think of income inequalities as a cause of health inequalities, but income inequality as a measure of the dispersion of income, measured so as to be unaffected by average income. The argument is that high levels of income inequality are associated with low levels of social support and cohesion and so sicken everyone, rich and poor alike. If so, income redistribution toward the poor, which narrows income inequality, will have a direct positive affect on population health. The hypothesis was originally supported by comparisons of life expectancy and inequality across wealthy countries and more recently by comparisons of mortality and income inequality across U.S. states and cities. However, the best recent data support none of the original international correlations, and the U.S. evidence is spurious: There is no relationship between income inequality and mortality once we control for the racial composition of American states and cities.[32] More generally, inequality almost certainly affects health, but income inequality is not the key.

Should Economic Policy Be Health Policy?

Should the United States follow Britain in deemphasizing health care or health insurance as the primary determinant of health and focusing more on the roles of poverty and education? Is it good health policy to raise the incomes of the poor? Is the current British focus on health inequalities well founded?

To answer these questions coherently, I need a framework for thinking about what is desirable. I have found it consistently helpful to think in terms of individual well-being within a broad, equity-preferring social objective, but also to follow Amartya Sen in noting that this welfarist approach by itself is insufficient and that we need to respect other considerations, one of which is process in access to health care.[33] Just what this means is best illustrated by applying the framework to the policy implications of the gradient.

Components of Individual Welfare

Perhaps the most important point is that individual welfare is neither health nor wealth but depends upon both. The gradient means that people who are deprived in terms of income and wealth are also deprived in terms of morbidity and mortality. If the urgency of redistribution depends on the degree of deprivation of the poor, as it surely must, the gradient strengthens the case for redistribution. When thinking about such redistribution, we need to think about improving well-being at the bottom, not just about improving health or income. While improvements in either are clearly a good thing, we must be careful about not improving health at the expense of income or improving income at the expense of health. A policy that does not involve any such conflict is one that improves the quality or quantity of education. More and better education improves both earnings and health, making it doubly attractive.

Pareto Criterion

A second important issue is respect for the Pareto criterion: that a policy that harms no one while making at least some people better off is a good thing. Although such an argument seems obvious, it is often denied in the public health and epidemiological literatures, and it sharply divides economists from other writers on health inequalities.

Consider a technical innovation—for example, a new life-saving procedure or new health-related knowledge. Coronary artery bypass grafts or neonatal intensive care units are good examples of the former; for the latter, think of the surgeon general's report on smoking in 1964 or the application at the turn of the twentieth century of the germ theory of disease to personal and medical hygiene. Better-educated people will be quicker to adopt or benefit from the innovation; if the innovation is not immediately available to everyone, money might help, too. Because the innovations are beneficial to health, some people's health is improved, and other people's health stays the same or is improved less. Because of the role of education and income, the gradient steepens; the health of the rich and well educated improves more.

The Pareto criterion says that such innovations are beneficial and are to be encouraged. To many in the public health community, this is the wrong answer; inequalities are inherently bad, and innovations that increase them are to be discouraged. Policies based on such arguments are misconceived; they result in some people dying who could have lived, without preventing any other deaths. They also abort the start of what is often a diffusion of knowledge or technology that in most cases (hygiene if not smoking) will benefit poorer people, too, albeit with some delay. Apart from the possible exception of sulfa drugs and antibiotics, whose introduction benefited the health of blacks more than that of whites in the United States, most innovations do appear to initially favor the better-off, so that a concern with preventing health inequalities is likely to be a real barrier to life-saving innovation.[34]

Pros and Cons of Targeting the Poor

What about a more general policy that targets those whose low income, poor education, or social standing makes them more prone to disease? Such a policy is to be welcomed to the extent that it improves the lot of those suffering the greatest burdens of income and health deprivation. But it is not clear that such policies are likely to be effective. Most of the variation in health is within social groups, not between them, so that targeting according to position on the gradient is unlikely to be an effective way of reaching people in need of care compared with simply treating people who are sick or at the high risk of being so. Also, for some groups, notably the elderly, the gradient is relatively weak and offers little power as a diagnostic aid.

Targeting Specific Diseases and Groups

We must also take care not to violate the process whereby people who are sick gain access to health care. Current British discussions on such policies provide disconcerting examples. It is hard to see why it is desirable to focus antismoking campaigns on manual workers or to focus on the mortality of infants of mothers whose spouses are manual workers, as opposed to single mothers, whose infants are much more likely to die but whose social class cannot be established because they do not have husbands (whose occupation would define their social class).[35] We should not deny people care because their social status is too high, any more than we should deny them care because their status is too low. More generally, it makes no sense to focus on a particular disease only because its prevalence is higher among the poor or among "those suffering inequalities," although there may well be diseases that are readily controlled and that fall most heavily on the poor. One of the most obvious and largest health inequalities is the longer life expectancy of women, yet it is hard to imagine public policy assigning priority in treatment to men.[36]

Targeting the Gradient Itself

If targeting the health of particular social groups has its problems, targeting the gradient itself is even less appropriate. Recent data from Britain show that the difference in life expectancy between the top and bottom social classes has increased from 5 to 9 years, and to many this statistic calls for a policy response.[37] Not necessarily. The appropriate response, if one is called for at all, depends on whether such a policy would actually improve the lot of the most disadvantaged, whose life expectancy has also been increasing, albeit not as rapidly as that of the most privileged. As I have already argued, the gradient is in part driven by rapid technical progress in health knowledge, something that is good, not bad. An increase in the quality of education, for example, by improving teacher skills or providing more resources to schools, will benefit more those who have many years of schooling: those with higher incomes and better health. Once again, something that is clearly desirable will increase the gradient.

Nor do we have measures of the gradient or its rate of change that are adequate to support such policies. The gradient is usually measured by ratios of mortality rates for different groups. Yet it is far from clear why the ratio of mortality rates is a better measure of inequality than the ratio of survival rates; inequality can be measured for the living just as well as for the dead. It is quite possible, and indeed likely at current mortality rates, for the mortality measure to show a widening of inequalities while the survival measure is simultaneously narrowing.[38] Without an overall framework for judging improvements in well-being, the choice of measure of the steepness of the gradient is arbitrary, and the policy implications of targeting it are obscure.

Directing Policy at Both Wealth and Health

I come finally to perhaps the most important point, which is the need to frame policy in the light of wealth and health simultaneously. There is great danger from those who emphasize health without adequate attention to other aspects of well-being. One example is the current debate over smoking, something that is often seen as a "health inequalities" issue because smoking rates are higher among the poor and less-educated. Policies that rely on increases in taxation or prices to pay for settlements that ostensibly punish tobacco companies transfer income from those who continue to smoke to people who are more advantaged. Some people smoke because it is good for them in a broad sense, if not for their health, so that policies that raise the price of cigarettes, often justified in terms of improving the health of the poor, actually make them worse off to the benefit of those who would otherwise pay higher property and income taxes. The appropriate policy is to relax the constraints on poor people by tackling low incomes and poor education. Health is an important component of well-being, but it is not the only component.

Another important case is the trade-off between income and health for the elderly. Victor Fuchs has recently emphasized that expansions of Medicare coverage, for example, to cover a wider range of pharmaceuticals, will be paid for, at least in part, by reductions in Social Security. As a result, at least some older people will find themselves health-rich but wealth-poor, entitled to expensive medical care but unable to afford everyday necessities that they might value as or more highly.[39]

It is not hard to imagine a policy in which health innovations, such as the availability of new procedures or new drugs on Medicare or Medicaid, would be vetted by a panel that examined the likely consequences. While it would be clearly an excellent idea for such a panel to consider whether such innovations were likely to improve the overall well-being of recipients, taking both health and other income into account, it would be an equally poor idea for it to turn back any innovation on the grounds that it would widen health inequalities. Policy should be concerned with well-being, not with health or income alone.

Need for More General Health Policies

What about more general health policies that refocus attention away from health care and health-related behavior and toward education and income? This seems a much easier case to make, and it is hard not to believe that the current U.S. system pays too much attention to health care delivery and to drugs and too little to the effects on health of the "upstream" social and economic arrangements. The case for education is surely stronger than that for income, at least in the United States, and it is time that the educational debate was more cognizant of health benefits. As for income, there is a very strong case in poor countries and among the poor in rich countries, for whom nutrition, nutrition-linked disease, and poor housing are important determinants of adult and child health. These factors are directly affected by income, and a policy of income provision to the poor may well be more effective than spending the same amount of public funds on a weak health care delivery system.[40]

This paper was presented 4 October 2001 at the conference, "Nonmedical Determinants of Health," sponsored by Princeton University's Center for Health and Well-being. The author thanks Anne Case, Victor Fuchs, Jon Gruber, Sandy Jencks, Adriana Lleras-Muney, Michael Marmot, David Mechanic, Jon Skinner, Jim Smith, and three anonymous referees for comments and suggestions. He is grateful for financial support from the John D. and Catherine T. MacArthur Foundation and the National Institute of Aging through the National Bureau of Economic Research. He also appreciates the support of the Woodrow Wilson School, Center for Health and Wellbeing, at Princeton.

Notes

1. R. Porter, *The Greatest Benefit to Mankind: A Medical History of Humanity* (New York: Norton, 1997); and N. Krieger, "Theories for Social Epidemiology in the Twenty-first Century: An Ecosocial Perspective," *International Journal of Epidemiology* 30, no. 4 (August 2001): 668–677.

2. E. M. Kitagawa and P. M. Hauser, *Differential Mortality in the United States: A Study in Socio-Economic Epidemiology* (Cambridge, MA: Harvard University Press, 1973).

3. E. Rogot et al., eds., *A Mortality Study of 1.3 Million Persons by Demographic, Social, and Economic Factors: 1979–1985 Follow-up* (Bethesda, MD: National Institutes of Health, 1992).

4. M. G. Marmot, M. J. Shipley, and G. Rose, "Inequalities in Death—Specific Explanations of a General Pattern?" *Lancet* (5 May 1984): 1003–1006; and M. G. Marmot et al., "Health Inequalities among British Civil Servants: The Whitehall II Study," *Lancet* (8 June 1991): 1387–1393.

5. See C. J. L. Murray et al., "U.S. Patterns of Mortality by County and Race, 1965–1994" (Cambridge, MA: Harvard Center for Population and Development Studies, 1998), quoted in M. G. Marmot, "Editorial: Inequalities in Health," *New England Journal of Medicine* (12 July 2001): 134–136.

6. *Independent Inquiry into Inequalities in Health: Report* (London: Stationery Office, 1998).

7. J. P. Smith, "Healthy Bodies and Thick Wallets," *Journal of Economic Perspectives* (Spring 1999): 145–166.

8. J. Gruber and D. A. Wise, eds., *Social Security and Retirement around the World,* NBER Conference Report Series (Chicago: University of Chicago Press, 1999).

9. J. Currie and R. Hyson, "Is the Impact of Health Shocks Cushioned by Socioeconomic Status?" *American Economic Review* (papers and proceedings) (May 1999): 245–250; S. M. Montgomery et al., "Health and Social Precursors of Unemployment in Young Men in Britain," *Journal of Epidemiology and Community Health* (August 1996): 415–422; N. Goldman, "Marriage Selection and Mortality Patterns: Inferences and Fallacies," *Demography* (May 1993): 189–208; D. I. W. Phillips et al., "Prenatal Growth and Subsequent Marital Status: Longitudinal Study," *British Medical Journal* (31 March 2001): 771; and D. J. P. Barker, "Maternal Nutrition, Fetal Nutrition, and Diseases in Later Life," *Nutrition* (September 1997): 807–813.

10. R. G. Wilkinson, *Class and Health: Research and Longitudinal Data* (London: Tavistock Press, 1986).

11. Calculated from Table 4.5 in A. Deaton and C. Paxson, "Mortality, Education, Income, and Inequality among American Cohorts," in *Themes in the Economics of Aging,* ed. D. A. Wise (Chicago: University of Chicago Press for the National Bureau of Economic Research, 2001), 129–165.

12. T. McKeown, *The Role of Medicine: Dream, Mirage, or Nemesis* (Princeton, NJ: Princeton University Press, 1979).

13. R. W. Fogel, "New Findings on Secular Trends in Nutrition and Mortality: Some Implications for Population Theory," in *Handbook of Population and Family Economics,* vol. 1A, ed. M. Rosenzweig and O. Stark (Amsterdam: Elsevier, 1997), 433–481.

14. P. Farmer, *Infections and Inequalities: The Modern Plagues* (Berkeley: University of California Press, 1999); and D. Goldman and J. P. Smith, "Can Patient Self-Management Explain the SES Health Gradient?" RAND Working Paper (Santa Monica, CA: RAND, June 2001).

15. M. G. Marmot, "Social Differences in Health within and between Populations," *Daedalus* (Fall 1994): 197–216.

16. A. M. Garber, "Pursuing the Links between Socioeconomic Factors and Health: Critique, Policy Implications, and Directions for Future Research," in *Pathways to Health: The Role of Social Factors,* ed. J. P. Bunker, D. S. Gombey, and B. Kehrer (Menlo Park, CA: Kaiser Family Foundation, 1989), 271–315.

17. D. R. Williams, "Socioeconomic Differences in Health: A Review and Redirec-

tion," *Social Psychology Quarterly* (June 1990): 81–99; and B. G. Link and J. C. Phelan, "Social Conditions as Fundamental Causes of Diseases," *Journal of Health and Social Behavior* (Extra Issue, 1995): 80–94; and B. G. Link et al., "Social Epidemiology and the Fundamental Cause Concept: On the Structuring of Effective Cancer Screens by Socioeconomic Status," *Milbank Quarterly* 76, no. 3 (1998): 375–402.

18. J. M. Muurinen and J. Le Grand, "The Economic Analysis of Inequalities in Health," *Social Science and Medicine* 20, no. 10 (1985): 1029–1035.

19. N. S. Scrimshaw, C. E. Taylor, and J. E. Gordon, *Interactions of Nutrition and Infection* (Geneva: World Health Organization, 1968).

20. J. Cassel, "The Contribution of the Social Environment to Host Resistance," *American Journal of Epidemiology* (August 1976): 107–123; R. M. Sapolsky, "Endocrinology Alfresco: Psychoendocrine Studies of Wild Baboons," *Recent Progress in Hormone Research* 48 (1993): 437–468; and B. S. McEwen, "Protective and Damaging Effects of Stress Mediators," *New England Journal of Medicine* (15 January 1998): 171–179.

21. S. Cohen et al., "Chronic Social Stress, Social Status, and Susceptibility to Upper Respiratory Infections in Nonhuman Primates," *Psychosomatic Medicine* (May–June 1997): 213–221; and S. Cohen, "Social Status and Susceptibility to Upper Respiratory Infection," in "Socioeconomic Status and Health in Industrialized Nations: Social, Psychological, and Biological Pathways," ed. N. Adler et al., *Annals of the New York Academy of Sciences*, 896 (1999), 246–253.

22. Much of the economic literature on health status traces back to M. Grossman, "On the Concept of Health Capital and the Demand for Health," *Journal of Political Economy* (March–April 1972): 223–255.

23. I. Elo and S. H. Preston, "Educational Differentials in Mortality: United States, 1979–1985," *Social Science and Medicine* (January 1996): 47–57.

24. Ibid.

25. V. R. Fuchs, "Poverty and Health: Asking the Right Questions," in *Medical Care and the Health of the Poor,* ed. D. E. Rogers and E. Ginzburg (Boulder, CO: Westview Press, 1993); and P. Farrell and V. R. Fuchs, "Schooling and Health: The Cigarette Connection," *Journal of Health Economics* (December 1982): 217–230.

26. A. Lleras-Muney, "The Relationship between Education and Mortality: An Analysis Using a Unique Social Experiment" (unpublished manuscript, Columbia University, Department of Economics, 2001).

27. D. S. Kenkel, "Health Behavior, Health Knowledge, and Schooling," *Journal of Political Economy* (April 1991): 287–305.

28. A. Deaton and C. Paxson, "Mortality, Income, and Income Inequality over Time in Britain and the United States" (working paper, Princeton University, Center for Health and Wellbeing, August 2001), http://www.wws.princeton.edu/~chw/papersframe.html.

29. M. G. Marmot et al., "Contribution of Job Control and Other Risk Factors to Social Variations in Coronary Heart Disease," *Lancet* (26 July 1997): 235–239.

30. V. Navarro, "World Health Report 2000: Responses to Murray and Frenk," *Lancet* (26 May 2001): 1701–1702.

31. R. G. Wilkinson, *Unhealthy Societies: The Affliction of Inequality* (London: Routledge, 1997); R. G. Wilkinson, *Mind the Gap: Hierarchies, Health, and Human Evolution* (London: Weidenfeld and Nicholson, 2000); and I. Kawachi, B. P. Kennedy, and R. G. Wilkinson, eds., *The Society and Population Health Reader, Vol. 1: Income Inequality and Health* (New York: New Press, 1999).

32. A. Deaton and D. Lubotsky, "Mortality, Inequality, and Race in American Cities

and States" (working paper, Princeton University, Center for Health and Wellbeing, June 2001); and A. Deaton, "Health, Inequality, and Economic Development" (Working paper, Princeton University, Center for Health and Wellbeing, May 2001). Both papers are available at http://www.wws.princeton. edu/~chw/papersframe.html.

33. A. K. Sen, "Why Health Equity?" (Keynote Address, International Health Economics Association, York, England, July 2001).

34. W. McDermott, "Medicine: The Public Good and One's Own," *Perspectives in Biology and Medicine* (Winter 1978): 167–187.

35. U.K. Department of Health, *Tackling Health Inequalities: Consultation on a Plan for Delivery,* 2001, http://www.doh.gov.uk/healthinequalities (accessed 11 December 2001).

36. Sen, "Why Health Equity?"

37. L. Hattersley, "Trends in Life Expectancy by Social Class—An Update," *Health Statistics Quarterly* (Summer 1999): 16–24.

38. See S. H. Preston and P. Taubman, "Socioeconomic Differences in Adult Mortality and Health Status," in *Demography of Aging,* ed. L. G. Martin and S. H. Preston (Washington, DC: National Academy Press, 1994), who attribute the point to M. C. Sheps, "Shall We Count the Living or the Dead?" *New England Journal of Medicine* 250 (1958): 1210–1219.

39. V. Fuchs, "The Financial Problems of the Elderly: A Holistic Approach," NBER Working Paper no. 8236 (Cambridge, MA: NBER, April 2001).

40. A. Case, "Health, Income, and Economic Development" (working paper, Princeton University Research Program in Development Studies, May 2001, for presentation at the World Bank's Annual Bank Conference on Development Economics, 1–2 May 2001); and A. Case, "Does Money Protect Health Status? Evidence from South African Pensions" (working paper, Princeton University Research Program in Development Studies, August 2001). Both papers are available at http://www.wws.princeton.edu/~rpds/working.htm (accessed 11 December 2001).

12

Putting the Picture Together

Prosperity, Redistribution,
Health, and Welfare

Richard G. Wilkinson

Introduction

Given the strong statistical associations between people's material circumstances and their health, it may seem that the soundest approach to improving public health would be to increase everyone's prosperity by maximizing economic growth rates while ensuring that some degree of "trickle down" spreads the health benefits to the poor. Indeed, a possible dilemma facing public health policy in the context of the social gradient in health is that redistributive policies may appear to achieve no more than a redistribution of a finite quantity of health-producing goods and services from the rich to the poor. Perhaps health gains for some would be canceled out by health losses for others. And if levels of unemployment and educational opportunities are regarded as fixed, it is possible that programs designed to improve the opportunities of disadvantaged individuals may seem to do little more than redistribute the scarce opportunities among the disadvantaged.

While this last point rightly underlines the need for structural policies aimed at decreasing unemployment levels and increasing the number of educational opportunities, the health implications of economic growth and of redistribution are more surprising. The well-known problems of drawing inferences from ecological data and assuming they tell us about causal processes at the individual level (the ecological fallacy) are matched by the problems of making inferences the other way round—from individual-level data to societal policies (the individualistic fallacy). Part of the association between people's material circumstances and their health appears to be not so much a direct relationship between exposure to unhealthy material circumstances, as a relationship between relative income, or social position, and health. If what matters causally is socioeconomic status rather than increased levels of consumption *per se,* then it may be wrong to assume that societal improvements in income or educational standards will improve health as much as the individual associations with either income or education seem to suggest.

What, then, is the solution if projects designed to improve individual job and educational prospects are flawed because they do not change the sum total of disadvantage, and societal policies to improve overall incomes and educational standards may mistake the effects of social position for an effect of absolute material standards? Fortunately, there is a solution. Evidence from a number of sources suggests that in more egalitarian societies, where differences in incomes and in social status are smaller, the average health standards of the population may be substantially improved. But as well as more egalitarian societies having a smaller burden of relative deprivation pressing down on health standards, they also seem to be more socially cohesive. Complementing the picture of better health among more egalitarian populations is evidence that, at least among the rich developed countries, health is indeed related to relative rather than absolute income, and that, as a consequence, health may not be strongly related to economic growth. This chapter will summarize some of this evidence and offer some tentative explanations before returning to the policy implications.

Relative Income

The main *material* and behavioral determinants of health—diet, absolute poverty, unemployment, exercise, drug abuse, housing, etc.—tend to be more widely recognized than the contribution to ill health from psychosocial sources. But research suggests increasingly that many of the socioeconomic determinants of health have their effects through psychosocial pathways. . . . Here I will first describe some indications of the overall importance to population health of the kinds of psychosocial pathways they describe, and then suggest how key psychosocial risk factors, such as social affiliations, early emotional development, and social status, are related to each other.

There are two important pieces of ecological (or macro-) level evidence which suggest that psychosocial pathways may exert a more powerful influence on health in the developed world than do pathways involving direct exposure to material hazards. Both suggest that correlations between income and health should be interpreted primarily as correlations between health and relative—rather than absolute—income or material standards. The implication is that what is important is not what your absolute level of material prosperity is, but how it compares, or where it places you, in relation to others in society. Interestingly, this accords well with the original basis on which the British registrar general ranked occupations according to their "general social standing" in order to show the social gradient in death rates.

Relationships between the average income and average health of developed countries are much weaker than the relationships found when using grouped data on income and health differences within them. Thus the United States has a gross domestic product per capita (GDPpc) which is well over twice as high as that of Greece, yet life expectancy is higher in Greece than in the United States. Among the developed countries this is not an exception to a more general relationship. The cross-sectional correlation between life expectancy among the 23 richest member countries of the Organization for Economic Cooperation and Development (OECD) (the rich market democracies) and GDPpc (converted at purchasing power parities) is very weak (in 1993, $r = .08$). Although we tend to assume that the gradual increase in life expectancy is a direct reflection of increasing prosperity, in fact the association even between long-term economic growth rates per capita and changes in life expectancy is also weak: The correlation coefficient between the percentage increase in GDPpc and the increase in life expectancy among the same group of rich countries over the period 1970–1993 was only .30. (Although life expectancy rises with economic development in developing countries, this relationship almost disappears among the developed countries. Among them, continued increases in life expectancy have little relation to economic growth.[1] This contrasts sharply with the very close relationships between income and mortality rates found using grouped data *within* countries, where correlations as strong as .8 or .9 are not uncommon. Indeed, mortality rates for small areas or occupations are usually almost perfectly rank ordered by income within countries. This is, of course, an expression of the relationship between a wide variety of measures of socioeconomic status and health within countries—known as "health inequalities" or the "social gradient" in health. . . .

Dealing as we are with whole nations, the much weaker or nonexistent income-health relationships between countries cannot be attributed to sampling error; nor is it attributable to differences in national cultures. For instance, among the 50 states in the United States, where cultural differences are smaller and people shop at many of the same chain stores selling the same range of goods throughout the country, the correlation between median state income and mortality is only .28, and even this weak relation disappears when it is controlled for income inequality ($r = .06$).[2]

This suggests that income is related to health not so much through its role as a determinant of material living standards, but rather as a marker for social status. Where (as within countries) income differences map onto differences in social status, they are closely related to health. Where (as between countries) they have no significance for social status, they are not closely related to health. The implication is that the bulk of the relation between income and health, at least in the developed countries, is a relation between health and relative income or socioeconomic status. Health appears to be related less to people's absolute material living standards than to their position in society, as expressed by their income.

This interpretation finds strong support in the association between a society's income distribution and population health. More egalitarian societies, that is societies with smaller differences in income between rich and poor, tend to have better health and increased longevity. There have been numerous reports of an association between income distribution and measures of health.[3] As well as evidence from international comparisons, studies within countries also suggest that more egalitarian areas tend to have better health. Thus, although mortality in U.S. states is not related to median state income,[4] it has been shown to be closely related to measures of income inequality within those states[5] and to income inequality among the 282 Standard Metropolitan Areas of the United States.[6] Indeed, the relation between income distribution and health now seems safe: alongside the 20 or so reports of an association between measures of income inequality and population health, there are only two reports (using the same data set) suggesting that the relation is weak or nonexistent.

There has been some discussion as to whether the relation of income distribution to health is simply a reflection of a tendency for the health of the poor to be more sensitive to changes in income than the rich, and could be accounted for by the relationships between individual incomes and health. There have now been a number of studies which have looked at the effects of different degrees of income inequality after controlling for individual incomes. All but one concluded that greater income equality has a beneficial effect on health even after taking individual incomes into account.[7] The methods of the one study which produced results at odds with the others[8] have been criticized.[9] However, the distinction between the health effects of individual income and the societal effects of income inequality is more important for those who believe that it coincides with the distinction between the effects of individual absolute income (as a determinant of material living standards) and the effects of societal social processes related to inequality. In the light of the preceding discussion, it seems more likely that the distinction is the less fundamental one between the psychosocial effects of individual relative income—or social position—and the societal effects of inequality. As we shall see, both are likely to involve similar pathways to do with issues of social status and social relations. The distinction may therefore be less important than first thought.

Having seen that among populations where there are greater income differences, implying greater disparities of socioeconomic status and a correspondingly greater burden of relative deprivation, health tends to be less good, we shall now go on to outline two powerful routes through which relative income and income inequality are likely to affect health. One is through the direct psychosocial effects of low social status, and the other is through the poorer quality of social relations found in more hierarchical societies.

Inequality and Psychosocial Welfare

The strongest evidence that there are psychosocial health effects attributable directly to low social status itself comes from work on the physiological effects of social status among nonhuman primates. Work on baboons in the wild and on macaques in captivity indicates important psychosocial pathways linking the chronic anxiety of subordinate social status to raised basal cortisol levels and attenuated responses to acute stress, increased atherosclerosis, worse HDL:LDL [high-density lipoprotein:low-density lipoprotein] ratios, central obesity, depression, and poorer immune function.[10] The effects of chronic anxiety and the consequent rise in basal cortisol levels appear to be so far-reaching that they have been likened to a process of more rapid ageing.[11] Many of the physiological risk factors which are also associated with social status among humans . . . seem, among nonhuman primates, to be directly attributable to the psychosocial effects of subordinate social status itself. In experiments on captive animals,[12] it is possible to manipulate social status by moving animals between cages with different groups, while at the same time controlling diet and the environment. This means that there is almost no way of explaining the physiological correlates of social status except to say that they are the direct result of subordinate social status. Important biological effects of social status differences remain among the monkeys even after the effects of factors like poor housing and diet, smoking, and job insecurity have been excluded. (That is not to suggest that the excluded factors do not have an important influence on the health of people exposed to them: The evidence shows quite clearly that they do. What it does mean is that there is also a substantial direct psychosocial effect of social status on health.)

Not only are the common physiological correlates of social status in humans unlikely to derive from totally different sources in species which are so closely related to us genetically, but there are a number of suggestions in the psychological literature that issues to do with shame, inferiority, subordination, people being put down and not respected, etc. are extremely important—if largely unrecognized—sources of recurrent anxiety resulting from hierarchy. The possible centrality of shame, fears of incompetence, and inferiority in relation to people in superior positions needs to be emphasized for two reasons. First, because a central part of the research task is to identify the most potent sources of recurrent anxiety related to low social status and, secondly, because these issues go beyond health: The same psychosocial processes may also contribute to a number of other social problems associated with relative deprivation.

Crucially important here is the evidence that the social environment becomes less supportive and more conflictual where income differences are bigger. Both Kaplan et al.[13] and Kennedy et al.[14] have shown close relationships between homicide and income inequality. We also have the benefit of a meta-analysis of some 34 papers, based on data comparing countries as well as areas within countries, which suggest that this is a robust relationship.[15] Kawachi et al.[16] have shown that the proportion of people who feel they can trust others declines sharply where income differences are bigger. Also closely related to income inequality are the differences in the average hostility scores for 10 U.S. cities, which were measured by Williams et al.:[17] The wider the income differences, the greater are the hostility scores. These measures of the social environment were all closely related to mortality as well as to income inequality; correlations were commonly as high as .7 or higher.

In his study of people's engagement in community life in the regions of Italy, Putnam notes that income inequality is strongly related to his index of "civic community" and says (referring here more to an egalitarian social ethos rather than to income distribution) that "Equality is an essential feature of the civic community."[18] I have also pointed to qualitative evidence suggesting that societies which were unusually egalitarian and unusually healthy were also unusually cohesive.[19] The examples I discussed included Britain during the two world wars, postwar Japan, Roseto in Pennsylvania,[20] and eastern Europe during the 1970s and 1980s. The more recent quantitative evidence (above), which includes a path analysis,[21] strongly suggests that the pathway is from income distribution, through the quality of social relations, to health.

. . . [I]t is now well established that the quality of people's social relations seems to have a powerful influence on their health. Several studies have reported death rates two or three times as high among people with low levels of social integration compared to people with high levels.[22] In valiant attempts to avoid psychosocial explanations, some people have suggested that the health benefits of friendship may result primarily from the gains that come from practical material support, overlooking the fact that the most common things which friends share or give each other are cigarettes, alcoholic drinks, and the proverbial "cup of sugar" borrowed from neighbors—not to mention AIDS. Hardly a recipe for good health! Much more plausible is that it is the psychosocial effect of the social relation itself which is important to health. Once more confirming the psychosocial pathway, studies of nonhuman primates have now shown that animals with fewer social affiliations have the familiar pattern of reduced basal cortisol levels and attenuated stress responses associated with chronic anxiety.[23]

Here it is conceptually helpful to see that friendship and social hierarchy are linked as opposite types of social relation: They may be thought of as opposite sides of the same coin. Friendship is about mutuality, reciprocity, and the recognition that the needs of friends are needs for us. In contrast, hierarchy, dominance, and subordination is a pecking order based on power, coercion, and access to resources regardless of the needs of others. Putnam refers to them as horizontal and vertical relations. He contrasts the horizontal relations between equals which are conducive to civic community with the vertical patron/client relations which predominate in the areas where community life is weaker. In studies of animal social behavior it is also clear that horizontal affiliations (based largely on grooming) not only confer obligations of mutual aid and reciprocity, but are used to improve or defend positions in the vertical dominance hierarchy.

The incompatibility of friendship and inequality has often been noted. Indeed, Plato remarked, "How correct the old saying is, that equality leads to friendship! It's right enough and it rings true."[24] In this context it is interesting to note that the current Cambridge Scale for ranking occupations in hierarchical order uses information on friendships as a measure of social distance.[25] It is based on data from a sample of the population who are asked details of their own occupations and those of six friends. Occupations with many friendships between them are regarded as being at a similar social level, whereas those with few friendships between them are assumed to be separated by a large social distance. So great is the friction between inequality and friendship that research has been undertaken to see "how individuals maintain or repair a close social bond when a perceived difference in status . . . has disrupted a close relationship."[26]

If increased income inequality is closely accompanied by a weakening of social bonds, the combination of the two can hardly fail to have a potent effect on health. Partly because of the large proportion of the population exposed to these risks, low social status and poor social relations are probably two of the most powerful risk factors influencing population health.

Reading between the lines of the evidence, we can see that a crucial source of chronic anxiety, related both to social hierarchy and inversely to friendship, is likely to center on feelings aroused by social comparisons to do with confidence, insecurity, and fears of inadequacy. Social hierarchy induces worries about possible incompetence and inadequacy, feelings of insecurity, and fears [of] inferiority. In contrast, the experience of friendship is primarily about the sense of being accepted and appreciated and of having a positive, confidence-boosting self-image reflected back.

The importance of social comparisons in inducing stress has been demonstrated in research which involves exposing people to experimentally induced stressors. Having to do a difficult and demanding task in isolation does not in itself seem enough to raise cortisol levels. But cortisol levels do rise when the same tasks are performed in a situation where failure is experimentally induced and people's results are publicly compared with others at frequent intervals.[27]

A third pointer (in addition to the health impact of social status and friendship) which seems to confirm the centrality of these basic issues of confidence and insecurity comes from the effects of early childhood emotional development on health. Because of the inherent methodological difficulties of collecting data during early life and relating [them] to disease in adulthood, there is still a serious shortage of evidence on the relationship between the emotional environment in early childhood and poor health in later life. However, all the pointers are there. Using retrospective data, Lundberg[28] found that "family dissension" in childhood was associated with a 52 per cent increase in mortality risk among Swedish adults 30–75 years old, and was a more important determinant of health in later life than economic hardship. Similarly, Montgomery et al.[29] found that domestic conflict in early childhood predicted slow growth and unemployment in adulthood. In addition, lack of secure attachment in early life, domestic conflict, and family instability have been shown to be related to the behavioral, developmental, psychosocial, and physiological markers suggesting that the early emotional environment is strongly related to adult disease. . . .

In a review paper, Fonagy[30] says that domestic conflict and poor early attachment lead to a lower IQ and less good educational achievement, antisocial behavior, depression, and aggression. Power et al.[31] reported that in the National Child Development Study the best predictors of health in early adulthood were teachers' assessments of the behavior of children when they were 16 years old. A review by Hertzman and Wiens,[32] which shows that various psychosocial interventions in early childhood can be effective in preventing or overcoming these difficulties, also confirms the importance of emotional development.

There is now strong evidence, mainly from animal studies, that the psychosocial effects of early emotional trauma are partly mediated by the activation of the hypothalamic–pituitary–adrenal axis and raised basal cortisol levels. Experiments on several species have shown that early handling, maternal licking in infancy, and good mothering results in lower cortisol levels throughout life.[33]

The emerging picture seems to combine two large bodies of apparently separate sociological and psychological literature. The mass of sociological literature on social stratification and social class contrasts sharply with the minor importance accorded to these issues in the psychological literature. Yet, for its part, psychology has an enormous literature on the importance of early childhood which is not matched in sociology. From our point of view these sociological and psychological literatures are closely related. The basic confidence or insecurity which comes from emotional experience in early childhood affects people's vulnerability to the insecurity induced by low social status in the social hierarchy. The social hierarchy seems to present itself to us as if it were a hierarchy of human adequacy, from the most superior, successful, and capable, at the top, to the most incapable at the bottom. Indeed, that people with low social status take that as an indication of their own incompetence and lack of ability was the central message of Sennett and Cobb's *The Hidden Injuries of Class.*[34] While the nature of society and the extent of inequality are likely to be the primary determinants of the proportion of the population made to feel inferior, the security or insecurity of people's early attachments is likely to determine which individuals are most likely to succumb to status insecurities.

The health risks associated with low social status, lack of social ties, and early emotional insecurity may then all point to the same source of anxiety at the heart of social life. Thomas Scheff, working on the emotional complex involving a sense of inferiority, shame, and embarrassment which he calls the *deference-emotion system*, notes that "there has been a continuing suggestion in the literature that shame is *the* primary social emotion, generated by the virtually constant monitoring of the self in relation to others."[35] Similarly, Goffman[36] argued that embarrassment played a prominent role in every social encounter; Gilbert and McGuire[37] have suggested that "shame" is distantly related to an evolved "submission" response of subordinate animals to superiors in the social hierarchy; and Darwin devoted a whole chapter to blushing (and its relation to shame), which he said "depends in all cases on . . . a sensitive regard for the opinion, more particularly the depreciation of others."[38] In Scheff et al.'s words:

> [S]hame involves painful feelings that are not identified as shame by the person experiencing them. Rather they are labeled with a wide variety of terms that serve to disguise the experience of shame: having low self-esteem, feeling foolish, stupid, ridiculous, inadequate, defective, incompetent, awkward, exposed, vulnerable, insecure, helpless. Our culture provides a great many such code words. Lewis classifies all these terms as shame markers, because they occurred only in a context [which] always involved a perception of self as negatively evaluated, by either self or other—the basic context for shame.[39]
>
> In these instances, the negative evaluation of self appears to cause so much pain that it interferes with the fluent production of thought or speech, even though the pain is mislabeled.[40]

The scene in TV soaps in which the boss and his wife come to dinner with the junior executive who is thereby reduced to a clumsy, gibbering idiot, unable to put a foot or a word right, is the comic representation of this process.

What is at stake is the sense of pride and need for self-confirmation on the one hand and shame, humiliation, and rejection on the other. It is the unacknowledged or repressed nature of shame which "explains how shame might be ubiquitous, yet usually escape notice."[41] So important are these processes in social life that it has been suggested that shame is the key to social conformity. The results of a number of social psychology experiments on people's tendency to conform (rather than sticking out from a group) are best explained in terms of their desire to avoid embarrassment, of being thought different, inadequate, or stupid: "[U]nacknowledged shame plays a central role in causing subjects to yield to group influence, even when it contradicts their own direct perceptions."[42]

These processes, triggered by invidious social comparisons, seem the most plausible source of the chronic stress related to low social status, to lack of friendship, and to poor emotional attachment early in life—all of which have been shown to lead to raised basal cortisol levels and attenuated responses to experimental stressors. Although few studies have investigated the role of cortisol in health differences in human populations, the first to have done so provides strong evidence of its importance.[43]

A Culture of Inequality

Given the close relationship between income inequality and both homicide and violent crime,[44] it is important to note that Scheff et al. also suggest that unacknowledged shame "leads to anger, disrespectful communication and a spiral of exchanges between the parties [which] results in anger and further hostile communication"—the "shame rage spiral." "As humiliation increases, rage and hostility increase proportionally to defend against loss of self-esteem . . . hostility can be viewed as an attempt to ward off feelings of humiliation (shame) generated by inept, ineffectual moves, a sense of incompetence, insults, and a lack of power to defend against insults."[45] The close accord between this and literature on violence and disrespect suggests an explanation for the link between violence and greater inequality. Gilligan, who was a prison psychiatrist for 25 years, said: "I have yet to see a serious act of violence that was not provoked by the experience of feeling shamed and humiliated, disrespected and ridiculed, and that did not represent the attempt to prevent or undo this 'loss of face'—no matter how severe the punishment."[46] A paper examining the common links between inequality, health, and violence argued that as greater inequality cuts more people off from other sources of status, we become increasingly sensitive to status issues, ready to defend ourselves against being looked down on, thought incompetent, treated as inferior, and disrespected.[47]

The indications are that there is a culture of inequality which is less supportive, more aggressive, and usually more macho or "laddish." Not only is this suggested by the relation we have seen between income inequality and various measures of the social environment, but it is also suggested by the causes of death which are most closely related to differences in inequality. Although not accounting for the largest number of excess deaths in more unequal places, the death rates which usually show the biggest percentage differences between more and less egalitarian places seem to include violence, accidents, and alcohol-related deaths.[48] Because deaths from these causes affect men (particularly young men) more than women, greater income inequality is often associated with bigger differences between male and female mortality rates.[49]

The stresses of hierarchy and the effects of more hierarchical relations, of institutional structures of power and subordination, are passed downward. The violence associated with wider income differences is not principally between rich and poor; it is most pronounced in the inner cities and among the poor themselves. People subordinated by their social or institutional superiors and threatened with humiliation attempt to regain their sense of control and restore their self-esteem by asserting authority and control over those below them. At intermediate levels in the hierarchy this can be done through institutional sources of authority rather than through personal physical violence. But at the bottom, where people lack other ways of regaining their self-respect, the tendency is to try to regain it by asserting superiority over whatever minorities are most vulnerable. Hence the well-known pattern for discrimination and scapegoating of minorities to increase in times of high unemployment and economic hardship. Kennedy et al.[50] have shown that there is more racial discrimination in those U.S. states where income differences are bigger.

That men who have been humiliated are more likely to try to regain a sense of themselves by taking it out on women is likely to account for the connection between income inequality and the status of women.[51] Gloria Anzaldua, who grew up where the word *macho* gained its modern meaning, gives a graphic description of how machismo is predicated on hierarchy and leads to the oppression of women:

> For men like my father, being "macho" meant being strong enough to protect and support my mother and us, yet being able to show love. Today's macho has doubts about his ability to feed and protect his family. His "machismo" is an adaptation to oppression and poverty and low self-esteem. It is the result of hierarchical male dominance. The Anglo, feeling inadequate and inferior and powerless, displaces or transfers these feelings to the Chicano by shaming him. In the Gringo world, the Chicano suffers from excessive humility and self-effacement, shame of self and self-deprecation.
>
> The loss of a sense of dignity and respect in the macho breeds a false machismo which leads him to put down women and even to brutalize them. Coexisting with his sexist behavior is a love of the mother which takes precedence over that of all others. Devoted son, macho pig. To wash down the shame of his acts, of his very being, and to handle the brute in the mirror, he takes to the bottle, the snort, the needle and the fist.[52]

Much the same processes are likely to lie behind the association between greater inequality and more racial discrimination in the United States.[53]

In a different cultural context, but where some of the same forces operate, James[54] has reviewed evidence showing that greater inequality and relative poverty increase the stresses on family life, so leading to more domestic violence and to more children growing up to become violent adults.

Conclusions

Returning to the issues raised at the beginning of this chapter about the policy conundrum round the dangers of both ecological and individualistic fallacies, the solution involves tackling the structural determinants of the social environment. This does not mean relying on economic growth, which, even with "trickle down," improves everyone's material prosperity in parallel while leaving social relations unchanged. Nor does it mean pursuing policies that simply affect which individuals suffer various forms of disadvantage without affecting the total burden of disadvantage in the population. Instead, policies need to aim at reducing the overall burden of disadvantage—tackling the structural sources of inequality through policies on employment, incomes, and education. (In Britain disparities in the educational achievements of 16-year-olds have been increasing.) In order to decrease socioeconomic inequality, we need to reduce both the proportion of the population who fall behind and the distance they fall behind, on each of these core criteria.

The admittedly speculative picture which has been suggested here is that greater income inequality is one of the major influences on the proportion of the population who find themselves in situations that deny them a sense of dignity, situations that increase the insecurity they feel about their personal worth and competence, and that carry connotations of inferiority in which few can feel respected, valued, and confident. Instead of offsetting some of this damage, friendships and social networks atrophy as people feel increasingly vulnerable to the way they are seen by others. Working through the kind of deference-emotion system described by Scheff, people become more vulnerable to feelings of shame and more likely to use violence to gain respect. As well as increased violence, accidents, and alcohol-related deaths, these feelings are plausibly one of the most powerful and recurrent sources of the chronic stress that increases people's vulnerability to a wide range of infectious and cardiovascular diseases. This provides the most plausible model we have of why low social status, weak social networks, and poor early attachment should be related not only to worse health but also to raised basal cortisol levels and attenuated cortisol responses to experimental stressors. The biological processes set in train by chronic anxiety appear to provide a plausible candidate for the hypothesized "general vulnerability factor" which could explain why so many causes of death become more common further down the social hierarchy.[55] Because they act cumulatively, they are also compatible with the additive effects of lifetime exposure to adverse circumstances. . . .

The importance to health of the social environment and psychosocial welfare does not, however, mean that we can ignore the material inequalities which are its foundations. The strength of the statistical relationships suggest that something between one-third and two-thirds of the differences in measures of the social environment, in mortality and in violence may be attributable to the extent of income inequality alone. Nor is improvement a matter of reaching some utopian state of perfect equality. On the contrary, rather than pointing to something unattainable, the statistical analyses show the importance of the differences in inequality which currently exist between developed market democracies or among the 50 states of the United States.

There are, of course, many other important sources of the relationship between socioeconomic circumstances and health. Diet, housing, job control, exercise, social support, smoking, unemployment, job insecurity, and many others all play a role. However, many of these risk factors will be influenced by—or work through—a number of different processes. For instance, unemployment, low income, substantial income reductions,[56] and lack of educational qualifications can all be experienced as a threat to pride and dignity and are potentially shaming. Income inequality is important partly because it is indicative of a number of these different contributions to the scale of disadvantage in a society. But even apparently independent risk factors, such as smoking and obesity, may not be completely unaffected by this axis: There is some evidence to suggest that self-esteem and a sense of control may make it easier to keep to resolutions about giving up smoking.[57] The same might be true of those who, despite their best intentions, continue to "eat for comfort." This might explain why behavioral risk factors such as body mass index, smoking, and sedentarism appear to be related to the extent of inequality.[58]

There are numerous complimentary policy approaches to the issues . . . and effective measures will probably mean bringing several of them together. Take obesity as an example:

1. A necessary but not sufficient condition for effective policy is a public awareness of its health risks and an understanding of the contribution of diet and exercise. That knowledge is probably fairly widespread already.
2. On top of that is the need to tackle the food industry, which promotes, particularly to children, refined foods containing concentrated fats and sugars. . . .
3. The problem of low incomes: Refined foods undoubtedly provide cheap calories, and diets that conform to nutritional recommendations usually cost more. This is an important part of the reason why more harmful diets are so much more common among poorer people.
4. The amount of exercise people take is influenced not only by individual choice, but also by a society's transport policies. . . .
5. It looks as if there is a direct contribution to central obesity and the "metabolic syndrome" from chronic stress.[59] . . .
6. There is little doubt that the tendency to eat (or drink) "for comfort" will be stronger among those whose circumstances do not provide them with the social sources of that comfort. People who feel depressed and trapped, who lack the resources and opportunities that allow them to experience a sense of control over their circumstances, will find it hardest to make (and keep to) resolutions to take more exercise and go without comfort foods: That is easiest when you feel on top of things and life is going well.

Greater equality is likely to make a contribution to the third, fifth, and sixth of these approaches to reducing obesity. If a more egalitarian ethos also contributes to people's willingness to fund and use public transport, it will also contribute to the fourth. Examples of other health problems would have shown a similarly wide range of policy approaches, including ways in which a reduction in relative deprivation and in the hierarchical differentiation of the population would lead to improvements.

In a nutshell, then, the health importance of greater income equality, and of the improved social environment that comes with it, is that it enhances the population's psychosocial welfare. By improving social functioning, it increases the effectiveness of a wide range of public health and social policy initiatives—including the reduction in cardiovascular risk factors.[60] Without tackling material inequalities, progress is likely to be slower and the quality of life poorer.

But it is not just health that is related to the extent of relative deprivation. We have already seen the links with violence and a less supportive social environment; equally strong is the association between deprivation and poorer educational performance of schoolchildren,[61] and of course a number of other social problems are also recognized to be more common in deprived areas. It seems likely that the powerful psychosocial effects of relative deprivation and low social status can explain why a variety of social problems share roots in relative poverty. The implication is that there may be multiple benefits to policies that address the underlying causes.

Finally, if a range of health and other social problems are related to relative income rather than absolute living standards, and income inequality is associated, as we have seen, with ill health, violence, and a poorer social environment, it suggests that part of the almost universal desire for higher incomes may be a desire for improved social status. This has been suggested by several economists, including Frank[62] and Schor,[63] both of whom argue that consumption is competitive and fueled by a concern to maintain or improve social status. Indeed, their views are reminiscent of Adam Smith's when he said:

> What is the end of avarice and ambition, of the pursuit of wealth, of power and preeminence? Is it to supply the necessities of nature? The wages of the meanest laborer can supply them . . . what are the advantages which we would propose to gain by that great purpose of human life which we call bettering our condition? To be observed, to be attended to, to be taken notice of with sympathy, complacency, and approbation, are all the advantages which we can propose to derive from it.[64]

Schor describes how American "aspirational" incomes increased during the 1980s when income differences were widening. She says that in 1980 people used to aspire to lifestyles pegged to about 20 percent above their prevailing standard of living, but then "A shift took place in that comparative process—everyone, especially the entire middle class—began to compare themselves with the top 20 percent of the income distribution," drastically widening the aspiration gap. She describes how a Roper poll in 1986 asked people "How much money would you need to make all your dreams come true?" and found a mean reply of U.S. $50,000. By 1994, that "dream-fulfilling" level had doubled to U.S. $102,000, and those earning U.S. $50,000 or more felt they would need U.S. $200,000. As a result, Americans spent higher fractions of their income, their savings declined, and they took on record levels of debt. She also presents data showing that the more television people watch, the less money they save, and the more they spend.

These trends are what one might expect if status differences are important in fueling consumption. The implication is that it may not be legitimate to assume that individual desires for higher incomes can be summed into a societal demand for economic growth. Because it does nothing about relative social status, economic growth may be less important to welfare in the developed world than is often supposed. This means that if we are to move toward environmentally sustainable levels of consumption, it may be necessary to reduce the status differences which drive the competitive element in consumption. But, as Schor says, "We live with high levels of psychological denial about the connection between our buying habits and the social statements they make."

Professor Wilkinson's research is supported by a grant from the Medical Research Council.

Notes

1. Wilkinson, R. G. (1996). *Unhealthy societies: The afflictions of inequality.* London: Routledge.

2. Kaplan, G. A., Pamuk, E., Lynch, J. W, Cohen, R. D., and Balfour, J. L. (1996). Inequality in income and mortality in the United States: Analysis of mortality and potential pathways. *BMJ* 312, 999–1003.

3. Kawachi, I., Kennedy, B., and Wilkinson, R. G. (eds.). (1999). *The society and population health reader: Income inequality and health.* New York: New Press.

4. Kaplan, G. A., Pamuk, E., Lynch, J. W., Cohen, R. D., and Balfour, J. L. (1996). Inequality in income and mortality in the United States: Analysis of mortality and potential pathways. *BMJ* 312, 999–1003.

5. Kennedy, B. P., Kawachi, I., and Prothrow-Stith, D. (1996). Income distribution and mortality: Cross sectional ecological study of the Robin Hood index in the United States. *BMJ* 312, 1004–1007. See also an important correction: *BMJ* 312, 1194.

6. Lynch, J., Kaplan, G. A., Pamuk, E. R., et al. (1998). Income inequality and mortality in metropolitan areas of the United States. *Am. J. Public Health* 88, 1074–1080.

7. Kennedy, B. P., Kawachi, I., Glass, R., and Prothrow-Stith, D. (1998). Income distribution, socioeconomic status, and self rated health: A U.S. multi-level analysis. *BMJ* 317, 917–921; Soobader, M.-J., and LeClere, F. B. (1999). Aggregation and the measurement of income inequality: Effects on morbidity. *Soc. Sci. Med.* 48:6, 773–744; Diez-Roux, A. V., Link, B., and Northridge, M. E. (1999). A multilevel analysis of income inequality and cardiovascular disease risk factors. *Soc. Sci. Med.* 50:5, 673–687.

8. Fiscella, K., and Franks, P. (1997). Poverty or income inequality as predictors of mortality: Longitudinal cohort study. *BMJ* 314, 1724–1728.

9. Kennedy, B. P., Kawachi, I., Glass, R., and Prothrow-Stith, D. (1998). Income distribution, socioeconomic status, and self rated health: A U.S. multi-level analysis. *BMJ* 317, 917–921; Diez-Roux, A. V., Link, B., and Northridge, M. E. (1999). A multilevel analysis of income inequality and cardiovascular disease risk factors. *Soc. Sci. Med.* 50:5, 673–687.

10. Sapolsky, R. M. (1993). Endocrinology alfresco: Psychoendocrine studies of wild baboons. *Recent Prog. Horm. Res.* 48, 437–468; Shively, C. A., and Clarkson, T. B. (1994). Social status and coronary artery atherosclerosis in female monkeys. *Arterioscler. Thromb.* 14, 721–726; Sapolsky, R. M., Alberts, S. C., and Altmann, J. (1997). Hypercortisolism associated with social subordinance or social isolation among wild baboons. *Arch. Gen. Psychiatry* 54(12), 1137–1143; Shively, C. A., Laird, K. L., and Anton, R. F. (1997). The behavior and physiology of social stress and depression in female cynomolgus monkeys. *Biol. Psychiatry* 41, 871–882.

11. Sapolsky, R. M. (1998). *Why zebras don't get ulcers: A guide to stress, stress related disease and coping.* 2nd ed. New York: Freeman

12. Shively, C. A., and Clarkson, T. B. (1994). Social status and coronary artery atherosclerosis in female monkeys. *Arterioscler. Thromb.* 14, 721–726; Shively, C. A., Laird, K. L., and Anton, R. F. (1997). The behavior and physiology of social stress and depression in female cynomolgus monkeys. *Biol. Psychiatry* 41, 871–882.

13. Kaplan, G. A., Pamuk, E., Lynch, J. W, Cohen, R. D., and Balfour, J. L. (1996). Inequality in income and mortality in the United States: Analysis of mortality and potential pathways. *BMJ* 312, 999–1003.

14. Kennedy, B., Kawachi, I., Prothrow-Stith, D., Lochner, K., and Gibbs, B. (1998). Social capital, income inequality, and firearm violent crime. *Soc. Sci. Med.* 47, 7–17.

15. Hsieh, C. C., and Pugh, M. D. (1993). Poverty, income inequality, and violent crime: A meta-analysis of recent aggregate data studies. *Criminal Justice Rev.* 18, 182–202.

16. Kawachi, I., Kennedy, B. P., Lochner, K., and Prothrow Stith, D. (1997). Social capital, income inequality and mortality. *Am. J. Public Health* 87, 1491–1498.

17. Williams, R. B., Feaganes, J., and Barefoot, J. C. (1995). Hostility and death rates in 10 U.S. cities. *Psychosom. Med.* 57:1, 94.

18. Putnam, R. D., Leonardi, R., and Nanetti, R. Y. (1993). *Making democracy work: Civic traditions in modern Italy.* Princeton, NJ: Princeton University Press, citing p. 105.

19. Wilkinson, R. G. (1996). *Unhealthy societies: The afflictions of inequality.* London: Routledge.

20. Bruhn, J. G., and Wolf, S. (1979). *The Roseto story.* Norman: University of Oklahoma Press.

21. Kawachi, I., Kennedy, B. P., Lochner, K., and Prothrow Stith, D. (1997). Social capital, income inequality and mortality. *Am. J. Public Health* 87, 1491–1498.

22. House, J. S., Landis, K. R., and Umberson, D. (1988). Social relationships and health. *Science* 241, 540–545; Berkman, L. F. (1995). The role of social relations in health promotion. *Psychosom. Res.* 57, 245–254.

23. Sapolsky, R. M., Alberts, S. C., and Altmann, J. (1997). Hypercortisolism associated with social subordinance or social isolation among wild baboons. *Arch. Gen. Psychiatry* 54(12), 1137–1143.

24. Plato. (1970). *The laws* (trans. T. J. Saunders). Harmondsworth, UK: Penguin, citing p. 229.

25. Prandy, K. (1990). The revised Cambridge Scale of Occupations. *Sociology* 24(4), 629–655.

26. Harris, S. R. (1997). Status inequality and close relationships: An integrative typology of bond saving strategies. *Symbolic Interaction* 20(1), 1–20.

27. Pruessner, J. C., Hellhammer, D. H., and Kirschbaum, C. (1999). Low self-esteem, induced failure and the adrenocortical stress response. *Pers. Individ. Dif.* 27:3, 1999, 477–489.

28. Lundberg, O. (1993). The impact of childhood living conditions on illness and mortality in adulthood. *Soc. Sci. Med.* 36, 1047–1052.

29. Montgomery, S. M., Bartley, M. J., and Wilkinson, R. G. (1997). Family conflict and slow growth. *Arch. Dis. Child.* 77, 326–330.

30. Fonagy, P. (1998). *Early influences on development and social inequalities: An attachment theory perspective.* Paper presented at the Kansas Conference on Health and Its Social Determinants, Wichita, KS.

31. Power, C., Manor, O., and Fox, J. (1991). *Health and class: The early years.* London: Chapman and Hall.

32. Hertzman, C., and Wiens, M. (1996). Child development and long-term outcomes: A population health perspective and summary of successful interventions. *Soc. Sci. Med.* 43, 1083–1095.

33. Meaney, M. J., Aitken, D. H., van Berkel, C., Bhatnagar, S., and Sapolsky, R. M. (1988). Effect of neonatal handling on age related impairments associated with the hippocampus. *Science* 239, 766–768; Suomi, S. J. (1991). Early stress and adult emotional reactivity in rhesus monkeys. In: *The childhood environment and adult disease* (ed. Ciba Foundation), pp. 171–186. Wiley, Chichester, UK; Liu, D., Diorio, J., Tannenbaum, B., et al. (1997). Maternal care, hippocampal glucocorticoid receptors, and hypothalamic pituitary adrenal responses to stress. *Science* 277, 1659–1662; Fonagy, P. (1998). *Early influences on development and social inequalities: An attachment theory perspective.* Paper presented at the Kansas Conference on Health and Its Social Determinants, Wichita, KS.

34. Sennett, R., and Cobb, J. (1973). *The hidden injuries of class.* New York: Knopf.

35. Scheff, T. J. (1988). Shame and conformity: The deference-emotion system. *Am. Sociol. Rev.* 53, 395–406, citing p. 397.

36. Goffman, E. (1967). *Interaction ritual.* Garden City, NY: Anchor Doubleday.

37. Gilbert, P., and McGuire, M. T. (1998). Shame, status, and social roles: Psychobiology and evolution. In: *Shame: interpersonal behavior, psychopathology, and culture* (ed. P. Gilbert and B. Andrews). New York: Oxford University Press.

38. Darwin, C. (1872). *The expression of emotion in men and animals.* London: Murray.

39. Scheff, T. J., Retzinger, S. M., and Ryan, M. T. (1989). Crime, violence, and self-esteem: Review and proposals. In: *The social importance of self-esteem* (ed. A. M. Mecca, N. J. Smelser, and J. Vasconcellos). Berkeley: University of California Press, citing p. 181.

40. Ibid., citing p. 182.

41. Ibid., citing p. 183.

42. Ibid.

43. Kristenson, M., Orth-Gomer, K., Kucinskiene, Z., et al. (1998). Attenuated cortisol response to a standardized stress test in Lithuanian versus Swedish men: The LiVicordia Study. *Int. J. Behav. Med.* 5:1, 17–30.

44. Hsieh, C. C., and Pugh, M. D. (1993). Poverty, income inequality, and violent crime: A meta-analysis of recent aggregate data studies. *Criminal Justice Rev.* 18, 182–202; Kaplan, G. A., Pamuk, E., Lynch, J. W., Cohen, R. D., and Balfour, J. L. (1996). Inequality in income and mortality in the United States: Analysis of mortality and potential pathways. *BMJ* 312, 999–1003; Kennedy, B., Kawachi, I., Prothrow-Stith, D., Lochner, K., and Gibbs, B. (1998). Social capital, income inequality, and firearm violent crime. *Soc. Sci. Med.* 47, 7–17.

45. Scheff, T. J., Retzinger, S. M., and Ryan, M. T. (1989). Crime, violence, and self-esteem: Review and proposals. In: *The social importance of self-esteem* (ed. A. M. Mecca, N. J. Smelser, and J. Vasconcellos). Berkeley: University of California Press, citing p. 188.

46. Gilligan, J. (1996). *Violence: Our deadly epidemic and its causes.* New York: Putnam, citing p. 110.

47. Wilkinson, R. G., Kawachi, I., and Kennedy, B. (1998). Mortality, the social environment, crime and violence. *Sociol. Health Illn.* 20, 578–597.

48. McIsaac, S. J., and Wilkinson, R. G. (1997). Income distribution and cause specific mortality. *Eur. J. Public Health,* 7, 45–53; Walberg, P., McKee, M., Shkolnikov, V., Chenet, L., and Leon, D. A. (1998). Economic change, crime, and mortality crisis in Russia: Regional analysis. *BMJ* 317, 312–318.

49. Kawachi, I., Kennedy, B. P., Gupta, V., and Prothrow-Stith, D. (1999). Women's status and the health of women: A view from the States. *Soc. Sci. Med.* 48:1, 21–32; Wilkinson, R. G., Kennedy, B., and Kawachi, I. (1999). Women's status and men's health in a culture of inequality.

50. Kennedy, B. P., Kawachi, I., Lochner, K., Jones, C. P., and Prothrow-Stith, D. (1997). (Dis)respect and black mortality. *Ethnic. Dis.* 7, 207–214.

51. Kawachi et al. 1998.

52. Anzaldua, G. (1987). *Borderlands.* San Francisco: Aunt Lute Books, citing p. 83.

53. Kennedy, B. P., Kawachi, I., Lochner, K., Jones, C. P., and Prothrow-Stith, D. (1997). (Dis)respect and black mortality. *Ethnic. Dis.* 7, 207–214.

54. James, O. (1995). *Juvenile violence in a winner-looser culture.* London: Free Association Books.

55. Marmot, M. G., Shipley, M. J., and Rose, G. (1984). Inequalities in death—specific explanations of a general pattern? *Lancet* 5 May, 1003–1006.

56. McDonough, P., Duncan, G. J., Williams, D., and House, J. (1997). Income dynamics and adult mortality in the U.S. 1972–1989. *Am. J. Public Health* 87, 1476–1483.

57. Action on Smoking and Health. (1993). *Her share of misfortune.* London: ASH; Marsh, A., and McKay, S. (1994). *Poor smokers.* London: Policy Studies Institute.

58. Diez-Roux, A. V., Link, B., and Northridge, M. E. (1999). A multilevel analysis of income inequality and cardiovascular disease risk factors. *Soc. Sci. Med.* 50:5, 673–687.

59. Shively, C. A., and Clarkson, T. B. (1988). Regional obesity and coronary artery atherosclerosis in females: A non-human primate model. *Acta Med. Scand. Suppl.* 723, 71–78; Brunner, E. J., Marmot, M. G., Nanchahal, K., et al. (1997). Social inequality in coronary risk: Central obesity and the metabolic syndrome. Evidence from the Whitehall II study. *Diabetologia* 40(11), 1341–1349.

60. Diez-Roux, A. V., Link, B., and Northridge, M. E. (1999). A multilevel analysis of income inequality and cardiovascular disease risk factors. *Soc. Sci. Med.* 50:5, 673–687.

61. Blane, D., White, I., and Morris, J. (1996). Education, social circumstances and mortality. In: *Health and social organization* (ed. D. Blane, E. Brunner, and R. Wilkinson). London: Routledge, pp. 171–187.

62. Frank, R. H. (1999). *Luxury fever.* New York: Free Press.

63. Schor, J. (1998). *The overspent American: When buying becomes you.* New York: Basic Books.

64. Smith, A. (2002). *Theory of the moral sentiments.* Book i, ch. ii. 1. Cambridge: Cambridge University Press, citing p. 50.

13

Why Justice Is Good
for Our Health

The Social Determinants
of Health Inequalities

Norman Daniels, Bruce P. Kennedy,
and Ichiro Kawachi

Justice and Health Inequalities

We have known for over 150 years that an individual's chances of life and death are patterned according to social class: The more affluent and educated people are, the longer and healthier their lives.[1] These patterns persist even when there is universal access to health care—a fact quite surprising to those who think financial access to medical services is the primary determinant of health status. In fact, recent cross-national evidence suggests that the greater the degree of socioeconomic inequality that exists within a society, the steeper the *gradient* of health inequality. As a result, middle-income groups in a less-equal society will have worse health than comparable or even poorer groups in a society with greater equality. Of course, one cannot infer causation from correlation, but there are plausible hypotheses about pathways that link social inequalities to health. Even if more work remains to be done to clarify the exact mechanisms, it is not unreasonable to talk here about the social "determinants" of health.[2]

When is an inequality in health status between different socioeconomic groups unjust?[3] An account of justice should help us determine which inequalities are unjust and which are tolerable. Many who are untroubled by some kinds of inequality are particularly troubled by health inequalities. They believe a socioeconomic inequality that otherwise seems just becomes unjust if it contributes to inequalities in health. But is every health inequality that results from unequally distributed social goods unjust? If there is an irreducible health gradient across socioeconomic groups, does that make the very existence of those inequalities unjust? Alternatively, are some health inequalities the result of acceptable trade-offs? Perhaps they are simply an unfortunate by-product of inequalities that work in other ways to help worse-off groups. For example, it is often claimed that permitting economic inequality provides incentives to work harder, thereby stimulating growth that will ultimately benefit the poorest groups. To whom must these trade-offs be acceptable if we are to consider them just? Are they acceptable only if they are part of a strategy aimed at moving the situation toward a more just arrangement? Does it matter in our judgments about justice exactly how social determinants produce inequalities in health status?

These are hard questions. Unfortunately, they have been almost completely ignored within the field of bioethics, as well as within ethics and political philosophy more generally. Bioethics has been quick to focus on exotic new medical technologies and how they might affect our lives. It has paid considerable attention to the doctor-patient relationship and how changes in the health care system affect it. With some significant exceptions, it has not looked "upstream" from the point of delivery of medical services to the role of the health care system in delivering improved population health. It has even more rarely looked further upstream to social arrangements that determine the health achievement of societies.[4]

This omission is quite striking since a concern about "health equity" and its social determinants has emerged as an important consideration in the policies of several European countries over the last two decades.[5] The World Health Organization (WHO) has devoted increasing attention to inequalities in health status and the policies that cause or mitigate them. So have research initiatives, such as the Global Health Equity Initiative, funded by the Swedish International Development Agency and the Rockefeller Foundation.

In what follows, we attempt to fill this bioethical gap by addressing some of these questions about justice and health inequalities. Rather than canvass answers that might be extracted from various competing theories of justice, however, we shall work primarily within the framework of John Rawls's theory of "justice as fairness" and the extension one of us has made of it to health care, probing the resources of that theory to address these issues.[6] Our contention is that Rawls's (extended) theory provides, albeit unintentionally, a defensible account of how to distribute the social determinants of health fairly. If we are right, this unexpected application to a novel problem demonstrates a fruitful generalizability of the theory analogous to the extension in scope or power of a nonmoral theory and permits us to think more systematically across the disciplines of public health, medicine, and political philosophy.

The theory of justice as fairness was formulated to specify terms of social cooperation that free and equal citizens can accept as fair. Specifically, it assures people of equal basic liberties, including equal access to political participation; guarantees a robust form of equal opportunity; and imposes significant constraints on inequalities. Together, these principles aim at meeting the "needs of free and equal citizens," a form of egalitarianism Rawls calls "democratic equality."[7] A crucial component of democratic equality is providing all with the social bases of self-respect and a conviction that prospects in life are fair. As the empirical literature demonstrates, institutions conforming to these principles together focus on several crucial pathways through which many researchers believe inequality works to produce health inequality. Of course, this theory does not answer all of our questions about justice and health inequality since there are some crucial points on which it is silent, but it does provide considerable guidance on central issues.

Social Determinants of Health: Some Basic Findings

There are four central findings in the literature on the social determinants of health, each of which has implications for an account of justice and health inequalities. First, the income/health gradients we observe are not the result of some fixed or determinate laws of economic development, but are influenced by policy choices. Second, the income/health gradients are not just the result of the deprivation of the poorest groups. Rather, a gradient in health operates across the whole socioeconomic spectrum within societies, such that the slope or steepness of the income/health gradient is affected by the degree of inequality in a society. Third, relative income or socioeconomic status (SES) is as important as, and may be more important than, the absolute level of income in determining health status, at least once societies have passed a certain threshold. Fourth, there are identifiable social and psychosocial pathways through which inequality produces its effects on health (and only modest support for "health selection," the claim that health status determines economic position).[8] These causal pathways are amenable to specific policy choices that should be guided by considerations of justice.

Cross-National Evidence on Health Inequalities

The pervasive finding that prosperity is related to health, whether measured at the level of nations or at the level of individuals, might lead one to the conclusion that these "income/health gradients" are inevitable. They might seem to reflect the natural ordering of societies along some fixed, idealized teleology of economic development. At the individual level, the gradient might appear to be the result of the natural selection of the most "fit" members within a society who are thus better able to garner socioeconomic advantage.

Despite the appeal and power of these ideas, they run counter to the evidence. Figure 13.1 shows the relationship between the wealth and health of nations as measured by per capita gross domestic product (GDPpc) and life expectancy. There is a clear association between GDPpc and life expectancy, but only up to a point. The relationship levels off beyond about $8,000–$10,000 GDPpc, with virtually no further gains in life expectancy.

This leveling effect is most apparent among the advanced industrial economies (see figure 13.2), which largely account for the upper tail of the curve in figure 13.1. The leveling of the relationship between wealth and health is true *within* individual countries as well.

Closer inspection of these two figures points out some startling discrepancies. Though Cuba and Iraq are equally poor (GDPpc about $3,100), life expectancy in Cuba exceeds that in Iraq by 17.2 years. The difference between the GDPpc for Costa Rica and the United States, for example, is enormous (about $21,000), yet Costa Rica's

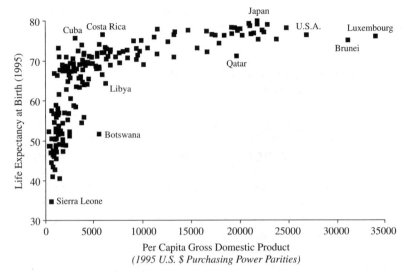

Figure 13.1 Relationship between country wealth and life expectancy.
Source: United Nations Human Development Report Statistics, 1998.

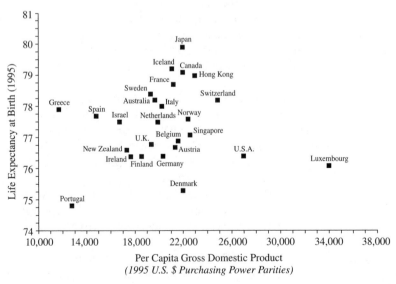

Figure 13.2 Per capita gross domestic product, 1995 U.S. $ purchasing-power parities.
Source: United Nations Human Development Report Statistics, 1998.

life expectancy exceeds that of the United States (76.6 versus 76.4). In fact, despite being one of the richest nations on the globe, the United States performs rather poorly on health indicators.

Taken together, these observations support the notion that the relationship between economic development and health is not fixed, and that the health achievement of nations is mediated by processes other than wealth. To account for the cross-national variations in health, it is apparent that other factors—such as culture, social organization, and government policies—are significantly involved in the determination of population health, and that variations in these factors may go some distance toward explaining the differences in health outcomes between nations.

If we are right that the health of nations does not reflect some inevitable natural order, but that it reflects policy choices—or features of society that are amenable to change via policies—then we must ask which of these policies are just.

Individual Socioeconomic Status and Health

At the individual level, numerous studies have documented what has come to be known as the "socioeconomic gradient." On this gradient, each increment up the socioeconomic hierarchy is associated with improved health outcomes over the rung below.[9] It is important to observe that this relationship is not simply a contrast between the health of the rich and the poor but is observed across all levels of socioeconomic status. What is particularly notable about the SES gradient is that it does not appear to be explained by differences in access to health care. Steep gradients have been observed even among groups of individuals, such as British civil servants, with adequate access to health care, housing, and transport.[10]

Importantly, the steepness of the gradient varies substantially across societies. Some societies show a relatively shallow gradient in mortality across SES groups. Others, with comparable or even higher levels of economic development, show much steeper gradients in mortality rates across the socioeconomic hierarchy. The determining factor in the steepness of the gradient appears to be the extent of income inequality in a society. Thus, middle-income groups in a country with high income inequality may have lower health status than comparable or even poorer groups in a society with less income inequality. We find the same pattern within the United States when we examine state and metropolitan area variations in inequality and health outcomes.[11]

Relative Income and Health

The apparent connection between the distribution of income in a society and the level of health achievement of its members is a relatively recent finding.[12] Simply stated, it is not just the size of the economic pie but how the pie is shared that matters for population health. It is not the absolute deprivation associated with low economic development (lack of access to the basic material conditions necessary for health such as clean water, adequate nutrition and housing, and general sanitary living conditions) that explains health differences between developed nations, but the degree of *relative* deprivation within them. Relative deprivation refers not to a lack of the "goods" that are basic to survival, but rather to a lack of sources of self-respect that are deemed essential for full participation in society.

Numerous studies have provided support for the relative-income hypothesis, both between and within nations.[13] This finding helps to explain the anomalies highlighted in figures 13.1 and 13.2. Much of the variation in life expectancy for the wealthy countries in the upper tail of figure 13.1 is explained by income distribution: Countries with more equal income distributions, such as Sweden and Japan, have higher life expectancies than do countries such as the United States, regardless of GDPpc. Furthermore, countries with much lower GDPpc, such as Costa Rica, appear to be able to obtain their remarkably high life expectancy through a more equitable distribution of income.

Within the United States, income inequality accounts for about 25 percent of the between-state variance in age-adjusted mortality rates independent of state median income.[14] Moreover, the size of this relationship is not trivial. A recent study across U.S. metropolitan areas, rather than states, found that areas with high income inequality had an excess of death compared to areas of low inequality that was equivalent in magnitude to all deaths due to heart disease.[15]

While most of the evidence so far has been accumulated from cross-sectional data, time-trend data support similar conclusions. Widening income differentials in the United States and the United Kingdom appear to be related to a slowing down of life expectancy improvements. In many of the poorest areas of the United Kingdom, mortality for younger age cohorts has actually increased during the same period that income inequality widened.[16] In the United States, states with the highest income inequality showed slower rates of life expectancy improvement compared to states with more equitable income distributions between 1980 and 1990.[17]

As we noted above, income distribution appears to affect the health of populations by shifting the slope of the curve relating individual income to health. This can be clearly seen in figure 13.3, where the prevalence of self-reported fair/poor health is higher (and the gradient steeper) in almost every income group for those living in states with the highest income inequality.[18] Nearly identical patterns have been found for individual mortality rates.[19]

Pathways Linking Social Inequalities to Health Inequalities

Our final contention is that there are plausible and identifiable pathways through which social inequalities produce inequalities in health. Some of these occur at the societal level, where income inequality creates a pattern for the distribution of social goods, such as public education, thereby affecting access to life opportunities—which are, in turn, strong determinants of health.

The evidence for these associations, while fairly new, is quite striking. In the United States, the most inegalitarian states with respect to income distribution invest less in public education, have larger uninsured populations, and spend less on social safety nets.[20] Differences in human capital investment, typically measured in terms of educational spending and (more important) educational outcomes, are particularly striking. Even when controlling for median income, income inequality explains about 40

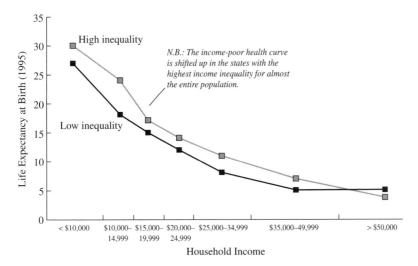

Figure 13.3 Self-related health and individual household income in the U.S.
Source: Ichiro Kawachi and Bruce P. Kennedy, "Income Inequality and Health: Pathways and Mechanisms," *Health Services Research* 34 (1999): 215–227.

percent of the between-state variation in the percentage of children in the fourth grade who fall below the basic reading level. Similarly strong associations are seen in the percentage of high school dropout rates. It is quite evident from these data that educational opportunities for children in high income inequality states are quite different from those in states with more egalitarian distributions.

Differential investment in human capital is also a strong predictor of health across nations. Indeed, one of the strongest predictors of life expectancy among developing countries is adult literacy, particularly the disparity between male and female adult literacy. For example, among the 125 developing countries with GDPpc less than $10,000, the difference between male and female literacy accounts for 40 percent of the variance in life expectancy after factoring out the effect of GDPpc. The fact that gender disparities in access to basic education drive the level of health achievement emphasizes further the role of broader social inequalities in patterning health inequalities. Indeed, in the United States, differences between the states in women's status—measured in terms of their economic autonomy and political participation—are strongly correlated with female mortality rates.[21]

These societal mechanisms are tightly linked to the political processes that influence government policy. One way that income inequality affects health and social welfare appears to be through its role in undermining civil society. Income inequality erodes social cohesion, as measured by levels of social mistrust and participation in civic organizations, both of which are features of civil society.[22] Lack of social cohesion is in turn reflected in significantly lower participation in political activity (e.g., voting, serving in local government, volunteering for political campaigns, etc.), thus undermining the responsiveness of government institutions in addressing the needs of the worst off in society. This is demonstrated by the human capital investment data presented earlier, but it is also reflected by the lack of investment in human security. States with the highest income inequality, and thus the lowest levels of social capital and political participation, are far less generous in the provision of social safety nets. For example, the correlation between social capital, as measured by low interpersonal trust, and the maximum welfare grant as a percent of state per capita income is –0.76.[23]

How can the points we have highlighted from scientific literature on social determinants be integrated into our views about the moral acceptability of health inequalities? Historically, disciplinary boundaries have stood as an obstacle to an integrated perspective. The social science and public health literature sharpens our understanding of the causes of health inequalities, but it contains no systematic way to evaluate the overall fairness of those inequalities and the socioeconomic inequalities that produce them. The philosophical literature has produced theories aimed at evaluating socioeconomic inequalities, but it has tended to ignore health inequalities and their causes. To produce an integrated view, we shall need the resources of a more general theory of justice. We can better see the need for such a theory if we first examine an analysis of "health inequities" that has been developed within a policy-oriented public health literature.

Health Inequalities and Inequities

When is a health inequality between two groups "inequitable"? This version of our earlier question about health inequalities and justice has been the focus of European and WHO efforts, as noted above. One initial answer that has been influential in the WHO programs is the claim, posited in writings by such researchers as Margaret Whitehead and Goran Dahlgren, that health inequalities count as inequities when they are *avoidable, unnecessary,* and *unfair.*[24] If we can agree on what is avoidable, unnecessary, and unfair—and if this analysis is correct—then we can agree on which inequalities are inequitable.

Age, gender, race, and ethnic differences in health status exist that are independent of socioeconomic differences, and they raise distinct questions about equity or justice. For example, should we view the lower life expectancy of men compared to women in developed countries as an inequity? If it is rooted in biological differences that we do not know how to overcome, then, according to this analysis, it is not avoidable and therefore not an inequity. This is not an idle controversy: Taking average, rather than gender-differentiated, life expectancy in developed countries as a benchmark will yield different estimates of the degree of inequity women face in some developing countries. In any case, the analysis of inequity is here only as good as our understanding of what is avoidable or unnecessary.

The same point applies to judgments about fairness. Is the poorer health status of some social classes or ethnic groups that engage in heavy tobacco and alcohol use unfair? We may be inclined to say it is not unfair, provided that participation in the risky behaviors or their avoidance is truly voluntary. But if many people in a cultural group or class behave similarly, there may also be factors at work that reduce how voluntary their behavior is and how much responsibility we should ascribe to them for it.[25] The analysis thus leaves us with the unresolved complexity of these judgments about responsibility and, as a result, with disagreements about fairness (or avoidability).

The poor in many countries lack access to clean water, sanitation, adequate shelter, basic education, vaccinations, and prenatal and maternal care. As a result of some or all of these factors, there are infant mortality differences between these and richer groups. Since social policies could supply the missing determinants of infant health, the inequalities must be regarded as avoidable. Are these inequalities also unfair? Most of us would immediately think they are, perhaps from a view that policies that not only countenance but sustain poverty are unjust. Social policies that compound poverty with a lack of access to the determinants of health may be viewed as doubly unfair. Of course, libertarians would disagree. They would insist that what is merely unfortunate is not unfair; in their view, society has no obligation of justice (as opposed to charity) to provide the poor with what they are missing.

Many of us might be inclined to reject the libertarian view as in itself unjust because of the dramatic conflict it opens with our beliefs about poverty and our social obligations to meet people's basic needs. The problem becomes more complicated, however, when we remember one of the basic findings from the literature on social determinants: We cannot eliminate health inequalities simply by eliminating poverty. Health inequalities persist even in societies that provide the poor with access to all of the determinants of health noted above, and they persist as a gradient of health throughout the social hierarchy, not just between the very poorest groups and those above them.

Faced with this realization, many of us may have to reexamine what we believe about the justice of other sorts of socioeconomic inequalities. Unless we believe that all socioeconomic inequalities (or at least all inequalities we did not choose) are unjust—and very few embrace such a radically egalitarian view—then we must consider more carefully the problem posed by the health gradient and the fact that it is made steeper under more unequal social arrangements. Judgments about fairness—to which many, rightly or wrongly, feel confident in appealing when rejecting the libertarian position—give less guidance than perhaps had been expected in thinking about the broader issue of the social determinants of health inequalities. Indeed, we may even believe that some degree of socioeconomic inequality is unavoidable or even necessary and therefore not unjust.

Justice as Fairness and Health Inequalities

One reason we develop general ethical theories, including theories of justice, is to provide a framework within which to resolve important disputes of the sort we have just raised about conflicting moral beliefs or intuitions. For example, in *A Theory of Justice* John Rawls sought to leverage the relatively broad liberal agreement on principles guaranteeing certain equal basic liberties into an agreement on a principle limiting socioeconomic inequalities—a matter on which liberals disagree considerably.[26] His strategy was to show that a social contract designed to be fair to free and equal people ("justice as [procedural] fairness") would not only justify the choice of those equal basic liberties but would also justify the choice of principles guaranteeing equal opportunity and limiting inequalities to those that work to make the worst-off groups fare as well as possible.

Our contention is that Rawls's account, though developed to answer this general question about social justice without specifically contending with issues of disease or health, turns out to provide useful principles for the just distribution of the social determinants of health. To simplify the construction of his theory, Rawls assumed his contractors would be fully functional over a normal life span—i.e., that no one would become ill or die prematurely.

This idealization itself provides a clue about how to extend this theory to the real world of illness and premature death. The goal of public health and medicine is to keep people as close as possible to the ideal of normal functioning, under reasonable resource constraints. (Resources are necessarily limited since maintaining health cannot be our only social good or goal.) Since the maintenance of normal functioning makes a limited but significant contribution to protecting the range of opportunities open to all individuals, it is plausible to see a principle guaranteeing equality of opportunity satisfying the condition of fairness as the appropriate principle to govern the distribution of health care, broadly construed to include primary and secondary preventive health as well as medical services.[27]

What is particularly appealing about examining the social determinants of health inequalities from the perspective of Rawls's theory is that the theory is egalitarian in orientation and yet justifies certain inequalities that might contribute to health inequalities. In addition, Norman Daniels's extension of Rawls links the protection of health to the protection of equality of opportunity, again setting up the potential for internal conflict. To see whether this combination of features leads to insight into the problem or simply to contradictions in the theory, we must examine the issue in more detail.

How does Rawls justify socioeconomic inequalities? Why would free and equal contractors not simply insist on strictly egalitarian distribution of all social goods, just as they insist on equal basic liberties and equal opportunity?

Rawls's answer is that it is irrational for contractors to insist on equality if doing so would make them worse off. Specifically, he argues that contractors would choose his Difference Principle, which permits inequalities provided that they work to make the worst-off groups in society as well off as possible.[28] The argument for the Difference Principle appears to suggest that relative inequality is less important than absolute well-being, a suggestion that is in tension with other aspects of Rawls's view. Thus he also insists that inequalities allowed by the Difference Principle should not undermine the value of political liberty and the requirements of fair equality of opportunity. The priority given these other principles over the Difference Principle thus limits the inference that Rawls has no concern about relative inequality. Specifically, as we shall see, these principles work together to constrain inequality and to preserve the social bases of self-respect for all.

Two points will help avoid misunderstanding of the Difference Principle and its justification. First, it is not a mere "trickle-down" principle but one that requires maximal flow in the direction of helping the worst-off groups. The worst off, and then the next worst off, and so on (Rawls calls this "chain connectedness"[29]) must be made as well off as possible, not merely just somewhat better off, as a trickle-down principle implies. The Difference Principle is thus much more demanding than a principle that would permit any degree of inequality provided there was some "trickle" of benefits to the worst off. Indeed, it is more egalitarian than alternative principles that merely assure the worse off a "decent" or "adequate" minimum. From what we have learned about the social determinants of health, the more demanding Difference Principle would also produce less health inequality than any proposed alternative principles that allow inequalities. By flattening the health gradient, it would also benefit middle-income groups, not simply the poorest. In this regard, its benefits are important beyond the level at which we have helped the worst off to achieve "sufficiency." This point provides a reply to those who suggest that the Difference Principle has no appeal once the worst off are sufficiently provided for.[30]

Second, when contractors evaluate how well off the principles they choose will make them, they judge their well-being by an index of "primary social goods."[31] The primary social goods, which Rawls thinks of as the "needs of citizens," include liberty, powers, opportunities, income and wealth, and the social bases of self-respect. (These objective measures of well-being should be contrasted with measures of happiness or desire-satisfaction that are familiar from utilitarian and welfare economic perspectives.) In his exposition of the Difference Principle, Rawls illustrates how it will work by asking us to consider only the simpler case of income inequalities. In doing so, he assumes that the level of income will correlate with the level of other social goods on the index.

This simplification should not mislead us, for, in crucial cases, the correlation may not obtain. For example, let us suppose that having "democratic" control over one's workplace is crucial to self-realization and the promotion of self-esteem.[32] Suppose further that hierarchical workplaces are more efficient than democratic ones, so that a system with hierarchical workplaces would have resources to redistribute that meant higher incomes for worst-off workers than democratic workplaces would permit. Then the Difference Principle does not clearly tell us whether the hierarchical workplace contains allowable inequalities since the worst off are better off in some ways but worse off in others. Without knowing the weighting of items in the index, we cannot use it to say clearly what inequalities are permitted. When we are evaluating which income inequalities are allowable, by asking which ones work to make the worst-off groups as well off as possible, we must, in any case, judge how well off groups are by reference to the whole index of primary goods—not simply the resulting income.

This point is of particular importance in the current discussion. Daniels's extension of Rawls treats health status as a determinant of the range of opportunity open to individuals. Since opportunity is included in the index, the effects of health inequalities are thereby included in the index.

Rawls says very little, however, about how items in the index are to be weighted. Therefore we have little guidance about how these primary goods are to be traded off against each other in its construction. This silence pertains not only to the use of the index in the contract situation, but also to its use, as we will examine more closely below, by a legislature trying to apply the principles of justice in a context in which many specific features of a society are known.

We can now say more directly why justice, as described by Rawls's principles, is good for our health. To understand this claim, let us start with the ideal case, a society governed by Rawls's principles of justice that seeks to achieve "democratic equality."[33] Consider what it requires with regard to the distribution of the social determinants of health. In such a society, all are guaranteed equal basic liberties, including the liberty of political participation. In addition, there are institutional safeguards aimed at assuring all, richer and poorer alike, the worth or value of political participation rights. Without such assurance, basic capabilities of citizens cannot develop. The recognition that all citizens must have these capabilities protected is critical to preserving self-esteem, in Rawls's view. Since there is evidence, as we have seen, that political participation is itself a social determinant of health, the Rawlsian ideal assures institutional protections that counter the usual effects of socioeconomic inequalities on participation and thus on health.

The Rawlsian ideal of democratic equality also involves conformity with a principle guaranteeing a fair distribution of equality of opportunity. Not only are discriminatory barriers prohibited by the principle; it requires as well robust measures aimed at mitigating the effects of socioeconomic inequalities and other social contingencies on opportunity. In addition to equitable public education, such measures would include the provision of developmentally appropriate day care and early childhood interventions intended to promote the development of capabilities independently of the advantages of family background. Such measures match or go beyond the best models we see in European efforts at day care and early childhood education. We also note that the strategic importance of education for protecting equal opportunity has implications for all levels of education, including access to graduate and professional education.

The equal opportunity principle also requires extensive public health, medical, and social support services aimed at promoting normal functioning for all.[34] It even provides a rationale for the social costs of reasonable accommodation to incurable disabilities, as required by the Americans with Disabilities Act.[35] Because the principle aims at promoting normal functioning for *all* as a way of protecting opportunity for all, it simultaneously aims at both improving population health and reducing health inequalities. Obviously, this focus requires the provision of universal access to comprehensive health care, including public health, primary health care, and medical and social support services.

To act justly in health policy, we must have knowledge about the causal pathways through which socioeconomic (and other) inequalities work to produce differential health outcomes. Suppose we learn, for example, that structural and organizational features of the workplace inducing stress and a sense of a loss of control tend to promote health inequalities. We should then view the modification of those features of workplace organization as a public health requirement of the equal opportunity principle in order to mitigate their negative effects on health. It would thus be placed on a par with the requirement that we reduce exposures to toxins in the workplace.[36]

Finally, in the ideal Rawlsian society, the Difference Principle places significant restrictions on allowable inequalities in income and wealth.[37] The inequalities allowed by this principle (in conjunction with the principles assuring equal opportunity and the value of political participation) are probably more constrained than those we observe in even the most industrialized societies. If so, then the inequalities that conform to the Difference Principle would produce a flatter gradient of health inequality than we currently observe in even the more extensive welfare systems of northern Europe.

In short, Rawls's principles of justice regulate the distribution of the key social determinants of health, including the social bases of self-respect. There is nothing about the theory, or Daniels's extension of it, that should make us focus narrowly on medical services. Properly understood, justice as fairness tells us what justice requires in the distribution of all socially controllable determinants of health.

We still face a theoretical issue of some interest. Even if the Rawlsian distribution of the determinants of health flattens health gradients further than what we observe in the most egalitarian, developed countries, we must still expect a residue of health inequalities. In part, this may happen because we may not have adequate knowledge of all the relevant causal pathways or interventions that are effective in modifying them. The theoretical issue is whether the theory requires us to reduce *further* those otherwise justifiable inequalities because of the inequalities in health status they create.

We should not further reduce those socioeconomic inequalities if doing so reduces productivity to the extent that we can no longer support the institutional measures we already employ to promote health and reduce health inequalities. Our commitment to reducing health inequality should not require steps that threaten to make health worse for those with less-than-equal health status. So the theoretical issue reduces to this: Would it ever be reasonable and rational for contractors to accept a trade-off in which some health inequality is allowed in order to produce some nonhealth benefits for those with the worst health prospects?

We know that in real life people routinely trade health risks for other benefits. They do so when they commute longer distances for a better job or take a ski vacation. Some such trades raise questions of fairness. For example, when is hazard pay a benefit workers gain only because their opportunities are unfairly restricted, and when is it an appropriate exercise of their autonomy?[38] Many such trades we would not restrict, thinking it unjustifiably paternalistic to do so; others we see as unfair.

Rawlsian contractors, however, cannot make such trades on the basis of any specific knowledge of their own values. They cannot decide that their enjoyment of skiing makes it worth the risks to their knees or necks. To make the contract fair to all participants, and to achieve impartiality, Rawls imposes a thick "veil of ignorance" that blinds them to all knowledge about themselves, including their specific views of the good life. Instead, they must judge their well-being by reference to an index of primary social goods (noted earlier) that includes a weighted measure of rights, opportunities, powers, income and wealth, and the social bases of self-respect. When Kenneth Arrow first reviewed Rawls's theory, he argued that this index was inadequate because it failed to tell us how to compare the ill rich with the well poor.[39] Amartya Sen has argued that the index is insensitive to the way in which disease, disability, or other individual variations would create inequalities in the capabilities of people who had the same primary social goods.[40] By extending Rawls's theory to include health care through the equal opportunity account, some of Arrow's (and Sen's) criticism is undercut.[41] But even raising our question about residual health inequalities reminds us that the theory says too little about the construction of the index to provide us with a clear answer.

One of Rawls's central arguments for singling out a principle protecting equal basic liberties and giving it (lexical) priority over his other principles of justice is his claim that once people achieve some threshold level of material well-being, they would not trade away the fundamental importance of liberty for other goods.[42] Making such a trade might deny them the liberty to pursue their most cherished ideals, including their religious beliefs, whatever they turn out to be. Can we make the same argument about trading health for other goods?

There is some plausibility to the claim that rational people would refrain from trades of health for other goods. Loss of health may preclude us from pursuing what we most value in life. We do, after all, see people willing to trade almost anything to regain health once they lose it. If we take this argument seriously, we might conclude that Rawls should give opportunity—considered as including the effects of health status—a heavier weighting in the construction of the index than income alone.[43] Such a weighting would mean that absolute increases in income that might otherwise have justified increasing relative income inequality, according to the Difference Principle, now fail to justify that inequality because of the negative effects on opportunity. Although the income of the worst off would increase, they would not be better off according to the whole (weighted) index of primary social goods, and so the greater inequality would not be permitted. Rawls's simplifying assumption about income correlating with other goods fails in this case (as it did in the hypothetical example about workplace democracy cited earlier).

Nevertheless, there is also strong reason to think that the priority given to health, and thus opportunity, is not as clear-cut as the previous argument implies—especially where the trade is between a *risk* to health and other goods that people highly value. Refusing to allow any (*ex ante*) trades of health risks for other goods, even when the background conditions on choice are otherwise fair, may seem unjustifiably paternalistic, perhaps in a way that refusing to allow trades of basic liberties is not.

We propose a pragmatic route around this problem, one that has a precedent elsewhere in Rawls. Fairness in equality opportunity, Rawls admits, is only approximated even in an ideally just system because we can only mitigate, not eliminate, the effects of family and other social contingencies.[44] For example, only if we were willing to violate widely respected parental liberties could we intrude into family life and "rescue" children from parental values that arguably interfere with equal opportunity. Similarly, though we give a general priority to equal opportunity over the Difference Principle, we cannot achieve complete equality in health any more than we can achieve completely equal opportunity. Even ideal theory does not produce perfect justice. Justice is always rough around the edges. Specifically, if we had good reason to think that "democratic equality" had flattened inequalities in accord with the principles of justice, then we might be inclined to think we had done as much as was reasonable to make health inequalities fair to all. The residual inequalities that emerge in conformance to the principles are not a "compromise" with what justice ideally requires; they are acceptable as just.

So far, we have been considering whether the theoretical question of a health trade-off can be resolved from the perspective of individual contractors. Instead, suppose that the decision about such a trade-off is to be made through the legislature in a society that conforms to Rawls's principles. Because those principles require effective political participation across all socioeconomic groups, we can suppose that groups most directly affected by any trade-off decision have a voice in the decision. Since there is a residual health *gradient,* groups affected by the trade-off include not only the worst off, but those in the middle as well. A democratic process that involved deliberation about the trade-off and its effects might be the best we could do to provide a resolution of the unanswered theoretical question.[45]

In contrast, where the fair value of political participation is not adequately assured—and we doubt it is so assured in even our most democratic societies—we have much less confidence in the fairness of a democratic decision about how to trade health against other goods. It is much more likely under actual conditions that those who benefit most from the inequalities, i.e., those who are better off, also wield disproportionate political power and will influence decisions about trade-offs to serve their interests. It may still be that the use of a democratic process in nonideal conditions is the fairest resolution we can practically achieve, but it still falls well short of what an ideally just democratic process involves.

We have focused on Rawlsian theory because it provides, however unintentionally, a developed account of how to distribute the social determinants of health. Other, competing theories of justice, including some recent proposals about "equal opportunity for welfare or advantage," offer no similarly developed framework for distributing the key social determinants of health.[46] On the other hand, Sen's account of the importance of an egalitarian distribution of "capabilities" actually resembles the account offered by Daniels (and others) of equal opportunity and normal functioning more than it seems at first.[47] Elizabeth Anderson has imaginatively focused the discussion of capabilities on those needed if citizens are to have "democratic equality."[48] The result is a striking convergence with Rawls's view of democratic equality—although Rawls's ability to talk about the fair distribution of social determinants of health follows directly from his principles, whereas Anderson must appeal intuitively to an account of the capabilities needed by citizens.

Policy Implications for a Just Distribution of the Social Determinants of Health

We earlier suggested that the analyses of Whitehead and Dahlgren of health inequities (inequalities that are avoidable and unfair) are useful, provided that we can agree on what counts as avoidable and unfair. We then suggested that the Rawlsian account of justice as fairness provides a fuller account of what is fair and unfair in the distribution of the social determinants of health. The theory provides a more systematic way to think about which health inequalities are inequities.

Compared to that ideal, most health inequalities that we now observe worldwide among socioeconomic and racial or ethnic groups are "inequities" that should be remedied. Even some countries with the shallowest health gradients, such as Sweden and England, have viewed their own health inequalities as unacceptable and have initiated policy measures to mitigate them. The broader efforts of the World Health

Organization in this direction are, probably without exception, also aimed at true inequities.

A central policy implication of our discussion is that reform efforts to improve health inequalities must be intersectoral and not focused just on the traditional health sector. Health is produced not just by having access to medical prevention and treatment, but, to a measurably greater extent, by the cumulative experience of social conditions across the life course. In other words, by the time a 60-year-old patient is brought to the emergency room to receive medical treatment for a heart attack, that encounter represents the result of bodily insults accumulated over a lifetime. Medical care is, figuratively speaking, "the ambulance waiting at the bottom of the cliff." Much of the contemporary discussion about increasing access to medical care as a means of reducing health inequalities misses this point. An emphasis on intersectoral reform will recognize the primacy of social conditions, such as access to basic education, levels of material deprivation, a healthy workplace environment, and equality of political participation in determining the health achievement of societies.[49]

Before saying more about intersectoral reform, we want to head off what from our view is a mistaken inference—namely, that we should ignore medical services and health sector reform because other steps have a bigger payoff. Even if we had a highly just distribution of the social determinants of health and of public health measures, people would still become ill and need medical services. The fair design of a health system should give weight to meeting actual medical needs.

We might think of those with known needs and those who are ill as "identified victims," whereas we might think of those whose lives would be spared illness by robust public health measures and a fair distribution of social determinants as "statistical victims." Several theoretical perspectives, both utilitarian and nonutilitarian, would hold that we should consider all these lives impartially, judging statistical lives saved to be just as valuable or important as identified victims. Utilitarian approaches would push us to maximize net benefit by allocating resources from saving identified lives to saving statistical ones.

Other reasonable considerations, however, temper our inclination to reallocate in such an impartial way from identified to statistical victims. Many of us give some extra moral weight to the urgent needs of those already ill. Others, through their roles as medical providers, may legitimately believe that the good that they can achieve through their control over the delivery of medical care has a greater claim on them than the good that would be brought about by more indirect measures beyond their control. More generally, many of us will be connected as family members and friends to the identified victims and will feel that we have "agent-relative" obligations to assist them that supersede the obligations we have to more distant, statistical victims.

It is impossible to dismiss the relevance of these other considerations. Consequently, we do not draw the inference that impartiality or rationality considerations might seem to support: namely, that we should immediately reallocate resources away from medical services to public health measures or a fairer distribution of social determinants in accordance with some algorithm based on the relative benefit, neutrally calculated, between statistical and identified lives. This is not to imply, however, that no reallocations are justifiable. No doubt some are, in light of what we have argued.[50]

What sorts of social policies should governments pursue in order to reduce health inequalities? Certainly, the menu of options should include equalizing access to medical care, but it should also include a broader set of policies aimed at equalizing individual life opportunities, such as investment in basic education, affordable housing, income security, and other forms of antipoverty policy. Though the connection between these broad social policies and health may seem somewhat remote, and though such policies are rarely linked to issues of health in our public policy discussions, growing evidence suggests that they should be so linked. The kinds of policies suggested by a social-determinants perspective encompass a much broader range of instruments than would be ordinarily considered for improving the health of the population. We discuss three such examples of social policies that hold promise of abating socioeconomic disparities in health: investment in early childhood development, improvement in the quality of the work environment, and reduction in income inequality.

The Case for Early Life Intervention

Growing evidence points to the importance of the early childhood environment in influencing the behavior, learning, and health of individuals later in the life course. Providing equal opportunities within a Rawlsian framework translates into intervening as early in life as possible. Several studies have demonstrated the benefits of early supportive environments for children. In the Perry High/Scope Project, children in poor economic circumstances were provided a high-quality early childhood development program between the ages of three and five.[51] Compared to the control group, those in the intervention group completed more schooling by age 27; were more likely to be employed, own a home, and be married with children; experienced fewer criminal problems and teenage pregnancies; and were far less likely to have mental-health problems.

Compensatory education and nutrition in the early years of life (as exemplified by the Head Start and WIC [Special Supplemental Nutrition Program for Women, Infants, and Children] programs) have been similarly shown to yield important gains for the most disadvantaged groups. As part of Lyndon Johnson's War on Poverty, the U.S. government introduced two small compensatory education programs—Head Start for preschoolers and Chapter 1 (now Title 1) for elementary school children. Evaluations of these programs indicate that children who enroll in them learn more than those who do not. In turn, educational achievement is a powerful predictor of health in later life, partly because education provides access to employment and income and partly because education has a direct influence on health behavior in adulthood, including diet, smoking, and physical activity.[52]

A similarly persuasive case can be made for nutritional supplementation in low-income women and children. An analysis of the National Maternal and Infant Health Survey found that participation of low-income pregnant women in the WIC program (the Special Supplemental Nutrition Program for Women, Infants, and Children) was associated with about a 40 percent reduction in the risk of subsequent infant death.[53] A mother's nutritional state affects her infant's chance of death not just in the first year of life but also throughout the life course. Thus, a woman's prepregnant weight is one of the strongest predictors of her child's birth weight, and, in turn, low birth weight has been linked with increased risks of coronary heart disease, hypertension, and diabetes in later life. It follows that investing in policies to reduce early adverse influences may produce benefits not only in the present, but also in the long run and for future generations.

The Case for Improving the Quality of the Work Environment

We alluded earlier to the finding that the health status of workers is closely linked to the quality of their work environment, specifically to the amount of control and autonomy available to workers on their jobs. Low-control work environments—such as monotonous, machine-paced work (e.g., factory assembly lines) or jobs involving little opportunity for learning and utilization of new skills (e.g., supermarket cashiers)—tend to be concentrated among low-income occupations. The work of Marmot and his colleagues has shown that social disparities in health arise partly as a consequence of the way labor markets sort individuals into positions of unequal authority and control.[54] Exposure to low-control, high-demand job conditions not only is more common in lower-status occupations, but also places workers at increased risk of hypertension, cardiovascular disease, mental illness, musculoskeletal disease, sickness absence, and physical disability.[55]

A growing number of international case studies has concluded that it is possible to improve the level of control in workplaces by several means: increasing the variety of different tasks in the production process; encouraging workforce participation in the production process; and allowing more flexible work arrangements, such as altering the patterns of shift work, to make them less disruptive of workers' lives.[56] In some cases it may even be possible to redesign the workplace and enhance worker autonomy without affecting productivity since sickness absence may diminish as a consequence of a healthier workplace.

The Case for Income Redistribution

Many of the measures suggested by the social determinants perspective tend to fall into the category of antipoverty policy. However, research on the social determinants of health warns us that antipoverty policies *do not go far enough* in reducing unjust health disparities. Though none would disagree about putting priority on reducing the plight of the worst off, the fact is that health inequalities occur as a gradient: The poor have worse health than the near-poor, the near-poor fare worse than the lower middle class, the lower middle class do worse than the upper middle class, and so on up the economic ladder. Addressing the social gradient in health requires action above and beyond the elimination of poverty.

To address comprehensively the problem of health inequalities, governments must begin to address the issue of economic inequalities *per se*. As we noted above, growing international and intranational evidence suggests that the extent of socioeconomic disparities—that is, the size of the gap in incomes and assets between the top and bottom of society—is itself an important determinant of the health achievement of society, independent of the average standard of living.[57] Most importantly, economic disparities seem to influence the degree of equality in political participation (in the form of voting, donating to campaigns, contacting elected officials, and other forms of political activity): The more unequal the distribution of incomes and assets, the more skewed the patterns of political participation, and, consequently, the greater the degree of political exclusion of disadvantaged groups.[58]

Inequalities in political participation in turn determine the kinds of policies passed by national and local governments. For example, Kim Hill and his colleagues carried out a pooled time-series analysis for the 50 U.S. states from 1978 to 1990 to examine the relationship between the degree of mobilization of lower-class voters at election time and the generosity of welfare benefits provided by state governments.[59] Even after adjusting for other factors that might predict state welfare policies—such as the degree of public liberalism in the state, the federal government's welfare cost-matching rate for individual states, the state unemployment rate and median income, and the state tax effort—robust relationships were found between the extent of political participation by lower-class voters and the degree of generosity of state welfare payments. In other words, *who participates* matters for political outcomes, and the resulting policies have an important impact on the opportunities for the poor to lead a healthy life.

For both of the foregoing reasons—that it yields a higher level of health achievement as well as greater political participation—the reduction of income disparity ought to be a priority of governments concerned about addressing social inequalities in health. Although the scope of this essay precludes further consideration here, a number of levers do exist by which governments could address the problem of income inequality, spanning from the radical (a commitment to sustained full employment, collective wage bargaining, and progressive taxation) to the incremental (expansion of the earned income tax credit, increased child care credit, and a raise in the minimum wage).[60]

Implications for International Development Theory

Our discussion has implications for international development theory, as well as for the economic choices confronted by industrialized countries. To the extent that income distribution matters for the health status of given populations, it is not obvious that giving strict priority to economic growth is the optimal strategy for maximizing social welfare. Raising everyone's income will improve the health status of the poor (the trickle-down approach), but not as much as paying attention to the *distribution* of the social product. Within the developing world, a comparison of the province of Kerala in India with more unequal countries like Brazil and South Africa illustrates this point. Despite having only a third to a quarter of the income of Brazil or South Africa (and thereby having a higher prevalence of poverty in the absolute sense), the citizens of Kerala nonetheless live longer, most likely as a result of the higher priority that the government of Kerala accords to a fair distribution of economic gains.[61]

The real issue for developing countries is what *kind* of economic growth is salutary. Hence, Dreze and Sen distinguish between two types of successes in the rapid reduction of mortality, which they term "growth-mediated" and "support-led" processes.[62]

The former works mainly *through* fast economic growth, exemplified by mortality reductions in places like South Korea and Hong Kong. Their successes depended on the growth process being wide based and participatory (for example, applying full employment policies) and on the gains from economic growth being utilized to expand relevant social services in the public sector, particularly in health care and education. The experiences of these states stand in stark contrast to the example of countries like Brazil, which have similarly achieved rapid economic growth but lagged behind in health improvements.

In contrast to growth-mediated processes, "support-led" processes operate not through fast economic growth but through governments giving high priority to the provision of social services that reduce mortality and enhance the quality of life. Examples include China, Costa Rica, and the Indian state of Kerala (mentioned above).

A similar choice, between policies emphasizing growth versus those promoting greater equality, applies to developed nations as well. Application of the Rawlsian Difference Principle suggests that a society like the United States has much room to move toward a more equitable (perhaps a more European) distribution of its national income without suffering a loss in productivity or growth. At the same time it would benefit from a gain in the health status of its citizens.

Some Concluding Remarks about Bioethics

We noted earlier that bioethics has generally tended to focus on medicine at the point of delivery, attending inadequately to determinants of health "upstream" from the medical system itself. We have tried to remedy that by putting together two elements: empirical findings about the social determinants of health and the result of a philosophical attempt to construct a theory of justice that might apply to any society. We arrive at the result that social justice, as defined by that theory, is good for our health. In a society that complies with its principles of justice, health inequalities will be minimized, and population health status will be improved. A theory of social justice turns out to be a theory about how to distribute health status in a just way, at least if the social science is correct.

The failure of bioethics to look at the social determinants of population health is not primarily a philosophical failing, nor is it simply disciplinary blindness to the social science or public health literature. People in bioethics, like the public more generally, concentrate on medical care rather than social determinants, for complex sociological, political, and ideological reasons that we can only mention here. The public, encouraged by scientists and the media, is fascinated by every new biomedical discovery and has come to believe that most of our "success" in improving population health is the result of exotic science. Vast economic interests benefit from this orientation of public and bioethical attention. Economic incentives for people in bioethics come largely from medicine and the scientific and policy institutions that interact with medical delivery. The idea that scientific medicine is responsible for our health blinds us to socioeconomic inequality as a source of inequity in the realization of opportunity for health across the population. Science, we are told, can rescue us all from our shared biological fate, and so we should all unite in supporting a focus on medicine and, if we care about justice, on the equitable access of all to its benefits. Challenging deeper inequalities in society, however, is divisive, not unifying; it threatens those with the greatest power and the most to lose. In the absence of well-organized social movements capable of challenging that inequality, the complaints of public health advocates pointing out the need for more basic change, rather than simply joining existing forces asking for more and better medical care, can seem utopian.

There may be more here than an extension of the scope of Rawlsian moral theory. Earlier, we suggested that challenging Rawls's construct to address questions about the fair distribution of the social determinants of health might show the theory to be generalizable in fruitful ways. This generalizability is analogous to the increase in scope and power of a nonmoral theory when we discover that it can explain phenomena beyond the domain for which its laws were initially developed. What exactly is the analogy?

When an empirical theory turns out to explain new phenomena that were not part of the evidentiary base for its laws, we tend to conclude that the concepts incorporated in it are "projectable" in a desired way. We may think of them as better confirmed as a way of dividing up or describing the world. Rawls begins with certain political concepts thought crucial to our well-being—to meeting our needs as free and equal citizens of a democracy. Using these ideas, the goal was to identify terms of cooperation that all free and equal citizens could agree are fair and reasonable. It then turns out, given the social science literature, that the aspects of well-being captured by these ideas expand to include the health of the population as well. Whatever controversy might have been thought to surround some of these political components of well-being, they do connect—albeit empirically—to some incontrovertibly objective components of our social well-being, namely, the health of the population. If this were an empirical rather than a normative theory, we would think the evidence of projectability counted in its favor, constituting support for the theory. Is there additional "support" for Rawls's theory?

It turns out that the support we now give the theory might not be greatly reduced even if the facts were different about the relationship between socioeconomic inequality and health. However, that does not mean we should not add to the support we think the theory has if it turns out to have the projectability described earlier. A lack of evidence of greater projectability is not evidence against a theory; it is and should be a neutral finding. If, however, we found that population health was undermined by greater political well-being of the sort the original theory talked about (before its extension), then we would have a puzzle to address: Why is one aspect of our well-being working in opposition to other elements of it?

This discussion is admittedly too brief to establish a firm conclusion, but we are inclined to think there is some corroborative support for Rawls's theory in the fact that it generalizes to the phenomena of population health in this way. It is the coherence among these different areas of evidence and principle that gives us grounds for thinking the theory has additional justification.[63] This does not mean, of course, that standing objections to the theory, which we have deliberately not addressed, should be ignored.

Another lesson is illustrated by our results. Ethical inquiry is not just one kind of inquiry involving one type of method. This is true for inquiry into practical ethical issues, including bioethics. Sometimes the inquiry requires the importation of tools from political philosophy, from ethical theory, and from the social sciences (as we have done). Sometimes, depending on the problem, we make better progress by examining specific cases carefully and then trying to move to the level of principles and theory. Sometimes we are better off deploying theory or theory-based considerations and refining and adapting them in light of what we learn about particular cases and social science (as we have also done). Since ethical inquiry answers many different kinds of questions, this variability in appropriate method should not surprise us.

Since it is the overall coherence of our system of beliefs that provides us with justification for specific parts of it, we should not become enamored of the tools developed for or appropriate to specific aspects of ethical inquiry and overgeneralize about their importance to all inquiry. In some areas of inquiry in bioethics (or ethics more generally), progress is doomed if we remain insensitive to the local texture of a problem, including the way in which a particular society's beliefs play a role in its policies. But this observation should not lead us to question the relevance of reasons, principles, or theory that purports to bear on issues more universally, despite local texture. We risk impoverishing our inquiry if we insist on limiting ourselves to tools that are best designed for certain specific tasks when our project involves integrating those tasks with others.[64]

No doubt an examination of what policy regarding the distribution of health in a particular population is fair or just will have to take into account some aspects of local beliefs and culture. The same inquiry into policy must also attend to the general implications of social science and political philosophy where they frame the problems raised by local policy.

Norman Daniels, Bruce P. Kennedy, and Ichiro Kawachi are recipients of Robert Wood Johnson Foundation investigator awards in health policy research.

Notes

1. Louis Rene Villerme, *Tableau de l'Etat Physique et Moral des Ouvriers,* vol. 2 (Paris: Renourard, 1840). Cited in Bruce G. Link et al., "Social Epidemiology and the Fundamental Cause Concept: On the Structuring of Effective Cancer Screens by Socioeconomic Status," *Milbank Quarterly* 76 (1998): 375–402. Throughout, we view disease and disability as departures from (species-typical) normal functioning and view health and normal functioning as equivalent.

2. Michael Marmot, "Social Causes of Social Inequalities in Health," Harvard Center for Population and Development Studies, Working Paper Series 99.01, January 1999.

3. To avoid additional complexity, in this essay we concentrate on class or socioeconomic inequalities, though many of our points generalize to race and gender inequalities in health as well.

4. Goran Dahlgren and Margaret Whitehead, *Policies and Strategies to Promote Social Equity in Health* (Stockholm: Institute of Future Studies, 1991). Michaela Benzeval,

Ken Judge, and Margaret Whitehead, eds., *Tackling Inequalities in Health: An Agenda for Action* (London: King's Fund, 1995). Sarah Marchand, Daniel Wikler, and Bruce Landesman, "Class, Health, and Justice," *Milbank Quarterly* 76 (1998): 449–468.

5. Benzeval, Judge, and Whitehead, eds., *Tackling Inequalities in Health: An Agenda for Action,* 1–9.

6. John Rawls, *A Theory of Justice* (Cambridge, MA: Belknap Press of Harvard University Press, 1971). Norman Daniels, "Health-Care Needs and Distributive Justice," *Philosophy and Public Affairs* 10 (1981): 146–179. Norman Daniels, *Just Health Care* (New York: Cambridge University Press, 1985).

7. Rawls, *A Theory of Justice,* secs. 12–13; Norman Daniels, "Democratic Equality: Rawls's Complex Egalitarianism," in Samuel Freeman, ed., *Cambridge Companion to Rawls* (New York: Cambridge University Press, 2002), 241–276.

8. Marmot, "Social Causes," 6–7; Michael G. Marmot, "Social Differentials in Health Within and Between Populations," *Daedalus* 123(4) (1994): 197–216.

9. Douglas Black et al., *Inequalities in Health: The Black Report; The Health Divide* (London: Penguin Group, 1988). George Davey-Smith, Martin J. Shipley, and Geoffrey Rose, "Magnitude and Causes of Socioeconomic Differentials in Mortality: Further Evidence from the Whitehall Study," *Journal of Epidemiology and Community Health* 44 (1990): 265–270. Gregory Pappas et al., "The Increasing Disparity in Mortality between Socioeconomic Groups in the United States, 1960 and 1986," *New England Journal of Medicine* 329 (1993): 103–109. Nancy E. Adler et al., "Socioeconomic Status and Health: The Challenge of the Gradient," *American Psychologist* 49 (1994): 15–24.

10. Davey-Smith, Shipley, and Rose, "Magnitude and Causes of Socioeconomic Differentials in Mortality." Michael G. Marmot et al., "Contribution of Psychosocial Factors to Socioeconomic Differences in Health," *Milbank Quarterly* 76 (1998): 403–408.

11. Bruce P. Kennedy et al., "Income Distribution, Socioeconomic Status, and Self-rated Health: A U.S. Multi-level Analysis," *British Medical Journal* 317 (1998): 917–921. John W. Lynch et al., "Income Inequality and Mortality in Metropolitan Areas of the United States," *American Journal of Public Health* 88 (1998): 1074–1080.

12. Richard G. Wilkinson, "Income Distribution and Life Expectancy," *British Medical Journal* 304 (1992): 165–168; "The Epidemiological Transition: From Material Scarcity to Social Disadvantage?" *Daedalus* 123(4) (1994): 61–77.

13. Wilkinson, "Income Distribution and Life Expectancy"; Richard G. Wilkinson, *Unhealthy Societies: The Afflictions of Inequality* (London: Routledge, 1996).

14. Bruce P. Kennedy, Ichiro Kawachi, and Deborah Prothrow-Stith, "Income Distribution and Mortality: Test of the Robin Hood Index in the United States," *British Medical Journal* 312 (1996): 1004–1008. Published erratum appears in *British Medical Journal* 312 (11 May 1996): 1194. George A. Kaplan et al., "Inequality in Income and Mortality in the United States: Analysis of Mortality and Potential Pathways," *British Medical Journal* 312 (1996): 999–1003.

15. Lynch et al., "Income Inequality and Mortality in Metropolitan Areas of the United States."

16. Wilkinson, *Unhealthy Societies: The Afflictions of Inequality.*

17. Ichiro Kawachi, Bruce P. Kennedy, and Richard G. Wilkinson, eds., *The Society and Population Health Reader: Income Inequality and Health: A Reader* (New York: New Press, 1999). Kaplan et al., "Inequality in Income and Mortality in the United States."

18. Kennedy et al., "Income Distribution, Socioeconomic Status, and Self-Rated Health."

19. Kimberly Lochner, "State Income Inequality and Individual Mortality Risk: A Prospective Multilevel Study," Ph.D. dissertation, Harvard University, 1999.

20. Kaplan et al., "Inequality in Income and Mortality in the United States." Ichiro Kawachi and Bruce P. Kennedy, "Health and Social Cohesion: Why Care about Income Inequality?" *British Medical Journal* 314 (1997): 1037–1040.

21. Ichiro Kawachi et al., "Women's Status and the Health of Women: A View from the States," *Social Science and Medicine* 48 (1999): 21–32. Richard G. Wilkinson, Bruce P. Kennedy, and Ichiro Kawachi, "Women's Status and Men's Health in a Culture of Inequality," *International Journal of Health Services Research* (under review).

22. Kawachi and Kennedy, "Health and Social Cohesion." Ichiro Kawachi et al., "Social Capital, Income Inequality and Mortality," *American Journal of Public Health* 87 (1997): 1491–1498.

23. Ichiro Kawachi and Bruce P. Kennedy, "Income Inequality and Health: Pathways and Mechanisms," *Health Services Research* 34 (1999): 215–227. The level of interpersonal trust at the state level was gauged by responses to the General Social Surveys conducted by the National Opinion Research Center, which asked citizens questions such as "Generally speaking, would you say that most people can be trusted or that you can't be too careful in dealing with people?" This approach to measure social trust is the same as the approach adopted by Robert D. Putnam in his work on social capital: "Bowling Alone: America's Declining Social Capital," *Journal of Democracy* 6 (1995): 65–78.

24. Margaret Whitehead, "The Concepts and Principles of Equity and Health," *International Journal of Health Services* 22 (1992): 429–445. Dahlgren and Whitehead, *Policies and Strategies to Promote Social Equity in Health.* Paula Braveman, *Monitoring Equity in Health: A Policy-Oriented Approach in Low-and Middle-income Countries* (Geneva: World Health Organization, 1999).

25. Daniel Wikler, "Persuasion and Coercion for Health: Issues in Government Efforts to Change Life Style," *Milbank Quarterly* 56 (1978): 303–338. John E. Roemer, *Equality of Opportunity* (Cambridge, MA: Harvard University Press, 1998).

26. Joshua Cohen, "Democratic Equality," *Ethics* 99 (1989): 727–754.

27. Daniels, *Just Health Care.* John Rawls, *Political Liberalism* (New York: Columbia University Press, 1993).

28. A careful discussion of Rawls's argument for the Difference Principle and the extensive critical literature it has generated is beyond the scope of this essay. It is important, however, to distinguish Rawls's own social contract argument from the many informal and intuitive reformulations of it. See Brian Barry, *Theories of Justice* (London: Harvester Wheatsheaf, 1989), 213–234; Gerald A. Cohen, "Incentives, Inequality, and Community," in *The Tanner Lectures on Human Values,* vol. 13, ed. G. B. Petersen (Salt Lake City: University of Utah Press, 1992), 262–329. Gerald A. Cohen, "The Pareto Argument for Inequality," *Social Philosophy and Policy* 12 (Winter 1995): 160–185. Cohen, "Democratic Equality," 727–751. Daniels, "Rawls's Egalitarianism."

29. Rawls, *A Theory of Justice.*

30. Amy Gutmann and Dennis Thompson, *Democratic Disagreement* (Cambridge, MA: Harvard University Press, 1995).

31. Rawls, *A Theory of Justice,* 62; *Political Liberalism.*

32. This example is taken from Joshua Cohen, "The Pareto Argument," unpublished manuscript.

33. Daniels, "Rawls's Egalitarianism."

34. Daniels, *Just Health Care.* Norman Daniels, Donald W. Light, and Ronald L. Caplan, *Benchmarks of Fairness for Health Care Reform* (New York: Oxford University Press, 1996), 41–44.

35. Norman Daniels, "Mental Disabilities, Equal Opportunity, and the ADA," in Richard J. Bonnie and John Monahan, eds., *Mental Disorder, Work Disability, and the Law* (Chicago: University of Chicago Press, 1996), 282–297.

36. Daniels, *Just Health Care,* chaps. 7–8.

37. Cohen ("Incentives, Inequality, and Community") has argued that a *strict* interpretation of the Difference Principle would allow few incentive-based inequalities; for a more permissive view, see Daniels, "Rawls's Egalitarianism."

38. Daniels, *Just Health Care,* chap. 7.

39. Kenneth Arrow, "Uncertainty and the Welfare Economics of Medical Care," *American Economic Review* 53 (1963): 941–973.

40. Amartya K. Sen, "Equality of What?" in Sterling M. McMurrin, ed., *Tanner Lectures on Human Values,* vol. 1 (Cambridge: Cambridge University Press, 1980). Amartya K. Sen, *Inequality Reexamined* (Cambridge, MA: Harvard University Press, 1992).

41. Norman Daniels, "Equality of What: Welfare, Resources, or Capabilities?" *Philosophy and Phenomenological Research* 50 (1990): 273–296.

42. Rawls, *A Theory of Justice,* 243–251.

43. Rawls does suggest, since fair equality of opportunity is given priority over the Difference Principle, that within the index, we can assume opportunity has a heavier weighting. Rawls, *A Theory of Justice,* 93.

44. James Fishkin, *Justice, Equal Opportunity, and the Family* (New Haven, CT: Yale University Press, 1983).

45. Norman Daniels and James E. Sabin, "Limits to Health Care: Fair Procedures, Democratic Deliberation, and the Legitimacy Problem for Insurers," *Philosophy and Public Affairs* 26 (1997): 303–350.

46. Richard J. Arneson, "Equality and Equal Opportunity for Welfare," *Philosophical Studies* 54 (1988): 79–95. Gerald A. Cohen, "On the Currency of Egalitarian Justice," *Ethics* 99 (1989): 906–944. Roemer, *Equality of Opportunity,* chaps. 12–13.

47. For Sen's account, see Sen, *Inequality Reexamined,* chaps. 1–5, 9. For the account offered by Daniels and others, see Daniels, "Equality of What: Welfare, Resources, or Capabilities?"; A. Buchanan et al., *From Chance to Choice: Genetics and the Just Society* (New York: Cambridge University Press, 2000).

48. Elizabeth Anderson, "What Is the Point of Equality?" *Ethics* 109(2) (January 1999): 287–337; cf. Daniels, "Rawls's Egalitarianism."

49. John N. Lavis and Gregory L. Stoddart, "Can We Have Too Much Health Care?" *Daedalus* 123(4) (1994): 43–60.

50. Ibid.

51. Lawrence J. Schweinhart, Helen V. Barnes, and David P. Weikart, *Significant Benefits: The High/Scope Project Perry Preschool Study through Age 27* (Ypsilanti, MI: High/Scope Press, 1993).

52. Donald Acheson et al., *Report of the Independent Inquiry into Inequalities in Health* (London: Stationery Office, 1998).

53. Nancy E. Moss and Karen Carver, "The Effect of WIC and Medicaid on Infant Mortality in the United States," *American Journal of Public Health* 88 (1998): 1354–1361.

54. Michael G. Marmot et al., "Contribution of Job Control and Other Risk Factors to Social Variations in Coronary Heart Disease Incidence," *Lancet* 350 (1997): 235–239.

55. Robert A. Karasek and Tores Theorell, *Health Work* (New York: Basic Books, 1990), 83–157.

56. Acheson et al., *Report of the Independent Inquiry into Inequalities in Health,* 48–50.

57. Kawachi et al., *Income Inequality and Health.*

58. Kawachi and Kennedy, "Health and Social Cohesion"; "Income Inequality and Health."

59. Kim Quaile Hill, Jan E. Leighley, and Angela Hinton-Andersson, "Lower-Class Mobilization and Policy Linkage in the U.S. States," *American Journal of Political Science* 39 (1995): 75–86.

60. Kawachi et al., *Income Inequality and Health,* xxviii–xxx.

61. Amartya K. Sen, "Mortality as an Indicator of Economic Success and Failure," *The Economic Journal* 108 (1998): 1–25.

62. Jean Dreze and Amartya Sen, *Hunger and Public Action* (Oxford, U.K.: Clarendon Press, 1989), 183–187.

63. Norman Daniels, "Wide Reflective Equilibrium and Theory Acceptance in Ethics," *Journal of Philosophy* 76 (1979): 256–282.

64. Daniels, *Justice and Justification,* 333–352.

14

Health Policy in a New Key

Setting Democratic Priorities

Bruce Jennings

This is a time of transition and transformation in the American health care system. The question is not *whether* it will change in some fundamental ways in the coming decade, but *whither* it is going—what direction the change will take, what interests and ends it will serve, and what values will be promoted by those ends.

In this essay I am particularly concerned with two facets of this exceedingly large and complex problem. The first concerns the general issue of allocation in the health care system as a whole. The era when interest group liberalism predicated on the assumption of expanding resources worked tolerably well in health politics is over. An era of scarcity and the politics of hard choices and redistribution has begun, and in this new era more explicit value-laden policy rationales grounded on considerations of justice and equity must come to the fore. At this stage of the debate, we need to consider various conceptual maps and various ways of sorting out the allocation issues. In what follows I offer and explore one such map.

The second cluster of problems involves the process of reaching some type of value consensus adequate to guide health policymaking in an era of scarcity and the contribution that democratic values and grassroots participation can make to that process. Civic or participatory democratic activity is actually more widespread and vital in the United States today than is generally acknowledged in the national media or the policy science literature. Nonetheless, it is hard to imagine how participatory democracy could play any meaningful role in a policy domain so technically complex and so fraught with deeply entrenched economic interests as health care—the largest single sector of the U.S. economy.

This is certainly the conventional wisdom on the matter. And yet the conventional wisdom may eventually be startled—if not completely overturned—by the importance of grassroots democracy in future health policymaking. Eroded on almost every front by low voter turnout, the decline of political parties, media-dominated and image-oriented campaigns, the influence of political action committees (PACs), and the rest, democratic politics may find in the coming restructuring of the health care system and health policy a new vitality and a new lease on life. And so, too, the dilemmas of legitimacy and public morality in health policy allocation may find their only viable solution, not in ethical or economic theory, but in the public process and the political imagination embodied in a democratic consensus.

The Coming Politics of Allocation

In 1989 Americans spent $604.1 billion (11.1% of gross national product) on health care.[1] In 1992 that figure rose to $838.5 billion, and by 1994 health care costs may reach $1 trillion and over 16% of gross national product. Other Western nations with comparable or even better health indices than the United States spend one-third to one-half less than we do on their health care systems, while providing nearly universal access to basic medical care.[2]

The United States, by contrast, offers state-of-the-art medical technology and care to those well insured or supported by government benefits, but at the cost of denying access to basic, timely care to over 35 million persons. These so-called medically indigent people are largely the working poor and their families or those who make too much to qualify for Medicaid in their state even though their income is well below the federal poverty line. One in four children under age 18 lack adequate insurance coverage, a state of affairs that hampers their getting preventive and timely care. Nearly 30 percent of African Americans are uninsured, as are 41 percent of Hispanic Americans.[3] Persons without adequate health care coverage typically utilize medical services in a way that is not cost-effective, and they place a burden on hospitals for uncompensated care that has reverberations throughout the entire health care financing system. For far too many Americans in urban areas the emergency room door may be their first and only portal into the health care system; in rural areas even this entry is sometimes lacking.

These financial problems are but one facet of a profound malaise in the health care system and the health professions. The mission of health care institutions is being redefined. The respective responsibilities of the individual, the family, and the government to pay for needed health care are shifting. Providers find themselves faced with new patterns of employment and reimbursement, with new forms of utilization review, group practice, price controls, and the ever-present specter of legal liability. Finally, the ends and scope of medicine are changing as science and technology allow us to intervene in biologic processes that only yesterday were beyond our comprehension and control.

In the face of all this, there can simply be no doubt that in the coming years health policymakers will have to make many fundamental decisions affecting the future shape of the health care system. They will have to determine—much more carefully, self-consciously, and systematically than ever before—what types of care will be available, to whom, in what setting, at what cost, and who will pay for them. These are what I shall refer to generically as *allocation decisions.* (Sometimes they are called "rationing" decisions, but that is a term probably best avoided due to the confusion it causes.) There is no purely scientific or value-neutral way to make them; ethical and value questions will impinge upon these decisions every step of the way. But what kind of public understanding and support will influence these decisions? What kind of public understanding will be needed if rational health policy initiatives in the future are to succeed? How can particular communities—and the country as a whole—forge an agreement about what is fair, what is wise, what is affordable?

The state of Oregon, where one of the most comprehensive experiments in health care priority setting has been attempted, offers one model of the promise—and the difficulties—of taking a systematic and publicly accountable approach to reform. In the aftermath of a 1987 legislative decision to move Medicaid funds away from organ transplantation coverage (which affected about 30 people per year) to prenatal care (expanding services for over 1,500 women), there was a tremendous public controversy surrounding the case of a young boy with leukemia who was denied coverage for a bone marrow transplant. This controversy made it clear that setting one isolated treatment modality off against another in this piecemeal fashion was not a politically viable (or medically sensible) approach to priority setting, and in any case it did little to address systemic problems.

In 1989 the Oregon legislature passed important legislation that begins a multi-faceted approach to health policy reform designed to universalize basic health care coverage and to rationalize the utilization of medical services. The Oregon strategy was designed to be phased in several stages over a number of years. It attacked the allocation problem on several fronts. It extended Medicaid eligibility up to the federal poverty line and creates an 11-member Oregon Health Services Commission (OHSC) charged with constructing a prioritized list of health services on the basis of which the legislature would establish and fund a basic benefits package for Medicaid. It included the working poor in the system of health care coverage by requiring that virtually all employers in the state provide their employees and their dependents coverage at least equivalent to the basic benefits package of the Medicaid program. It also set up a state fund to cover those who would be otherwise uninsurable because of preexisting medical conditions.

Aspects of the master plan never were implemented, including a system of discounted prescription drugs and medical supplies made possible by centralized purchasing and the incorporation of all state employees into the basic health insurance system mandated of private employers and offered to the Medicaid population. If it had taken place, this could have important political consequences by reducing the isolation and stigmatization of the Medicaid program and by merging middle-class interests with those of the poor so as to protect the basic benefits package from excessively limited funding decisions by the legislature in the future.

To be implemented and financed, the Oregon reform plan required a waiver from the federal government's Medicare and Medicaid program requirements. In 1992 the Bush administration denied Oregon's request for a waiver, citing concerns that the Oregon plan may constitute discrimination against persons with certain types of disabilities. Policymakers in Salem were able to overcome these objections and received a more positive response from the Clinton administration, which granted the waiver in 1993.

For the purposes of this discussion, one of the most noteworthy features of the Oregon experiment is that there has been a substantial grassroots component to the work of the OHSC. After experimenting with several different methods of prioritizing services, based on the number of persons affected, the quality of life restored by the service, and cost, the commission constructed a list of 17 categories of health services into which 714 diagnosis-treatment pairs were placed.[4] The priority ranking of these categories was guided by the findings of several public outreach activities–public hearings; specially commissioned public surveys designed to reach low-income, minority, and disabled populations; and 47 town meetings held throughout the state by Oregon Health Decisions, a private, nonprofit community education group. When asked to deliberate about and articulate the basic values or human goods a health care system ought to serve, the grassroots process in Oregon revealed an emphasis on equity, quality of life, cost-effectiveness, functional independence, and community compassion.[5] The public did not rank order medical services directly in these town hall meetings and opinion surveys, but their deliberations did offer value orientations and definitions of quality of life that guided the OHSC as they put together their list.

Equally important, perhaps, the very grassroots process and its attendant publicity helped produce a climate of public discussion and education on health policy questions in the state that is unusual for this or any other public policy issue. It was a first step in a process that one could envision as a spreading and ongoing one. That, and not the specifics of its Medicaid program, may yet be Oregon's most important contribution to health policy reform. Parallel grassroots discussion projects on health care priorities are taking place in many states throughout the country, including California, Georgia, Michigan, New Jersey, and Vermont, where comprehensive health care reform legislation was passed in 1992.[6]

Rational, comprehensive planning is not the strong suit of our health care system. Yet we know that priorities are set, allocations are made, "rationing" does take place— these things are happening now; they are not simply questions for the future. Yet these are "quiet" allocation decisions that have not been publicly debated or endorsed. They grow out of cost-containment efforts, market forces, and other factors that influence health care utilization, leading providers and consumers alike to postpone or forgo care. In all likelihood, however, much more severe and explicit modes of priority setting and allocation choices lie ahead. In this respect, Oregon is now giving us a glimpse of a public debate that awaits most states and the federal government eventually. In the face of this prospect, current attempts to undertake public education and citizen involvement campaigns come none too soon. For surely it will be essential to develop some broad public consensus to guide public officials and others charged with designing a new system of health care delivery and finance.

And yet, as clearly predictable as these developments are, a serious, substantive public debate on the ethics of health care access and priorities has not yet begun in earnest in this country. Some initial efforts to enhance public understanding of the problem of health care priorities have been made, to be sure. Occasionally, rationing issues are addressed, fleetingly, in the mass media, particularly when some identifiable and sympathetic victim of a denial of benefits becomes the focus of attention. But these efforts are only a beginning. The time has come to move the public discussion of health care allocation to a new, more substantive level, and to create the resources and a process for doing so.

The Scope of the Allocation Question

As I use the term here, health care allocation encompasses three distinct, yet intertwined, sets of issues: (1) setting limits to the routine utilization of expensive new medical procedures of uncertain efficacy; (2) setting priorities among currently recognized health care needs and health goals; and (3) determining how access to medical resources should be distributed—how equitable should access be, and what should everyone be entitled to have access to?

1. *Allocation as setting limits.* Allocation decisions made by society through the mechanism of public policy and financing arrangements involve the setting of justifiable limits to new health care possibilities opened up by advancing science and technology. In the past, we have very rarely said no to any potentially promising medical or technological advance. In the future, it will be necessary to be more discerning and more discriminating about the new therapies and procedures we decide first to research, then to add to standard medical practice, and finally to make widely available through public financial support and private insurance coverage.

2. *Allocation as setting priorities.* Allocation also means establishing priorities among those forms of care that are already provided on a more or less routine basis to patients. In an aging society where acute and chronic illness are both bound to become more prevalent, we will inevitably face trade-offs between the goals of preventive and curative medicine, between acute and chronic care, between prolonging the life span and enhancing the quality of life. These hard choices will also arise between the conflicting needs of different age groups in society—a dilemma that is already being felt within state Medicaid programs, where the health care needs of poor children are competing for scarce funds with the long-term care needs of the elderly.

3. *Allocation as just access to health care.* The final broad component of the allocation issue is the just and equitable distribution of access to basic health care. This is an important component of the analysis because efforts to set explicit priorities run the risk of disproportionately burdening the least powerful and least well off, if we take the current pattern of health care access as a given and a starting point. Thus it is important to insist that the public policy problem of allocation is one of getting the currently disenfranchised into the health care system as well as one of deciding what they will be offered once they get there. In other words, priority setting is not simply a matter of cost containment. And the policy problem is a comprehensive one involving both private and governmental financing systems; it is not, and should not be, limited to state Medicaid program benefits.

Setting limits and setting priorities are particularly difficult, it is true, in medicine and health care.[7] They are difficult because the values at stake are so important and because Americans have come to expect so much from modern medicine. Thus far we have not engaged in a comprehensive and searching public discussion about the ethics of health care allocation. We have not engaged in that discussion because we have not had to. Until now. And even today when a growing chorus of physicians, professional associations, business leaders, and public officials are calling for a more rational, fairer, and less arbitrary system of utilizing our health care resources, there is still a great hesitancy and resistance in some quarters to taking priority setting seriously.

Some maintain that the ethical issues of allocation will not have to be faced because the problems we see today can be solved by greater efficiency. If we could "cut the fat" from the system, we would not have to ration at the clinical level or set limits or priorities at the level of the health care system as a whole. If we eliminate wasteful utilization, the argument goes, then we would have the necessary resources available to meet everyone's genuine, basic medical needs. In that case, no truly worthwhile—or even marginally useful—medical benefit would have to be denied anyone.

For the last 15 years or so, cost containment—the search for greater efficiency through market competition and financial incentives—has been the centerpiece of American health policy. The experiment with cost containment has shown that our ability to cut the fat is more limited overall than was expected, and it is more limited in some areas of medical care than in others. After a brief slowdown in the mid-1980s, health care expenditures have begun to accelerate once again, running about twice as high as the general rate of inflation. Reducing the length of hospital stays, as the prospective payment (DRG [diagnosis related group]) system has, for example, is clearly not a complete solution; the health care system is like a balloon—you contract it on one side, and it expands somewhere else. Also, cutbacks in Medicare and Medicaid reimbursements may temporarily reduce the amount of federal and state expenditures on health care, but they do little to control the aggregate spending from all sources on health care.

Unhappily, this leads to an especially fierce and counterproductive "beggar thy neighbor" form of health policy politics. Various payers and interest groups take steps to limit their liability and shift costs elsewhere. The federal government mandates increased Medicaid benefits while leaving it to the states to shoulder the cost. State governments slash their own budgets, leaving cities, already overwhelmed with fiscal crises of their own, to cope with staggering inner city health problems associated with AIDS and drug abuse. Companies attempt to offset huge premium increases by increasing copayments, raising deductibles, and increasing the cost of family coverage. Insurance underwriting practices shift from community rating to experience rating in an effort to screen out individuals who may become severely ill and present large claims. The list goes on and on. Something beyond our usual forms of interest group politics will be necessary to break out of this mold.

The troubling, but inescapable, conclusion is plain. Cost-containment strategies aimed at making the system more efficient have not succeeded. Faute de mieux, policymakers and legislators are beginning to look more closely at prioritizing the health needs and allocating funds only to those areas of medical care that are deemed most necessary and socially valuable. This means that for some patients, some medical interventions that would help them and that the present system would now give them will be denied in the future. But how necessary is "necessary"? How valuable is "valuable"? Valuable to whom, and according to whom?

Public Opinion and Wishful Thinking

Public officials who must make allocation decisions—or who must make public policy decisions that have allocational consequences—need public guidance and support. These decisions will be very controversial. In a democratic society these decisions should reflect the community's sense of value priorities and goals for health care; they should not be left up to elites and experts alone. And as a practical matter, any policy that strays too far from what is acceptable to a broad spectrum of health care consumers and providers and the general public will not succeed.

Hence, setting health care priorities is the kind of combined ethical and policy problem in health care that requires more than technical expertise and elite decision making. It requires a large measure of public input and the formation of a broad public consensus on the principles and processes that ought to govern decisions of a more technical kind. Unfortunately, however, policymakers are receiving some very confused and mixed signals from the public on these matters, and we seem quite far from any kind of workable consensus on the priorities that should be established in health care.

Research conducted by the Public Agenda Foundation[8] has shown a very high level of public support for expanding health care services for the working poor, those with a catastrophic acute illness, and those in need of long-term care. However, when presented with reasonable estimates about how much such programs will cost, as few as 10 percent were willing to pay the necessary amounts in increased taxes. This study found that there was a certain realism mixed with the idealistic and generous view that most Americans have about health care: Most people expected that rationing decisions would have to be made, that costs would continue to climb, and that we would not be able to afford everything that we might want. Nonetheless, this sober realism did not lead people to draw back from their moral conviction that individuals should have a right to all beneficial health care, regardless of its cost. Thus the Public Agenda study concludes:

> As concerned as they were about their vulnerability to the high cost of catastrophic illness and long-term care . . . most of the participants . . . remained unwilling either to lower their own expectations about what the government should provide or to pay what is necessary for even a modest level of government provided coverage. . . . While there is strong support for more government involvement in this area, there is no corresponding inclination to pay for it.[9]

Does health care allocation then pose a dilemma that is irresolvable in a democratic society? I believe it does not. Public understanding of the three sets of issues involved in allocation—setting limits, setting priorities, and just access—can be enhanced through participation in civic dialogues at the community level and through the media. A public consensus on the ethical framework for allocation can be developed to give policymakers the guidance they need to produce workable, acceptable policies. In principle, a considerably more open and democratic conversation than we now have can be comprised of sound arguments, solid factual information, and reasonable inferences about the consequences of alternative policy choices. The question is not whether this needs to be done, but how it can be done. The problem is a practical one of arranging the circumstances in such a way that this kind of civic conversation will ensue and of providing the community leaders and public officials (who will be ultimately responsible for creating these circumstances) with the advice and intellectual support they need in order to succeed.[10]

What steps can be taken toward this end? Here again the strategy to follow depends upon analysis of why, at present, health care allocation and priorities are not receiving the kind of public attention they deserve. A good deal more community-based research is needed to shed light on this question. At this point, though, I would argue that there are two principal reasons why this is the case today.

First, the moral issues have simply not yet been clearly defined. Much more systematic research and ethical argumentation is required on the substantive value issues raised by allocation. We need to look very closely, and on the basis of the best empirical information we can obtain, at the implications and ramifications of limiting certain kinds of medical technologies and of setting normative and financial priorities among various classes of competing health care needs and interests. Equally important, we need to listen closely and systematically to what community leaders and ordinary citizens have to say on these issues, and we need to create the settings and the occasions—through focus groups, community forums, and carefully planned public education and media campaigns—in which these voices can be heard.

A second important reason why a more serious and comprehensive discussion of allocation has been difficult to achieve is political and procedural. Existing political institutions and the prevailing interest group system in the health policy arena do not give key actors a sufficient incentive to promote a serious public dialogue on allocational issues. Questions about health care limits and priorities are widely perceived as "no win" issues. "Quiet" rationing rarely causes a fuss. And consensus is exceedingly difficult to achieve in an environment dominated by interest group competition for policy influence, constituency support, and scarce government funds.

This analysis suggests that existing institutions—such as health-planning agencies, professional societies, and consumer advocacy groups—will not readily provide the forums necessary for the kind of public conversation and deliberation that participatory democracy requires. It is necessary to actively seek out alternative channels of community discussion and civic education in order to provide the initial impetus and structure for forums on allocation issues.

Steps toward a Democratic Space and Conversation

In concluding this discussion I would like to outline several steps that are necessary to move toward an enhanced democratic dialogue in communities across the country. These steps require the cooperation of researchers from the fields of medicine, bioethics, the social sciences, and policy studies, together with the skills of community leaders and grassroots organizers. I regard the interchange between ethics specialists and policy specialists, on the one hand, and the architects of successful grassroots projects, on the other, as a key ingredient, indeed as the "new key" to health policy. Philosophical research on the ethics of allocation that is not accessible to, and does not reach, the informed public does little to promote better civic understanding or enlightened public policy. Likewise, simply more sensational publicity, rhetoric, and emotional debate are not constructive goals to be sought either. It is essential to couple substantive research with the creation of democratic forums for civic education on the problem of health care priorities.

Holding open community meetings on a subject as complex as this requires careful planning. It also requires a strategy that will intelligently inform and guide the citizen deliberation process without imposing a preconceived agenda from above. Thoughtful materials have to be produced that lay out the ethical and social issues and provide basic information about the current realities of our health care system. Moreover, a discussion process and strategy needs to be devised that will let thoughtful deliberation happen and will capture its results in a record that can be made available to community and political leaders. I suggest the following steps as an agenda for future research and development for grassroots health decisions projects.

Understanding Peoples' Values and Perceptions

It is essential to assess current public perceptions and attitudes concerning the health care priorities, to find patterns of special concern and areas of possible consensus. Here one may identify misunderstandings and misperceptions that impede the public's ability to think realistically about priorities in health care. However, when working in an area as complex and multifaceted as public opinion on health values, one may find that public values and priorities differ significantly from those of professionals or policy intellectuals.

One of the most complex aspects of the entire priority-setting debate is the close connection between empirical and normative assumptions. Here, as in other areas of so-called practical or applied ethics, factual information alone will not settle all value disputes. Indeed, particular normative orientations will themselves determine what empirical information should "count" in a discussion and what facts are relevant to the rationing problem in the first place. Even so, when a common basis of empirical data and factual information is available to all participants in a discussion, it can greatly facilitate a constructive dialogue on ethical and value questions. At present, particularly among the public at large, people come to discussions of health care limits and priorities with widely varying understandings of the costs, utilization patterns, and demonstrated efficacy of different forms of medical care.

It is no less important to assess where the public starts in thinking about health values and priorities. Research is needed that helps us understand the public's definition of both adequate and optimal care. It should strive to determine whether people believe hard choices and trade-offs have to be made in medicine and to identify the concerns, preconceptions, or misconceptions people may hold.

The following are the types of questions that might guide this research:

- Do people understand the degree of the nation's current health cost crisis? If not, what kinds of information will help people understand the problem?
- Do they understand that costs masked by insurance, or hidden in fringe benefits or taxes, are nevertheless real costs that they pay for, however indirectly?
- Do people think that not enough resources are available for health care and therefore rationing is necessary, or do they believe there would be sufficient funds if the system were less wasteful and more efficient?
- Do people's fears and sense of vulnerability about health costs impede their ability to think clearly and constructively about what kinds of care should be covered?
- Do people overestimate the chances for success for some kinds of care and thus assign them a higher priority than they would if they had a more realistic understanding of their effectiveness?
- Alternatively, do people understand, as many experts argue, that some kinds of care (e.g., prenatal care for disadvantaged mothers) may be highly cost-effective? Do people reevaluate their priorities for health care in light of this new information?
- Do people believe, as many experts propose, that the country should accept less than state-of-the-art ("first class") care for some in exchange for a more modest ("coach class") but universal health coverage for all Americans?
- Do people have a small number of "nonnegotiable" items—for example, being able to go to a cancer center if they have cancer—that, if accommodated, would make a less-inclusive basic plan far more acceptable to them?
- People are very concerned about the prevalence of what might be called "extended death" among the elderly and others with terminal illnesses. How does public concern, and in some cases anger, over this phenomenon affect thinking on what constitutes good and acceptable basic health care?

Developing a Conceptual Framework for Civic Discourse

A second key task is to develop an analytic framework of ethical principles and social values that can facilitate public deliberation on health care priorities. The dearth of sustained analyses of setting priorities in the current scholarly literature means that much basic, foundational work remains to be done.[11] The aim here should not be simply to produce a written study for an academic audience in the fields of health policy and bioethics. Instead, it should be to produce a comprehensive and rigorous treatment of the ethics of priority setting in a form that will be able to travel out into the "public square" and enter the ongoing civic conversation about our basic values and goals as a society.

Integral to such a study is an analysis of how moral ideals and conceptions structure perception of health care and expectations surrounding it. A large majority of

Americans, for example, view health care as a right, something to which each individual ought to be morally entitled. We need to understand better how people define and conceive key ethical notions such as rights, responsibilities, and moral desert and how people tend to apply these notions in their thinking about health care allocation. This, in turn, will enable us to identify and address misperceptions that political officials may have concerning public reactions to proposed allocational policies. In a similar vein, we need to gain better insight into the reasons why so many Americans seemingly fail to see the inconsistency between their support for expanding medical services, on the one hand, and their unwillingness to pay for those services, on the other.

A comprehensive ethical analysis must begin with a careful definition and examination of the notion of allocation. Important distinctions that affect the meaning of allocation and its ethical dimensions should be made, such as the distinctions noted earlier in this article, among allocation as setting limits, allocation as setting priorities, and allocation as access to basic medical care. In order to clarify terms and to fix ideas in any discussion of allocation, it is essential to comprehend the different senses of the term and the different kinds of social decisions and policies that are appropriate to allocation in each of its various manifestations. The allocation problem is not a one-dimensional problem; it is necessary to begin with a clear recognition of its many-faceted and multidimensional nature.

An ethical analysis of health care allocation has several distinct levels. At the most general level stand basic ethical *principles*. Examples of such principles include justice, equity, individual rights and liberty, beneficence, procedural impartiality, and respect for persons. These principles preside over an ethical evaluation of both the substance of a public policy or professional practice decision and the procedures, protocols, and processes that lead up to that decision.

On a second, more concrete level of analysis are ethical *criteria* for placing more weight on, or giving more value to, one thing than another. Ethical criteria should be compatible with more general ethical principles, but they must be developed in their own right. They do not automatically follow or become self-evident once one has accepted certain principles. Criteria are the considerations we employ to select between two mutually exclusive goals when both of those goals are morally legitimate from the point of view of basic principles; in such a case, obviously, recourse to principles alone will not help us make a choice.

It is here, at the level of ethical criteria, that the most basic work on the problem of health care priority setting remains to be done. To take this problem seriously is to recognize that hard choices between deserving persons and between beneficial forms of health care have to be made. Acknowledging patient wants—or even needs—is not enough; not all wants and needs can be met. Neither is it enough to rule out clearly useless and wasteful forms of care. Some therapies, diagnostic tests, procedures, and promising lines of research or technological developments that have real benefit to some individual patients will have to be forgone. For only in this way can resources be made available for other forms of care that are also beneficial but in different ways and to different individuals. It is here that ethical criteria enter into the very heart of the priority-setting debate and begin to guide decision making in specific ways that more general ethical principles such as justice, equality, and autonomy cannot.

It is not possible here to attempt a detailed exploration of potential ethical prioritizing criteria. Mention of a few notions that are often put forward will have to suffice. These include

- the numbers of people affected by a given form of care,
- the effect of care on preventing disease,
- the effect on curing disease,
- the effect on prolonging life,
- the effect on enhancing the quality of life,
- the worthiness of the typical patient served by a given form of care,
- the social and cultural implications of the widespread acceptance and use of a given form of care.

Finally, the analysis I propose will move to the level of *procedural guidelines* concerning the development of specific policies that accord with general moral principles and justifiable ethical criteria for setting limits and priorities and for allocating access to care. Ethical principles and criteria cannot specify one single "best" or "right" allocational pattern or priorities for health care; they can only set parameters within which somewhat different allocations may be judged acceptable.[12]

Principles and criteria can enable us to spot clearly wrong or unjust allocations, but they cannot pick out the single right answer. Perhaps, as I believe to be the case, there is no one right answer. When there is not (or when we do not know what it is), we must turn to ethical considerations about process—not what is selected, but how it is selected: how openly, how thoughtfully, how fairly. This is where guidelines are relevant. During this stage of the analysis the nature of the policymaking process and procedural values that should govern it will come to the fore. Then the central aim becomes ensuring that policymaking in this area is as open and as democratically well informed as possible.

Creating a Process for Grassroots Participation

The final key task is to develop a model process and educational materials for organizing community dialogue on values underlying health priority and allocational choices. This is what is being attempted in the community health decisions process in several parts of the country.[13] One of its goals is to open new lines of communication on priorities between government and corporate policymakers, physicians and other health professionals, the media, and the general public.

But this kind of participatory democratic forum on health values and policy is not valuable solely because it can sometimes facilitate coalition building and grease the gears of interest group politics at the local or state level. Far more important, in my view, is the role that the practice of democratic deliberation can have on the cultural and moral ethos that informs existing political expectations in health policy. Ultimately it seems to me that Callahan, Churchill, and others are right when they argue that a just and affordable health care system will require not so much a new payment system as a public re-vision of personal aspiration and a transformation in our habits of the heart.

Of course, that will not come quickly—perhaps not quickly enough in view of our current situation. And it will not come automatically as people read or hear about rising costs in the media, or even as they experience the pinch of out-of-pocket expenses and the insult of quiet rationing in their own personal encounters with the high-tech health care system. The cultural transformation in question involves what I have been calling a democratic or civic consensus on the basic values that should guide specific policy decisions that have redistributive and allocational effects. It involves, that is to say, a common sense that allocation decisions in health policy have a bearing on the shape of our public life together in a community of shared purpose, common endeavor, and common human frailty and vulnerability in the face of aging, disability, dependency, and disease. It involves a political education and a political consciousness, in the classical sense of the term *political*—a common sense of shared problems and goods and a sense of what we have in common.

Only through active involvement in settings designed to orient attention toward these public dimensions of the issue can this kind of political education and sensibility be nurtured. So long as individuals confront the problems of our health care system only in their own personal, private, or occupational capacities as consumers, patients, and particularistically self-interested persons, it is unlikely that they will be motivated to see the system and their own involvement in it from a public perspective as citizens who have communal, civic interests as well as particular, private interests. It is this perspective, and citizenship in this sense, that the transformative experience of direct democratic participation in a properly planned setting can provide.[14]

When the representative mechanisms of liberal or pluralist democracy do not seem responsive to a manifestly growing crisis, or when the policymaking process seems paralyzed and stymied by the pushing and hauling of narrowly interested parties, it takes a recrudescence of citizenship to produce and give voice to a different dimension of interests. It takes participatory democracy to provide citizens for representative democracy to represent. It takes citizens who have an active, publicly forged vision of common interests and common needs to be a supporting constituency for political representatives and policymakers who must exercise leadership and vision and political courage of their own. These are lessons we seem to have somehow forgotten on all fronts of domestic policy. Health policy, at the moment, provides the best hope of a venue for relearning them.

The author gratefully acknowledges helpful advice from Daniel Callahan, Jean Johnson, Ellen Severoni, and Deborah Wadsworth in the preparation of this paper.

Notes

1. Friedman, E. (1991). The uninsured: From dilemma to crisis. *Journal of the American Medical Association, 265*, 2491–2495, citing p. 2493.

2. Pear, R. (1993, January 5). Health care costs up sharply again, posing new threat. *New York Times,* pp. A-1, A-10.

3. Friedman, E. (1991). The uninsured: From dilemma to crisis. *Journal of the American Medical Association, 265*, 2491–2495, citing p. 2491.

4. Hadorn, D. (1991). Setting health care priorities in Oregon: Cost-effectiveness meets the rule of rescue. *Journal of the American Medical Association, 265*, 2218–2225.

5. Garland, M. I., and Hasnain, R. (1990, September/October). Health care in common: Setting priorities in Oregon. *Hastings Center Report,* 20, 16–18; Kitzhaber, I. (1990–1991, Winter). A healthier approach to health care. *Issues in Science and Technology,* 59–65.

6. Colbert, T. (1990, September/October). Public input into health care policy: Controversy and contribution in California. *Hastings Center Report,* 20, 21; Hill, T. P. (1990, September/October). Giving voice to the pragmatic majority in New Jersey. *Hastings Center Report,* 20, 20; Leichter, H. M. (ed.). (1992). *Health policy reform in America: Innovation from the states.* New York: Sharpe; Wallace-Brodeur, P. (1990, September/October). Community values in Vermont health planning. *Hastings Center Report,* 20, 18–19.

7. Churchill, L. R. (1987). *Rationing health care in America.* Notre Dame, IN: Notre Dame University Press.

8. Melville, K., and Doble, I. (1988). *The public's perspective on social welfare reform.* New York: Public Agenda Foundation.

9. Ibid., citing p. 75.

10. Barber, B. (1984). *Strong democracy: Participatory politics for a new age.* Berkeley: University of California Press; Evans, S. M., and Boyte, H. C. (1986). *Free spaces: The sources of democratic change in America.* New York: Harper and Row.

11. Callahan, D. (1990). *What kind of life: The limits of medical progress.* New York: Simon and Schuster; Daniels, N. (1985). *Just health care.* Cambridge: Cambridge University Press.

12. Daniels, N. (1991). Is the Oregon rationing plan fair? *Journal of the American Medical Association,* 265, 2232–2235.

13. Jennings, B. (1988, June/July). Bioethics at the grassroots: Community health decisions. *Hastings Center Report,* 18 (Special Suppl.), 1–16; Jennings, B. (1990, September/October). Democracy and justice in health policy. *Hastings Center Report,* 20, 22–23.

14. Jennings, B. (1990, Spring). Bioethics and democracy. *Centennial Review,* 34, 207–226; Jennings, B. (1992). Democratic values and health policy reform. In H. M. Leichter (ed.), *Health policy reform in America: Innovation from the states* (pp. 191–205). New York: Sharpe.

Further Reading

Berkman, Lisa F., and Ichiro Kawachi, eds., *Social Epidemiology* (New York: Oxford University Press, 2000).

Buchanan, Allen, "The Right to a Decent Minimum of Health Care," in President's Commission for the Study of Ethical Problems in Medicine and Biomedical and Behavioral Research, *Securing Access to Health Care,* vol. 2 (Washington, DC: U.S. Government Printing Office, March 1983), pp. 207–238.

Evans, Robert G., Morris L. Barer, and Theodore R. Marmor, eds., *Why Are Some People Healthy and Others Not? The Determinants of Health of Populations* (New York: Aldine de Gruyter, 1994).

Evans, Timothy, Margaret Whitehead, Finn Diderichsen, Abbas Bhuiya, and Meg Wirth, eds., *Challenging Inequities in Health: From Ethics to Action* (Oxford: Oxford University Press, 2001).

Garland, Michael, and John Stull, "Public Health and Health System Reform," in Bruce Jennings, Jeffrey Kahn, Anna Mastroianni, and Lisa S. Parker, eds., *Ethics and Public Health: Model Curriculum* (Washington, DC: Association of Schools of Public Health, 2003), 241–267. Available at http://www.asph.org/document.cfm?page=782.

Gutmann, Amy, "For and Against Equal Access to Health Care," in President's Commission for the Study of Ethical Problems in Medicine and Biomedical and Behavioral Research, *Securing Access to Health Care,* vol. 2 (Washington, DC: U.S. Government Printing Office, March 1983), pp. 51–66.

Institute of Medicine, *Insuring America's Health: Principles and Recommendations* (Washington, DC: National Academies Press, 2004).

Kawachi, Ichiro, and Bruce P. Kennedy, *The Health of Nations: Why Inequality Is Harmful to Your Health* (New York: New Press, 2002).

President's Commission for the Study of Ethical Problems in Medicine and Biomedical and Behavioral Research, *Securing Access to Health Care,* 2 vols. (Washington, DC: U.S. Government Printing Office, March 1983).

Putnam, Robert D., *Bowling Alone* (New York: Simon and Schuster, 2000).

Rhodes, Rosamond, Margaret P. Battin, and Anita Silvers, eds., *Medicine and Social Justice: Essays on the Distribution of Health Care* (New York: Oxford University Press, 2002).

Tarlov, Alvin R., and Robert F. St. Peter, eds., *The Society and Population Health Reader, Vol. 2: A State and Community Perspective* (New York: New Press, 2000).

Wilkinson, Richard G., *Unhealthy Societies: The Afflictions of Inequality.* (London: Routledge, 1996).

PART IV

INFECTIOUS DISEASE: COERCION AND THE PROTECTION OF SOCIETY

Introduction

The public health authority to limit individual freedom when disease threatens has long been recognized in constitutional jurisprudence. One hundred years ago, in *Jacobson v. Massachusetts,* a case that centered on the question of compulsory vaccination, the Supreme Court held that the U.S. Constitution permits states to enact "such reasonable regulations [to] protect the public health and the public safety" as long as such efforts did not "contravene the Constitution of the United States, nor infringe any right guaranteed or secured by that instrument." *Jacobson* also underscored the belief that courts should give deference to the government's exercise of the police powers designed to protect the public.[1] Capturing the enormous scope afforded to the state acting in the name of public health, a treatise on constitutional law in 1900 asserted that before the demands of public health "all constitutionally guaranteed rights must give way."[2] From an ethical point of view, the warrant for state interventions to protect individuals from the dangers of infectious threats is provided by the "harm principle" famously given voice by the nineteenth-century philosopher John Stuart Mill, who said in *On Liberty*, "The only purpose for which power can be rightfully exercised over any member of a civilized community, against his will, is to prevent harm to others. His own good, either physical or moral, is not sufficient warrant."[3] Part IV examines the ethics of infectious disease control.

In the wake of the bacteriological revolution of the nineteenth century, which located the etiology of disease in microscopic agents, "germs," that could spread from the infected to the uninfected, the central pillars of public health practice were created. Screening, case reporting to public health departments, contact tracing, mandatory treatment, and quarantine would all be brought to bear on infectious threats, and each entailed the exercise of public health power backed by the threat of compulsion.

During the twentieth century, screening for the presence of disease and at times occult infection was a central feature of public health practice. Often, such screening was mandatory or legislated as a condition for undertaking a desired course of action. Screening for venereal disease prior to marriage was instituted as a way of protecting unsuspecting spouses from infection. Screening children for entry into public schools was instituted to protect classmates. Screening of newborns for inborn errors of metabolism was initiated to ensure that needed remedial actions, dietary or otherwise, were taken. And of course screening for tuberculosis by x-ray and skin test became widespread in schools and workplaces.

If mandatory screening raised questions about the circumstances under which the public health could justify intrusions on the body, public health surveillance posed questions about the tension between privacy, confidentiality, and the public good. It was not until the late nineteenth century that systematic reporting of cases of infectious disease to public health departments began. Since surveillance was undertaken not only to track patterns of morbidity and mortality but also to initiate other restrictive measures (e.g., compulsory treatment and quarantine), it provoked public and professional concern. Hence, physicians, on occasion, challenged the authority of the public health authorities to intrude on the sanctity of the doctor-patient relationship in the name of surveillance.

Eventually, despite such opposition, name-based case reporting was extended to a host of other conditions practically without any sign of protest. Recognizing that resistance could undermine their efforts, public health officials began to develop the legal and organizational capacity for protecting the confidentiality of names reporting to health departments.

Case-based surveillance served not only to monitor epidemiological patterns of disease but also as a trigger for contact tracing. In programs designed to treat and control sexually transmitted diseases (STDs), contact tracing has played a central role for more than six decades. Patients diagnosed with STDs are urged to reveal the names of their sexual partners so that they may be examined and, if infected, treated. Contact tracing thus serves two functions: case finding and interrupting the chain of transmission. To encourage individuals to provide the names of their partners, a guarantee of absolute anonymity is provided: Those who are notified are never informed of the identity of the person who provided their name. In this way, contact tracing has always been voluntary and has always rested on the foundation of confidentiality.

In the face of infectious disease threats, public health departments have also at times been involved in attempting to ensure that those who could spread disease had undergone appropriate treatment. Treatment in this instance had to be understood as serving both the interest of the individual as patient and the broader community that would be protected from the transmission of disease. In the late 1980s and early 1990s, the resurgence of tuberculosis in the United States and the pattern of drug resistance made it clear to public health officials that strategies for managing the disease had failed.[4] Those who had begun treatment but did not complete their therapy ran the risk not only of reactivation of their disease but also of developing resistance that could be very costly to treat and, in the case of those with compromised immune systems, could prove fatal. Of course, drug-resistant disease could be transmitted to others.

Among the strategies designed to enhance patient compliance with treatment is directly observed therapy, a practice that involves having the patient take his or her medication in the presence of health care providers or other responsible parties. First proposed for individuals with poor records of treatment adherence and for those whose demographic or psychological profile suggested a higher prospect of failure, directly observed therapy has emerged as the standard of care for all tuberculosis patients.

Finally, legal and constitutional principles have long recognized the authority of the state to confine individuals with dangerous infectious diseases because of the threat they posed to others. This power to deprive an individual of his or her liberty in the name of public health has vested officials with an authority that, from the perspective of the individual, may seem indistinguishable from that wielded by the criminal justice system. Yet, until relatively recently, the protections accorded to defendants in criminal prosecutions had not been extended to those viewed as a threat to the public health.

The past four decades of constitutional development, particularly in the area of involuntary confinement of psychiatric patients, have seen increasing scrutiny of the exercise of the police powers of the state, raising questions about the constitutionality of statues relating to communicable disease, many enacted before the profound shift in the balance between individual liberties and state authority.

As important to the transformations in the perspective on the state's public health authority was the impact of the AIDS epidemic.[5] In the early 1980s, when the United States like other democratic nations had to confront the public health challenge posed by the new epidemic, it was necessary to face a set of fundamental questions: Did the history of responses to lethal infectious disease provide lessons about how best to contain the spread of HIV itself, an ultimately deadly sexually transmitted and blood-borne virus? If AIDS were not to be so treated, what would justify such differential policies? It was the specter of the most coercive aspects of the public health tradition that concerned proponents of civil liberties and advocates of gay rights as they considered the potential direction of public health policy in the presence of AIDS. Bioethicists concerned about autonomy also sounded the alarm.

Although there were some public health traditionalists who pressed to have HIV infection brought under the broad statutory provisions established to control the spread of sexually transmitted and infectious disease, they were in a distinct minority. In the first decade of the AIDS epidemic, an alliance of gay leaders, civil libertarians, and public health officials began to shape policy for dealing with AIDS that reflected an "exceptionalist" perspective.[6] That perspective entailed the commitment to rely on preventive measures that were not coercive and respected the privacy and social rights of those who were at risk. In fact, it was argued that there was no tension between the rights of the individual and the protection of the public health. What shielded the former advanced the latter. Mass education, voluntary testing, and counseling were the centerpiece of the public health strategy that sought to avoid interventions that might "drive the epidemic underground." While the force of the exceptionalist perspective has waned since the 1990s, as AIDS has been "normalized," the issues posed by the challenge to conventional public health practice remain pertinent.

The first selection in this chapter, Ronald Bayer and Amy L. Fairchild's "Surveillance and Privacy," provides an analysis of the history of public health surveillance and poses questions about the limits of privacy. The second selection, Lawrence O. Gostin, Ronald Bayer, and Amy L. Fairchild's discussion of the severe acute respiratory syndrome (SARS) outbreak of 2003, underscores how, in the face of a threatening deadly outbreak, traditional public health measures were effectively brought to bear and highlights the ways in which infectious threats compel us to confront the questions of what threat, to whom, with what degree of certainty, and with what consequences justify intrusive public health interventions.

This part concludes with a selection on compulsory vaccination.

Immunization in the United States has attained all-time highs. In 1998 the rates had reached 90 percent for 19- to 35-month-old children for most vaccines.[7] To a very large extent, this achievement can be viewed as a consequence of both persuasion—physicians routinely urge parents to immunize their children—and compulsion. All states require evidence of vaccination against a host of diseases, including measles, polio, and diphtheria. Children who are not immunized may not attend school or be registered in licensed day care centers. There are exceptions for religious reasons, and 15 states permit "philosophic exemption." But such provisions affect only an extraordinarily small number of children.[8]

As a result of immunization programs, diseases that were formerly a common occurrence among children have declined by well over 99 percent. For example, in 1941 there were 890,000 cases of measles, and by the late 1990s the number had fallen to 89. In 1968, there were approximately 150,000 cases of mumps; by 1998 the number had fallen to 61.[9] These achievements have, ironically, set the stage for the emergence of challenges to mandatory childhood vaccination.

As the experience of disease has receded, what has emerged is concern about the limited prospect of adverse reactions. With the possibility of disease so small, why subject a child to any risk? The issue of vaccination places into sharp relief the clash between the rationality of public policy and the rationality of decision making on the part of individuals or by those they have a duty to protect. Because it typically involves children who cannot consent for themselves, the issue of compulsory vaccination also raises questions about when the state may substitute its judgment for that of parents.

In the selection by Douglas S. Diekema and Edgar K. Marcuse, three broad questions that need to be considered are identified:

- First, do parents who withhold vaccination from their children harm them to such an extent that parental refusal ought to be overridden?
- Second, what duties do parents owe others in the community to avoid causing harm through an unvaccinated child?
- Third, does the social value of having a vaccinated population—for the sake of herd immunity and the eradication of disease—justify coercive efforts to vaccinate all children?

Demonstrating the enduring nature of the issues addressed in this chapter is the very recent debate over the extent to which the threat of bioterrorism can justify the exercise of public health measures like case reporting to health departments, mandatory vaccination, and quarantine in situations defined as a public health emergency. The very determination of what constitutes an emergency warranting such measures is more than a technical matter. It is suffused with value questions regarding the balance of risks and benefits, tolerable uncertainties, and our conceptions of rights. Part IV's final selection by Ronald Bayer and James Colgrove examines these issues.

Notes

1. *Jacobson v. Massachusetts* 197 U.S. 11 (1905).

2. Cited in Deborah Merritt, "The Constitutional Balance Between Health and Liberty," *Hastings Center Report* 16: 1986, S2–S10.

3. Mill, John Stuart, *On Liberty* (New Haven, CT: Yale University Press, 2003).

4. Institute of Medicine, *Ending Neglect: The Elimination of Tuberculosis in the United States* (Washington, DC: National Academy Press, 2000).

5. Bayer, Ronald, *Private Acts, Social Consequences: AIDS and the Politics of Public Health* (New York: Free Press, 1989).

6. Bayer, Ronald, "Public Health Policy and the AIDS Epidemic: An End to HIV Exceptionalism," *New England Journal of Medicine* 324: 1991, 1500–1504.

7. Colgrove, James, *State of Immunity: The Politics of Vaccination in Twentieth Century America* (Berkeley: University of California Press, 2006).

8. Salmon, Daniel, Michael Haber, Eugene Gangarosa, et al. "Health Consequences of Religious and Philosophical Exemptions from Immunization Laws," *Journal of the American Medical Association* 282: 1999, 47–53.

9. Campos-Outcalt, Doug, and Mikel Aickin, "Incidence of Infectious Disease and the Licensure of Immunobiologics in the United States," *American Journal of Preventive Medicine* 13: 1997, 98–103.

15

Surveillance and Privacy

Ronald Bayer and Amy L. Fairchild

Surveillance has been critical for epidemiological and population-based research into patterns of morbidity and mortality for a wide variety of diseases and conditions. However, the prospect of measures such as long-term monitoring, contact tracing, and quarantine has provoked alarm and concern about the potential for the unwarranted use of surveillance data.

Ethical issues are raised by public health surveillance regarding the extent to which name-based reporting violates trust and assumptions that are made about how medical information will be treated. For a brief period, there was discussion about whether emerging rules and regulations for human subjects research should apply to epidemiological studies, whether the principle of informed consent for the use of records was necessary, and if this requirement would render such inquiries virtually impossible. Yet that discussion had no impact on public health surveillance. Although epidemiological research has been the subject of ethical review, it is remarkable that public health surveillance has not been subject to similar oversight.

It was not until the late nineteenth century that systematic reporting of infectious diseases began. Surveillance was also undertaken to initiate quarantine, isolation, or vaccination[1] and provoked public and professional concern. Physicians, on occasion, challenged the authority of public health professionals to breach the sanctity of the doctor-patient relationship in the name of surveillance. In New York City, for example, physician outrage over mandatory tuberculosis (TB) reporting beginning in 1897 resulted in an essentially voluntary reporting system in which doctors withheld the names of their private patients and reported the names of their poor, dispensary cases.[2]

Conflict also surrounded the reporting of sexually transmitted diseases.[3] Although names were used in some locales, venereal disease reporting was often attenuated by compromises like those that emerged in the TB conflict. Nonetheless, this was not always so. In 1911, Western Australia adopted a compulsory name-based notification system for infectious diseases that included venereal diseases, seemingly without incident. Sweden followed suit in 1915, coupling name-based notification with compulsory detention, treatment, and prohibitions against marriage among the infected.

Eventually, name-based reporting was extended to a host of other conditions, typically without any sign of protest.[4] But recognizing that resistance could undermine their efforts, public health officials began to develop the legal and organizational capacity for protecting the confidentiality of names.

Nonetheless, in the last part of the twentieth century, a protracted and furious debate about surveillance would again surface. The U.S. controversy over HIV name reporting, beginning in 1985, was radically affected by the circumstances under which it emerged, e.g., the special fears surrounding the AIDS epidemic, a transformed conception of the rights of privacy, constitutional limits on state authority exercised for benevolent purposes, the development of a vigorous debate about medical ethics, and the emergence of patient advocacy as a potent social force. An increasing number of public health officials, who believed they could protect the confidentiality of name-based reports, found themselves pitted against AIDS activists and proponents of civil liberties who focused on the potential for discrimination and coercion if names were sent to public health registries.

When it became clear that some form of HIV infection reporting was necessary, the debate shifted to the question of whether relying on unique identifiers in lieu of names could meet surveillance requirements. The coalition opposed to name-based reporting insisted that a uniquely stigmatized disease demanded policies uniquely protective of privacy. Although some public health officials [such as those in Maryland] supported the use of unique identifiers, most remained skeptical. The U.S. Centers for Disease Control and Prevention (CDC) had, by the 1990s, become convinced that name-based reporting was most efficient and accurate. When, in 1999, it mandated that all states adopt some form of HIV surveillance, it only reluctantly acknowledged that, under stringent performance criteria, unique identifiers could serve public health adequately.[5]

The emphasis on name reporting has been greater in the United States than in much of Europe. In February 1998, a meeting convened under the auspices of the European Centre for the Epidemiological Monitoring of AIDS concluded that, whereas HIV case reporting is essential, effective surveillance could be attained without the use of names.[6]

Vaccine registries provide a counterpoint to HIV. In response to sporadic disease outbreaks, poor coverage in inner-city communities, increasingly complex vaccine schedules, family mobility, and poor provider and patient awareness of immunization coverage levels, the National Vaccine Advisory Committee (NVAC) recommended in 1999 creation of a nationwide network of state and community immunization registries. *Healthy People 2010* included a goal for surveillance, aiming for 95 percent registration of children up to age 5.

In the face of considerable anxiety, the federal initiative to register immunization coverage put a premium on community participation and cooperation. Immigrant communities feared that registry information would be used to deny medical coverage or to make reports to the Immigration and Naturalization Service. Parents who opted against vaccination were concerned that they would suffer harassment or discrimination. Finally, providers with low immunization rates worried that they would be "punished" in some fashion. As a result, a central concern of the NVAC was to protect patient confidentiality.[7] The NVAC report recommended that, at a minimum, registries notify parents of the existence and content of the registry. Critically, it recommended that parents should be permitted to decide whether children would be included in registries.

Although cancer is historically a highly stigmatized disease and registration of cases in western Europe has in recent years been the subject of strict regulation, cancer registries in the United States, which have been in existence for 50 years, provide the primary example of a surveillance regimen that has not produced ethical controversy. In 1973, the National Cancer Institute recognized that its strategy of ascertaining data on cancer through periodic surveys was inadequate. It established the Surveillance, Epidemiology, and End Results (SEER) program to take advantage of cancer data already being collected at population-based tumor registries. Nineteen years later, Congress enacted the Cancer Registries Amendment Act, which authorized the CDC to establish a national program in support of cancer registries. Despite the wide array of medical information linked by name and the duration of surveillance for each case from the first pathology report through death, most patients are unaware that cancer registries exist or that they represent cases within these registries. Supporters have argued for using names as the basis for linking records, in the name of surveillance accuracy.[8] Those concerned with the needs and rights of breast cancer patients have supported cancer registries despite the commitment of the women's health movement to norms of privacy.

In 1997 it was estimated that as a result of occupational exposure, more than 800,000 individuals become sick and 60,000 die each year in the United States.[9] Advocates for workers' health have urged that occupational diseases be made reportable by name to permit work site interventions and investigations. Ultimately, the National Institute for Occupational Safety and Health (NIOSH) developed the Sentinel Event Notification System for Occupational Risks (SENSOR) in 1987. SENSOR helps state programs to expand their reporting capacity and to develop standardized case definitions. A number of European nations have also developed special surveillance programs to monitor the health status of workers, for example, those exposed to asbestos. Although occupational disease reporting by name is uncommon in less-developed nations, it does exist.

Birth defects registries emerged to meet environmental and teratogenic hazards to the fetus. Currently, the U.S. Birth Defects Monitoring Program, a multistate surveillance system based on hospital discharge reports, is the largest source of birth defects information in the nation.[10] Although the architects of birth defects registries endorse the use of names to facilitate follow-up studies and the linkage of infant, maternal, and paternal records, they have embraced parental choice. In that way, they are like vaccine registries in that parents retain the right to decide whether or not their children will be subject to reporting. Birth defects and vaccine registries thus stand as a challenge to the proposition that only universal, name-based reporting without consent is an adequate basis for surveillance.

Conclusions

Five themes emerge that help to explain the circumstances under which surveillance is contested and those under which it is accepted without debate.

First, the extent to which surveillance might trigger public health interventions and the way such interventions have been viewed have been central. Fear that those reported would be the targets of coercion or discrimination has energized opposition to name-based reporting. A recent Institute of Medicine report provoked concern because it recommended screening and surveillance of immigrants from countries with a high incidence of TB and proposed that infected individuals be compelled to undergo prophylactic therapy or lose their immigrant status.[11] In contrast, labor advocates have supported occupational disease reporting as a prelude to interventions that could protect workers from hazardous work site conditions. Similarly, cancer activists have viewed tumor registries as crucial to research that could lead to intervention or treatment.

A second theme is the extent to which proposals for reporting provoke resistance or alarm when they involve diseases carrying social stigma or touch those who view themselves as socially marginalized or vulnerable to social or economic injury. Affected individuals may find pledges that reported information will be protected from unwarranted disclosure hard to believe and, as a consequence, see themselves as endangered.

Third, special populations can elicit special protections. Thus, surveillance regimes involving children and reproduction have put a high premium on both confidentiality and informed consent.

Fourth, although constituencies have sometimes been highly alert to the potential imposition of a surveillance regime, that has not always been the case. In the case of tumor registries, the subjects of reporting remain largely unaware of ongoing reporting requirements. Without such awareness, the possibility of voicing privacy concerns remains out of reach.

Perhaps most important, changes in expectations regarding privacy have had a profound impact on the acceptability of name-based reporting systems and the willingness of policymakers to consider alternatives. Registries that have developed most recently (particularly birth defects registries and vaccination registries) have been more sensitive to a culture of privacy than older ones, which find themselves challenged. For example, concerns have emerged about how commitments to privacy might eventually impede the extent to which tumor registries can serve as the basis for critical research.

Every U.S. state has statutes or regulations developed over the course of the twentieth century that protect the confidentiality of names reported to disease registries. Nonetheless, existing state laws lack uniformity and make it difficult to define clearly the ways in which they will protect reported data from unwarranted disclosure. That the CDC supported the development of a model state public health privacy act to protect such information underscores the salience of this issue.

This is an opportune moment for analysis of ethical challenges posed by name-based reporting requirements. Such an effort would necessitate recognition that the protection of public health may require some limitations on privacy. The central ethical question posed by name-based reporting is whether an abrogation of medical privacy can be justified by public health benefits. Although medical privacy is a fundamental value, it is not an absolute.

Notes

1. M. L. Moro and A. McCormick, in W. J. Eylenbosch, N. D. Noah, eds., *Surveillance in Health and Disease* (Oxford University Press, New York, 1988), pp. 166–182.

2. D. M. Fox, *Bull. Hist. Med.* 49, 169 (1975).

3. A. Brandt, *No Magic Bullet* (Oxford University Press, New York, 1987).

4. W. F. Snow, *Proceedings Second Pan American Scientific Congress, 1915–1916* (American Social Hygiene Association, Washington, DC, 1917), sec. 8, pt. 1, vol. 9, p. 491.

5. CDC, *Guidelines for National Human Immunodeficiency Virus Case Surveillance* (CDC, Atlanta, 1999), pp. 1–28.

6. F. F. Hammers, *Eurosurveillance* 3, 51 (1998).

7. Report of the National Vaccine Advisory Committee (NVAC), *Development of Community- and State-Based Immunization Registries*, 12 January 1999.

8. C. S. Muir, E. Demaret, and P. Boyle, *IARC (Int. Agency Res. Cancer) Sci. Publ.* 66, 21 (1985).

9. J. P. Leigh et al., *Arch. Intern. Med.* 157, 1557 (1997).

10. M. C. Lynberg and L. D. Edmonds, in *Public Health Surveillance,* W. Halperin, E. L. Baker, eds. (Van Nostrand Reinhold, New York, 1992), pp. 157–177.

11. Institute of Medicine, *Ending Neglect: The Elimination of Tuberculosis in the United States* (National Academy Press, Washington, DC, 2000).

16

Ethical and Legal Challenges Posed by Severe Acute Respiratory Syndrome

Implications for the Control of Severe Infectious Disease Threats

Lawrence O. Gostin, Ronald Bayer, and Amy L. Fairchild

Not long after the first reports of what ultimately would be called severe acute respiratory syndrome (SARS) began to appear in February 2003[1,2] and as nations and the international community began to confront the spread of the new disease, it became clear that a host of ethical and legal issues had begun to surface. Indeed, not since the first years of the HIV/AIDS pandemic in the mid-1980s[3] and the alarm over multidrug-resistant tuberculosis in the early 1990s[4] did it seem that so many issues touching on the core ethical questions posed by public health had to be addressed simultaneously. In several respects, SARS took society back to a pretherapeutic era with no definitive diagnostic test, a nonspecific case definition, and no effective vaccine or treatment.[5] From 1 November 2002, to 1 July 2003, 8,445 cases were reported to the World Health Organization (WHO); among these, 5,327 (63%) were from China, 1,755 (20%) from Hong Kong, 678 (8%) from Taiwan, 252 (3%) from Canada, and 206 (2%) from Singapore. There were 812 deaths. Comparatively, the United States, with 73 cases (0.9%) and no deaths, was spared.[6]

Now that the first wave of cases has apparently ended, it is especially important to evaluate the global public health response to SARS, which focused on surveillance, isolation and quarantine, contact tracing, and travel advisories or restrictions.[1] Such an analysis provides the basis for thinking about the ethical and legal principles that should guide public health efforts if and when cases surface again.

Three values involving the ethics of public health were bought into tension: the duty to protect the public, which is a collective good, and the individual rights of privacy and liberty. A set of critical questions emerged:

- What limits on privacy are justified by surveillance designed to characterize SARS outbreaks, permit contact investigation, and open the way to other interventions?

- What limits on liberty are justified by isolation or quarantine designed to separate the healthy from the infected or exposed?
- What restrictions of movement and economic liberty are justified by travel advisories to and from areas with SARS?

It is now clear that SARS is caused by a corona virus that symptomatic individuals transmit through large airborne droplets. Those most at risk are individuals at close contact—family and health care workers.[7] However, the transmission to many patrons at a hotel in Hong Kong and the outcropping of disease among residents at a single apartment complex raise perplexing questions about modes of transmission.[8] There are also remaining questions about whether some individuals are especially infectious—so-called superspreaders.

These unresolved issues required sociopolitical judgments about the tolerability of risk and the role of the precautionary principle in public health. These issues similarly raised important questions about personal stigma, group prejudice, and the economic viability of businesses, cities, and countries. These questions will need to be addressed again in the event that SARS recurs or with the emergence of other airborne severe infectious threats.

The lessons learned from SARS in varying social and political contexts provide the backdrop for a set of recommendations designed primarily to inform public health decision making in all nations that share the central values of a liberal democracy, including respect for individual rights. They may have more universal applicability under international human rights law, which has global acceptance. Thus, these recommendations may serve as a standard to judge measures to impede disease transmission without unduly restricting the rights of individuals.

Surveillance and Contact Tracing

The identification and reporting of SARS cases by name to public health authorities have been central features of all national responses to the outbreak, bringing into focus the tension between surveillance as an essential public health strategy and the claims of privacy.[9,10] The function of surveillance, which is complicated when the case definition is uncertain and there is no diagnostic assay,[11] has been to identify disease clusters, map the spread of disease, understand the patterns of contagion, and detect lapses in hospital infection control practices. But, as the WHO explained, the SARS outbreak also represented "a test case" of whether name reporting, "rigorous contact tracing and other stringent public health measures can contain further spread even when very large numbers of persons may have been exposed."[12]

Some countries, using a highly sensitive case definition, undertook aggressive contact tracing, tracking social, hospital, and occupational contacts during the 10 days before presumed symptom onset.[13] In Singapore, responsibility for the conduct of tracing was assigned to the military and in Hong Kong to the police.[14-16] However, in Toronto, hospitals sometimes failed to meet stringent reporting obligations,[17] without which contact tracing cannot be conducted.

Most of the affected areas also undertook a form of surveillance more extensive than name reporting by requiring body temperatures to be taken in certain segments of the population. In Toronto and Singapore, hospital workers took their temperatures and answered health questionnaires twice a day.[18,19] In Singapore, taxi drivers, government workers, food servers, bank tellers, reporters, beauty parlor patrons, and hotel staff determined their body temperature once a day and wore "fever-free" stickers: The goal was that the entire population monitor their temperatures daily.[20] In Hong Kong, parents of schoolchildren were required to sign a daily certification that their child had no fever, and bus drivers and caretakers were monitored.[21] In the United States, surveillance and contact tracing efforts were less aggressive,[22] reflecting social and cultural norms and the limited nature of the SARS outbreak.

Although the broad tradition of disease reporting in constitutional democracies includes privacy safeguards, this has not always been a priority for authoritarian regimes. Hong Kong adopted intrusive measures to track the personal contacts of SARS patients, such as the use of police detectives to locate family members and close friends.[23] In Singapore, the names of superspreaders were made public; in contrast, Hong Kong kept its SARS-related data on a separate computer with the intention of ultimately destroying the records.[16] Even in countries with strong traditions of civil rights, it was inevitable that where tracing of all close contacts occurred that the identity of individuals with SARS became clear; when broad public health measures, such as hospital or school closure, were put into place, the public identification of contacts likewise became inevitable. In Toronto, for example, when hospitals were closed the identity of no one was disclosed; yet, by implication, every hospital employee was identified, and health care workers found themselves ostracized.[24]

SARS surveillance data also carried financial and social consequences for geographic and ethnic communities. The publication of surveillance data unwittingly called unwelcome and even injurious attention to people of particular racial or national backgrounds.[25] The origins of the disease in China fueled negative Chinese stereotypes. There was also evidence of overt discrimination and racism in North America.[26,27]

Isolation and Quarantine

Countries have used two of the oldest public health tools in response to SARS, isolation and quarantine, underscoring the tension between liberty and the imperative to protect the public's health.[15] Although the terms are often used interchangeably, there are technical distinctions. Isolation is the separation, for the period of communicability, of known infected persons in such places and under such conditions to prevent or limit the transmission of infection. In contrast, quarantine is the restriction of the activities of healthy persons who have been exposed to a communicable disease to prevent disease transmission during the incubation period if infection should occur.[28,29] Quarantines can operate at the individual or population level. Perimeter or geographic quarantines may involve restrictions on travel to and from designated geographic areas or places.

Public health authorities implemented containment strategies in countries with diverse sociopolitical and constitutional traditions, ranging from China, Hong Kong, Vietnam, and Singapore to Canada and the United States.[30] Most jurisdictions confined patients in their homes or general hospitals, but others considered the construction of special infectious disease hospitals, as in Guandong Province and Hong Kong.[31] In Asia and Canada, authorities ordered mass quarantines or closures for schools, hospitals, factories, hotels, restaurants, places of entertainment, or residential buildings.[32–35] In the United States, New York City issued a 10-day hospital quarantine order for a foreign tourist.[36] The city of San Jose, California, held an incoming flight from Tokyo on the tarmac for several hours to investigate a potential SARS case.[37]

Some countries, particularly the United States, sought voluntary separation of exposed patients,[38] but others used more intrusive forms of enforcement. In Singapore, where thousands were subjected to quarantine, authorities used thermal scanners, Web cameras, and electronic bracelets to enforce quarantine, supervised by a security agency.[39] In Hong Kong, the police department's electronic tracking system was used to enforce quarantine.[40] In Beijing and Taipei, hospitals with SARS cases quarantined staff and patients. In Canada, a high school was closed and 1,500 students ordered to home quarantine because of a single case involving a student with symptoms of SARS. Ontario's commissioner of public health warned that he had the authority to hospitalize those who failed to adhere to the order.[41]

Travel Restrictions

The role of a physician from Guandong Province, China, as a source of infection to hotel patrons in Hong Kong, who then carried the disease to Singapore, Toronto, and Vietnam, led to an early focus on the role of international travel in the spread of disease. In a striking observation, the WHO asserted that it "regard[ed] every country with an international airport, or bordering an area having recent local transmission, as a potential risk for an outbreak."[39]

As a consequence, the WHO issued "the toughest travel advisories in its 55-year history" when in April and May 2003 it recommended the postponement of all but essential travel to high-risk SARS areas.[39] At one time or another, advisories were issued for Hong Kong, the Guandong Province of China, Beijing, Shanxi Province, Toronto, Tianjin, Inner Mongolia, and Taiwan.[42] Such geographically specific travel advisories were historically unprecedented. To prevent the spread of SARS from outbreak areas, the WHO also recommended screening all international departing travelers for symptoms of SARS or exposure to those with the disease before embarkation. Individuals with fevers were "requested" to postpone their journeys.[43] In Vietnam, Hong Kong, and Singapore, air travelers were screened for high body temperatures with either digital thermometers or thermal-imaging scanners.[44–48] Thus, the imperative to interrupt the spread of SARS through travel restrictions placed limits on privacy, freedom of association, and liberty.

In the United States, President Bush added SARS to the list of quarantinable diseases in early April 2003,[49] and in May the Department of Homeland Security announced that immigration and customs agents were authorized to detain travelers who appeared to be ill with SARS-associated symptoms.[50] Reflecting the level of national anxiety, prominent universities sought to impose their own restrictions. In early May, the University of California at Berkeley, acting on the advice of a local health official, cancelled a summer program for students from China.[51] Some universities discouraged friends and families from traveling to commencement exercises. Harvard prohibited students and faculty from using university funds to travel to China, Hong Kong, Singapore, and Taiwan.[52]

Reflecting the rapidly changing understanding of the nature and tolerability of risk associated with casual contact, public health agencies ultimately cautioned against such restrictive measures. In mid-May, the Centers for Disease Control and Prevention (CDC) stated it would not "recommend . . . the cancellation or postponement of classes, meetings or other gatherings that would include travelers from areas with SARS."[53] The WHO, reflecting similar concerns, stated, "the best defense is not exclusion."[9]

Ethical and Legal Recommendations for Responding to Severe Infectious Disease Threats

The WHO concluded that the prompt reporting of cases involving symptoms suggestive of SARS, early identification and isolation of patients, "vigorous contact tracing," and the confinement of close contacts had effectively contained the outbreak: SARS had been curtailed and "driven back out of its new human host."[54] Whether this prognosis is correct—eradicationism has a troubled history—or whether the next flu season will witness a recrudescence of disease remains to be seen. But the fact that a rapidly spreading disease with high case fatality rates was quickly brought under control by some combination of these measures is beyond question.

That a common set of public health interventions worked in contexts as different as China, Vietnam, Singapore, Taiwan, Hong Kong, and Canada should not mask the fact that public health measures are embedded in broader sociopolitical contexts. Coercive strategies reflect conceptions of individual rights, the legitimacy of state intrusions, and the appropriate balance between security and liberty. Measures tolerable in an authoritarian regime would not be tolerated in a liberal democratic state. What then is acceptable in constitutional democracies? What ethical norms and legal principles should guide preparations for what may follow? The specific answers will, of course, depend on the scale of any future epidemic—a handful of cases may call for less rigorous measures than hundreds of cases. Nevertheless, the following principles should guide policymakers in the event of any outbreak.

We take as a starting point the centrality of the precautionary principle for the ethics of public health. The principle stipulates an obligation to protect populations against reasonably foreseeable threats, even under conditions of uncertainty.[55] First articulated in the context of environmental hazards, the precautionary principle seeks to forestall disasters and guide decision making in the context of incomplete knowledge. Given the potential costs of inaction, it is the failure to implement preventive measures that requires justification. Proponents of the precautionary principle explicitly defend their position by noting that entities that threaten the environment are best able to bear the burdens of regulation. Opponents warn that the imposition of such burdens may stifle economic progress and scientific innovation.[56] The principle has not been explicitly invoked in the context of epidemic threats where preemptive actions may burden individuals and impose limits on their freedoms. Nevertheless, the precautionary principle has implicitly guided public health interventions designed to limit or forestall epidemic outbreaks.

For nations that share the central values of a liberal democracy, safeguards of individual rights must bound the precautionary principle. Consequently, the least restrictive/intrusive alternative, fairness and justice (both procedural and substantive), and transparency provide the basis for effective public health actions that are not unduly burdensome on individual rights.

Requiring the least restrictive/intrusive alternative that can effectively achieve a legitimate public health goal represents a means to impose limits on state interventions consistent with the traditions of privacy, liberty, and freedom of association. The standard does not require public health authorities to adopt measures that are less effective but does require the least invasive intervention that will achieve the objective. How to strike the balance between degrees of efficacy and invasiveness will inevitably remain a matter of controversy.

Justice requires that the benefits and burdens of public health action be fairly distributed, thus precluding the unjustified targeting of already socially vulnerable populations. Therefore, a careful assessment of the burdens attendant on public health interventions is necessary. Procedural justice requires a fair and independent hearing for individuals who are subjected to burdensome public health action. Due process requirements are inherently important because fair hearings affirm the dignity of the person; due process is also instrumentally important because it best ensures accurate decision making.

Finally, transparency requires government officials to make decisions in an open and fully accountable manner. It further demands civic deliberation and public participation in the policymaking process. Individuals should understand the facts and reasons justifying public health interventions, the goals of intervention, and the steps taken to safeguard individual rights.

When taken together, the precautionary principle, the least intrusive/restrictive alternative, justice, and transparency underscore the importance of using voluntary rather than coercive measures whenever possible. Although mandatory measures and recourse to coercion may be necessary, efforts designed to elicit the voluntary cooperation of those at risk of acquiring or transmitting infectious diseases are preferable. Mass persuasion and public education to prevent panic and encourage risk avoidance are thus essential features of public health. From an ethical perspective, such efforts are desirable because they enhance the public's health without burdening personal interests in privacy and liberty. From a pragmatic perspective, such efforts reduce the necessity of invoking the coercive power of the state that may provoke resistance at a juncture when cooperation is essential. The following recommendations address the challenges that will be posed to public health by future outbreaks of SARS or other epidemic threats.

Surveillance and Contact Tracing:
The Limits of Privacy

Surveillance, as an epidemiological measure and a call to intervene, raises issues regarding the limits of privacy. The question of when, if ever, the confidentiality of the clinical relationship might be breached has challenged policymakers since the late nineteenth century, when health officials undertook modern disease surveillance. Although physicians have historically resisted public health intrusions, the absence of legal and ethical challenges to the practice in recent decades—the debates over reporting the names of patients with human immunodeficiency virus were a striking exception[57]—suggests that name-based surveillance has been recognized as an acceptable limit on privacy. The state, of course, has to meet rigorous standards: demonstrate an important need to know and intervene, make decisions openly, consult with the relevant communities, and use data only for legitimate public health purposes.

An Important Need to Know and Intervene

Name reporting is crucial in facilitating public health interventions such as contact tracing and isolation or quarantine, thus necessitating the subordination of privacy interests to the common good. In the context of a communicable disease such as SARS, which has a high case fatality rate, it is important to know who is infected and who was exposed to target interventions. Reporting SARS cases without names would be less intrusive but also ineffective. Consequently, name reporting would meet the least intrusive alternative standard.

Physicians and hospitals have a moral obligation to report all SARS cases to ensure the most effective public health interventions and that the benefits and burdens of privacy invasions are equitably distributed. Where public health authorities have so directed, such obligations may be required as a matter of law. The U.S. Supreme Court has held that mandatory name reporting constitutes "a reasonable exercise of the state's broad police powers" when people's names are stored in a secure manner.[58]

Transparency Regarding Uses, the Potential
for Disclosure, and Harm

The privacy-limiting nature of name reporting imposes on health departments an obligation to educate the public about the nature of ongoing surveillance and the way in which case reports will be used. It is imperative not only to determine how privacy will be protected but also to account for the practical limits of privacy, particularly as contact tracing is undertaken. When coworkers, neighbors, or classmates are told that they may have been exposed to SARS, the identity of the sick and missing index case may become apparent even if names are not used.

Those who are interviewed in contact tracing need to be given an appreciation of why they have a moral obligation to reveal the names of those they might have exposed. The willingness to cooperate may rest on their understanding of the public health needs and the practical limits of privacy. Protection of the needs and interests of those who are identified as sick or exposed is essential.

Consultation with the Community at Risk to Minimize Stigma

Diseases that may differentially affect segments of the population have usually imposed the additional burden of social opprobrium. Public health officials may inadvertently amplify the process as they conduct their surveillance activities.[59] Although they may not be able to prevent stigmatization, officials have an obligation to take steps to mitigate the suffering that may attend their efforts by underscoring the irrationality and inequity of ethnic stereotyping. Consultation with representatives of the communities most at risk will be important for instrumental reasons and as an expression of social solidarity.

Legitimacy of Public Health Purpose

The breach in privacy represented by mandatory notification can only be justified if systems are in place to ensure that reported data are used solely for legitimate public health purposes. Surveillance is warranted if it is directed, for example, to reducing morbidity and mortality or directing resources to those who require treatment but not to achieve punitive ends. Although it may prove appropriate for the health system to call on law enforcement to fulfill public health mandates (e.g., enforcing quarantines), health professionals should have exclusive responsibility for eliciting the names of contacts and instructing individuals about precautionary measures.

Just as physicians and hospitals have a moral obligation and may be legally required to report cases to public health authorities, nations have an obligation to report aggregate, nonidentified data on SARS outbreaks to the WHO to facilitate the coordination of international control efforts. It was the months-long failure of China to report its outbreak that delayed an effective international public health response. These obligations are also grounded in binding treaty obligations. The WHO's International Health Regulations (IHRs), originally adopted in 1951, require member states to notify the WHO of cases of cholera, plague, or yellow fever.[60] The WHO is currently revising the IHRs to include all public health emergencies of international concern through reliance on "global information networks."[61] SARS would likely be included in this broadened definition. In May 2003, the 56th World Health Assembly adopted a resolution that called SARS an international public health emergency and urged member states to report cases to the WHO "promptly and transparently."[1]

Isolation and Quarantine: The Limits of Liberty

Isolation and quarantine, as ancient measures to separate the healthy from those infected or exposed, raise questions about the limits of liberty.[62] Certainly, such separation is warranted to avert significant risks of transmission. But beyond that, there are questions of the level of risk that justifies loss of liberty, the social and economic harms, and potential for using public health as a subterfuge for discrimination. One U.S. court, for example, invalidated an early twentieth century quarantine in San Francisco, California, that operated exclusively against the Chinese community, concluding that public health officials had operated with an "evil eye and an unequal hand."[63] We recommend the following criteria to assess the ethical and legal justification for isolation and quarantine: scientific assessment of risk, targeting restrictive measures, a safe and humane environment, fair treatment and social justice, procedural due process, and the least restrictive alternative.

Scientific Assessment of Risk

We suggest a hierarchy of cases, ranging from the most easily justifiable to those that may be viewed as problematic, based on the scientific certainty that the patient is infectious and poses a risk to others. Isolation of a confirmed SARS case during the period of infectiousness is firmly supported by legal tradition and ethics.[64] All legal systems, as well as international human rights, permit governments to infringe on personal liberty to prevent a significant risk to the public.[65] In the liberal tradition, the harm principle justifies restrictions on liberty to avert tangible harms to third parties.[66] Since those with SARS pose a direct threat to close contacts, their liberty can be justifiably restrained. However, if a SARS case is unconfirmed or if the individual simply has been exposed or is suspected of being exposed, the justification for restricting liberty is less clear.

Faced with the prospect of a significant risk—measured in terms of the probability of transmission and the severity of harm—populations should be protected, even in the context of medical uncertainty. The precautionary principle provides a justification for such restrictions: Government may act to prevent tangible harms to the population even without complete scientific information. Consequently, from a public health perspective, individual movement can be restrained to avert transmission until potential infectiousness can be ruled out.

Targeting Restrictive Measures

In principle, restrictive measures should be limited to those known to be infectious. But in the case of SARS, the uncertainty about how wide to cast the net of quarantine for exposed, asymptomatic individuals is framed by the absence at this juncture of a diagnostic assay that can rapidly distinguish between the infected and merely exposed with high specificity. Were such a test available, it would be possible to screen exposed individuals, subjecting only those who were infected—but not yet symptomatic—to isolation. Under such circumstances, individuals would have the choice of being tested and, if test results are negative, being freed from the burden of quarantine; those choosing not to be tested would be subject to quarantine.

A Safe and Habitable Environment

Since isolation and quarantine are designed to promote well-being and not to punish the individual, public health authorities have the obligation to provide quarters that are decent and not degrading. Jails and prisons are unacceptable settings for confinement. Patients should have adequate health care, protection from further exposure to SARS, the necessities of life such as food and clothing, and means of communication with family, friends, and attorneys. For those diagnosed as having SARS, places of confinement should be safe for the patient, caregivers, and family members. Ideally, patients should be placed in hospitals or other health care settings that offer skilled medical and nursing care, infection control, and isolation facilities. Consequently, public health preparedness requires strengthening the health care system through planning and resources to ensure adequately trained staff, infection control methods and equipment, and negative pressure isolation rooms.[67]

Contemporary public health practice favors "sheltering in place," preferably in a person's home.[68] Home confinement is less restrictive, more humane, and more likely to achieve public acceptance. Nevertheless, home quarantines can only be morally justified in contexts where residential units permit exposed but asymptomatic individuals to remain confined without imposing risks on those with whom they live. Sheltering in place assumes voluntary compliance. Yet, enforcement of home quarantine may necessitate limits on privacy and may have an impact on dignity as well, involving, for example, surveillance cameras; electronic bracelets, placards, or notices; and the presence of police guards. Home quarantine also can create divisions based on social class because the poor may not have homes adequate to protect the unexposed.

Fair Treatment and Social Justice

Fairness may require consideration of compensation, particularly for the poor who lose vital income during isolation or quarantine. When public health authorities require people to forgo their freedom for the common good, equity requires that the financial burden be borne by the community as a whole. To do so will require a fundamental, and no doubt controversial, departure from historical practice. Such measures were taken in Taiwan, where "Persons who completed quarantine received the equivalent of U.S. $147. Quarantined persons could request other social services from local health and civil affairs departments."[69] There is currently an intense policy discussion about this matter in Canada. A broad public debate of how best to achieve equity is therefore necessary. Among the possibilities are ensuring that sick pay benefits—where they are contractually available—be guaranteed to those deprived of the ability to work because of quarantine; the provision of basic welfare benefits to those without access to sick pay; and an extension of disaster relief now available to communities faced with flood, storms, and earthquakes when the Federal Emergency Management Agency is called on. The potential cost of such measures should not be permitted to limit the capacity of officials to impose isolation and quarantine when necessary for the public's health.

Procedural Due Process

Due process requires the right to be heard by an independent tribunal in a timely manner with representation by an attorney. The U.S. Supreme Court has noted that civil confinement constitutes "a significant deprivation of liberty" that "can engender adverse social consequences."[70] Although some may argue that home quarantine need not trigger a full-blown hearing, we believe that anyone deprived of liberty under color of law, whatever the place of confinement, should have available a due process hearing. In a public health emergency, it may be necessary to confine individuals before a hearing is held, but a speedy hearing should, if requested, follow. We make these observations aware of the vast logistical complications of hearings in the event of mass quarantines. Ensuring a well-functioning judicial system with trained attorneys and knowledgeable judges will prove challenging.

The Least Restrictive Alternative

Even if all of the foregoing conditions are satisfied, public health authorities should resort to isolation or quarantine only if it is the least restrictive/intrusive alternative. During the first SARS outbreak, broad quarantines were justifiable because of the uncertainties of risk. If careful examination of that experience reveals that more circumscribed measures would serve the public good, more narrowly drawn quarantines would be appropriate.[70]

Travel Advisories and Restrictions: Limits on the Freedom of Movement

The right to travel within a nation or internationally is vitally important legally, economically, and politically. Travel is important to well-being because it enables people to pursue their goals, associate with their family and friends, and conduct business. The freedom of movement is recognized as a basic right within countries,[71] regionally,[72,73] and globally.[74] The U.S. Supreme Court declared, "[f]reedom of movement and of residence must be a fundamental right in a democratic State."[75] The United Nations similarly finds that "[l]iberty of movement is an indispensable condition for the free development of a person."[76]

International law affords a right to travel within one's country.[77] Individuals also have the human right to leave and return to their country of origin.[78] Yet, these rights may be permissibly restricted on public health grounds.[79] The right to travel, although fundamental, is not unlimited: "Freedom does not mean that areas ravaged by flood, fire or pestilence cannot be quarantined . . . [to protect] safety and welfare."[80] Countries may also restrict these rights to protect "public health or . . . the rights and freedoms of others."[73] Furthermore, IHRs (article 30.1.a) oblige health officials to take all practicable steps to prevent the departure of any individual known or suspected of being infected with a communicable disease that poses a serious public health threat.

Thus, we maintain that government cannot abridge the right to travel without a legitimate public health purpose, and that restrictions must be narrowly drawn and targeted. Although private entities such as universities are not bound by national constitutions or international law, they are bound by the basic moral considerations that should inform public policies that infringe the right to travel.

Limiting Travel Is Justified by a Legitimate Public Health Purpose

Restricting travel by those with SARS, and even those recently exposed to SARS, poses few moral quandaries. There is no right to board conveyances if in so doing one imposes ineliminable risks on others. Nor is there a right of entry into a country if one is sick with an infectious condition marked by high case fatality rates. Consequently, screening passengers before embarkation and at borders is legally and morally appropriate.

The Right of Return to a Person's Home Country Should Not Be Denied

International human rights law entitles individuals to return to their country of citizenship. The reasoning is that people have a right to a place to reside and should not suffer the indignity of forced exclusion from their home country. In emergency situations, however, this principle may be limited when infectious individuals pose a risk to others on international conveyances. As soon as it is safe to do so, individuals infected with or exposed to SARS should be permitted to return to their home countries.

Travel Advisories to SARS-Affected Areas Are Warranted to Accurately Inform the Public

Travel to areas marked by SARS outbreaks poses a different set of issues. Travel advisories or warnings that inform individuals about the risks of travel to certain locales are not problematic. Indeed, it would represent a failure of public health responsibility not to issue such warnings. Since they pose potentially severe economic consequences, travel warnings should be based on reliable epidemiological evidence.

Travel Restrictions to SARS-Affected Areas Are Justified Only Where Return Travel Imposes a Serious Risk to Others

More complex and troubling is the imposition of travel restrictions to SARS outbreak areas, such as those that were imposed by some U.S. universities. Competent adults, in general, have the right to assume risks once informed of the consequences of their decisions. However, when travel to an outbreak area poses a risk of acquiring a fatal illness and where return travel might impose hazards on others, the case for restrictions is enhanced by the harm principle. For example, in an uncontrolled generalized outbreak, travel restrictions could be justifiable. In such a situation, exceptions for scientists and health care workers who may be critical to disease control and for journalists providing news coverage should be made.

Nevertheless, where outbreaks are largely restricted to health care institutions, restrictions on travel would be overbroad.

Conclusion: Acting Under Scientific Uncertainty

The first reports of SARS from China, coming after months of delay, provided the occasion for an extraordinary international mobilization of public health resources. At the WHO there was consternation that if preventive measures were not put in place rapidly a worldwide pandemic might emerge.[15] It was necessary to take action despite the CDC's acknowledgment in April 2003 that the scientific community had an incomplete understanding of SARS and its mode of transmission.[81] It was appropriate for public health authorities to act on worst-case scenarios based on assumptions of how an airborne disease might spread. When a cluster of cases in a single apartment complex was identified in Hong Kong, the possibility of more efficient modes of transmission could not be discredited.

The precautionary principle—even when limited by the least restrictive/intrusive alternative, justice, and transparency—dictated that restrictive measures be imposed to halt the spread of SARS. It is not surprising that those primarily concerned with civil liberties would be troubled by the measures taken, that they would argue that in face of uncertainty greater deference be given to the rights of individuals. Nor is it surprising that those whose economic interests might have been harmed by travel advisories saw an "overblown" reaction that they feared would be ruinously costly.[15]

There is no way to avoid the dilemmas posed by acting without full scientific knowledge. Failure to move aggressively can have catastrophic consequences. Actions that prove to have been unnecessary will be viewed as draconian and based on hysteria. The only safeguard is transparency. International and national public health agencies must be willing to make clear the bases for restrictive measures and openly acknowledge when new evidence warrants reconsideration of policies. Adoption of ethical recommendations will be a necessary concomitant of epidemic control in democratic societies. Public health decisions will reflect in a profound way the manner in which societies both implicitly and explicitly balance values that are intimately related and inherently in tension.

Funding/Support: The Center for Law and the Public's Health at Georgetown University and Johns Hopkins University are supported by the CDC and the Alfred P. Sloan Foundation, New York, New York.

Disclaimer: The contents of this article do not necessarily represent the views of the CDC. Mr. Gostin, a health law and ethics editor for JAMA, was not involved in the editorial review or decision to publish this article.

Acknowledgment: We acknowledge support of the Office of the Dean at the Columbia University Mailman School of Public Health for hosting a meeting entitled "Ethical Challenges Posed by SARS" on 18 June 2003 and support by the Visiting Scholars Program at the Institute for the Medical Humanities, University of Texas Medical Branch, Galveston.

References

1. World Health Organization. Revision of the International Health Regulations—severe acute respiratory syndrome (SARS). Available at: http://www.who.int/gb/EB_WHA/PDF/WHA56/ea5648.pdf. Accessed 14 July 2003.

2. World Health Organization. Update 95-SARS: chronology of a serial killer. Available at: http://www.who.int/csr/don/2003_07_04/en/. Accessed 3 September 2003.

3. Bayer R, Levine C, Wolf SM. HIV antibody screening: an ethical framework for evaluating proposed programs. *JAMA*. 1986;256:1768–1774.

4. Fujiwara PI, Frieden TR. TB control in New York City: a recent history. Available at: http://www.cdc.gov/nchstp/tb/notes/TBN_1_00/TBN2000Fujiwara. Accessed 14 July 2003.

5. Gerberding JL. Faster . . . but fast enough? Responding to the epidemic of severe acute respiratory syndrome. *N Engl J Med.* 2003;348:2030.

6. World Health Organization. Cumulative number of reported probable cases of SARS. Available at: http://www.who.int/csr/sars/country/2003_07_01/en/. Accessed 3 September 2003.

7. Masur H, Emanuel E, Lane HC. Severe acute respiratory syndrome: providing care in the face of uncertainty. *JAMA.* 2003;289:2861–2863.

8. Kuepper GJ. The Hong Kong experience. Available at: http://www.emergency-management.net/pdf/sars_gjk.pdf. Accessed 14 July 2003.

9. Outbreak of severe acute respiratory syndrome-worldwide, 2003. *MMWR Morb Mortal Wkly Rep.* 2003;52:226–228.

10. World Health Organization. Guidance for mass gatherings: hosting persons arriving from an area with recent local transmission of SARS. Available at: http://www.who.int/csr/sars/guidelines/gatherings/en/print.html/html. Accessed 14 July 2003.

11. World Health Organization. Case definitions for surveillance of severe acute respiratory syndrome (SARS). Available at: http://www.who.int/csr/sars/casedefinition/en/. Accessed 14 July 2003.

12. Rider D. SARS infects "protected" medical staff: gloves, gowns, masks didn't stop outbreak at Sunnybrook. *Ottawa Citizen.* 20 April 2003:A1.

13. World Health Organization. Update 70—Singapore removed from list of areas with local SARS transmission. Available at: http://www.who.int/csr/don /2003_05_30a/en/.print.html. Accessed 30 May 2003.

14. Long S. Singapore at war. *The Straits Times (Singapore).* 11 May 2003. Available at: http://web.lexis-nexis.com. Accessed 16 September 2003.

15. Bradsher K, Altman L. Isolation, an old medical tool, has SARS fading. *New York Times.* 21 June 2003:A1.

16. Bradsher K. The SARS epidemic: Asia: to broad support, Hong Kong police take on an expanded role in fighting SARS. *New York Times.* 25 April 2003:A20.

17. Krauss C. Fifteen new cases of pneumonia near Toronto may be SARS. *New York Times.* 10 June 2003:A13.

18. Sternberg S. World health experts treat SARS as if it's the big one. *USA Today.* 24 April 2003:1A.

19. Battling a national crisis [extract of Deputy Prime Minister Lee Hsien Loong's May Day speech]. *The Straits Times (Singapore).* 25 April 2003. Available at: http://Iweb.lexis-nexis.com. Accessed 16 September 2003.

20. Paddock R. A hotbed of SARS warfare: mass temperature testing is just one of the tools that the autocratic city-state of Singapore is wielding in its winning assault on the disease. *Los Angeles Times.* 8 May 2003:1 (main news, part 1, foreign desk).

21. Cohn M. No end in sight in Hong Kong. *Toronto Star.* 21 April 2003:A1.

22. Donovan K. Suspected cases reported in U.S., Ireland, Bulgaria. *Toronto Star.* 25 April 2003:A14.

23. Police system tracking virus sources. Available at: http://www.news.gov.hk/en/category/issues/030425/html/030425en08002.htm. Accessed 14 July 2003.

24. Perl T. *A Report from Toronto: Ethical Challenges Posed by SARS.* Toronto, ON: Mailman School of Public Health, Columbia University; 18 June 2003.

25. Sorensen C. Chinese Canadians feeling backlash. *Toronto Star.* 4 April 2003: A6.

26. Cheng M. Sorry for snub: New Jersey schools apologize for SARS episode. *New York Newsday.* 17 May 2003:A4.

27. Rider D. Fear of virus fuels racism: Ontario must do more to stop return to days of "yellow peril" Asian leaders say. *Ottawa Citizen.* 4 April 2003:A10.

28. Benenson AS, ed. *Control of Communicable Diseases Manual.* Washington, DC: American Public Health Association; 1995.

29. Barbera J, Macintyre A, Gostin L, et al. Large-scale quarantine following biological terrorism in the United States: scientific examination, logistic and legal limits, and possible consequences. *JAMA.* 2001;286:2711–2717.

30. Bloom BR. Lessons from SARS. *Science.* 2003;300:701.

31. Hong Kong Economic and Trade Office Tokyo [press release]. Available at: http://www.hketotyo.or.jp/english/news_sars030605_e.html. Accessed 14 July 2003.

32. Kahn JB. Quarantine set in Beijing areas to fight SARS. *New York Times.* 25 April 2003:A1.

33. Centers for Disease Control and Prevention. Severe acute respiratory syndrome—Singapore 2003. *MMWR Morb Mortal Wkly Rep.* 2003;52:40–41.

34. Bradsher K. The SARS epidemic: economy; outbreak of disease brings big drop-off in China's economy. *New York Times.* 28 April 2003:A1.

35. Wayne A. In Singapore, 1970s law becomes weapon against SARS. *New York Times.* 10 June 2003:F4.

36. Altman LK. The SARS epidemic: New York; public health fears cause New York officials to detain foreign tourist. *New York Times.* 28 April 2003:A1.

37. McNeil DG Jr. A respiratory illness: tracking disease; worries over respiratory illness prompt quarantine of jet in California. *New York Times.* 2 April 2003:A1.

38. Cooper MH. Fighting SARS. *CQ Researcher.* 20 June 2003.

39. World Health Organization. Severe acute respiratory syndrome-Singapore, 2003. *Wkly Epidemiol Rec.* 2003;78:161.

40. World Health Organization. *Severe Acute Respiratory Syndrome (SARS): Status of the Outbreak and Lessons for the Immediate Future.* Geneva, Switzerland: World Health Organization; 2003.

41. Brown DL. Sick of quarantine in Toronto; after school's SARS scare, teens bored by week in isolation. *Washington Post.* 3 June 2003:A20.

42. World Health Organization. Update 95—chronology of travel recommendations, areas of local transmission. Available at: http://www.who.int/csr/don/2003_07_01/en/. Accessed 1 July 2003.

43. World Health Organization. WHO recommended measures for persons undertaking international travel from areas affected by severe acute respiratory syndrome (SARS). *Wkly Epidemiol Rec.* 2003;78:98.

44. Nakashima E. Vietnamese cautiously hail progress on SARS: strict measures planned to prevent new cases. *Washington Post.* 1 May 2003:A11.

45. Cohn MR. No end in sight in Hong Kong. *Toronto Star.* 21 April 2003:A1.

46. Marshall T, Paddock RC, Kuhn A. Vietnam first to contain SARS. *Los Angeles Times.* 28 April 2003:1 (main news, part 1, foreign desk).

47. Garrett L. Masks off—for now. *Newsday.* 29 June 2003:A5.

48. Maynard M. Passport, mask, thermometer. *New York Times.* 11 May 2003;5:6.

49. Public Health Service Act. 42 USC 264 (2003); Executive Order, signed 4 April 2003.

50. Sheldon P. U.S. approves force in detaining possible SARS carriers. *New York Times.* 7 May 2003:A10.

51. Murphy DE, Arenson KW. Students in SARS countries banned for Berkeley session. *New York Times.* 6 May 2003:A12.

52. Harvard University Health Services. University announces policies regarding visitors. summer residency at Harvard. Available at: http://www.uhs.harvard.edu/NewsFlash/SARSinfo.htm. Accessed 7 July 2003.

53. Centers for Disease Control. Update: severe acute respiratory syndrome—United States. 14 May 2003. *MMWR Morb Mortal Wkly Rep.* 2003;52:436.

54. World Health Organization. Update 58–first global consultation on SARS epidemiology. Travel recommendations for Hebei Province (China), situation in Singapore. Available at: http://www.who.int/csr/sars/archive/2003_05_17.html. Accessed 7 July 2003.

55. Applegate J. The precautionary preference: an American perspective on the precautionary principle. *Hum Ecol Risk Assess.* 2000;6:413–443.

56. Morris J. Defining the precautionary principle. In: *Rethinking Risk and the Precautionary Principle.* Boston, MA: Butterworth-Heinemann; 2000:1–21.

57. Gostin LO, Ward JW, Baker AC. National HIV case reporting for the United States: a defining moment in the history of the epidemic. *N Engl J Med.* 1997; 337:1162–1167.

58. *Whalen v. Roe.* 429 U.S. 589 (1977).

59. Council for International Organizations of Medical Sciences. International guidelines for ethical review of epidemiological studies. *Law Med Health Care.* 1991;19: 247–258.

60. World Health Organization. Current International Health Regulations (IHR). Available at: http://www.who.int/csr/ihr/current/en/. Accessed 14 July 2003.

61. Fidler DP. Emerging trends in international law concerning global infectious disease control. *Emerg Infed Dis.* 2003;9:285–290.

62. Gostin LO. *Public Health Law: Power. Duty. Restraint.* Berkeley, CA, and New York, NY: University of California Press and Milbank Memorial Fund; 2000.

63. *Jew Ho v. Williamson.* 103 F 10 (CCND Ca11900).

64. Gostin LO. Public health law in an age of terrorism: rethinking individual rights and common goods. *Health Aff (Millwood).* 2002;21:79–93.

65. United Nations Economic and Social Council. The Siracusa principles on the limitations and derogation provisions in the International Covenant on Civil and Political Rights. UN Doc. E/CN.4/1985/4, Annex. Available at: http://www1.umn.edu/humanrts/instree/siracusaprinciples.html. Accessed 7 July 2003.

66. Feinberg J. *The Moral Limits of the Criminal Law.* 4 vols. New York, NY: Oxford University Press; 1987–1990.

67. Wynia MK, Gostin L. The bioterrorist threat and access to health care. *Science.* 2002;296:1613.

68. Sheltering in place. Available at: http://www.avertdisasters.org/html/shelterinplace.html. Accessed 14 July 2003.

69. Use of quarantine to prevent transmission of severe acute respiratory syndrome—Taiwan. 2003. *MMWR Morb Mortal Wkly Rep.* 2003;52:680–683.

70. *Addington v. Texas,* 441 U.S. 418. 426 (1979).

71. *Shapiro v. Thompson,* 394 U.S. 618 (1969).

72. *EC Commission v. Netherlands,* 19932 CMLR 389 (1991).

73. *Peirmont v. France,* 20 ECHR 301 (1995).

74. Freedom of movement and transnational migrations: a legal survey. Available at: http://heiwww.unige.ch/cont/psio_230502/files/chetail.doc. Accessed 7 July 2003.

75. *Edwards v. California,* 314 U.S. 160 (1941).

76. Human Rights Committee. *General Comment No. 27 to Article 12 of the International Covenant on Civil and Political Rights.* New York, NY: United Nations; 1999.

77. *International Covenant on Civil and Political Rights.* New York, NY: United Nations; 1999:article 12, §1.

78. *International Covenant on Civil and Political Rights.* New York. NY: United Nations; 1999:article 12, §§2 and 4.

79. *International Covenant on Civil and Political Rights.* New York, NY: United Nations; 1999:article 12, §3.

80. *Zemel v. Rusk,* 381 U.S. 1 (1965).

81. Centers for Disease Control and Prevention. Update: outbreak of severe acute respiratory syndrome—worldwide. 2003. *MMWR Morb Mortal Wkly Rep.* 2003;52:270.

17

Ethical Issues in the Vaccination of Children

Douglas S. Diekema and
Edgar K. Marcuse

The vaccination of children against a multitude of infectious agents has been hailed by many as one of the most effective health interventions of the 20th century. Vaccination serves two goals.[1] The first is to prevent disease among individuals and within groups. This goal may be accomplished directly through the protection offered to vaccinated individuals and indirectly to unvaccinated individuals surrounded by vaccinated individuals who neither contract nor spread the agent in question—a phenomenon known as herd immunity.[2] A second goal of vaccination programs is the eradication of disease. The global eradication of smallpox in 1977 is an example of a vaccine program that attained the second goal, as a result eliminating the need for smallpox vaccination.

For vaccination programs to be successful either individuals must willingly agree to vaccination or vaccination must be coerced. Vaccination programs involving children pose three important and distinct issues that we will address. First, do parents who withhold vaccinations from their children harm them to such an extent that parental refusal ought to be overridden? Second, what duties do parents owe others in the community to avoid causing harm through an unvaccinated child? Third, does the social value of having a vaccinated population—for the sake of herd immunity and the eradication of disease—justify coercive efforts to vaccinate all children?

It is useful to look at the issues related to the vaccination of children in light of the maxim, *primum non nocere* (above all, do no harm). The phrase has often been used to convey that in practicing their art, physicians ought to benefit the patient when possible, and at least not make the situation worse.[3] Jonsen's examination of the maxim has revealed at least four different and not necessarily inconsistent ways in which *primum non nocere* has been interpreted.[4]

The first common use interprets the maxim to imply that medicine, as a practice, is a moral enterprise that ought to be applied for the benefit of the patient. In thinking about vaccination, the first use of the maxim would require that physicians vaccinate patients because of the benefit vaccination brings to those patients. Vaccination for reasons other than patient benefit would be suspect. A physician administering a vaccine to patients without their consent solely to meet an organizational quality assurance goal would be violating the maxim in its first sense.

The second use suggests that in practicing medicine for the benefit of the patient, physicians should take due care to prevent any harm that might arise from the practice of their art. This sense of the maxim is less rigid than the first, requiring only that the physician takes care not to harm their patient or others. Providing and encouraging vaccination of children should be done in a way that minimizes harm. For example, physicians should warn parents to avoid exposing a child who has received the oral polio vaccine to those who might be immunocompromised. Jonsen notes that the first and second meanings of the maxim are directed primarily at the physician as a moral agent. They direct the physician in how to practice their craft, for the benefit of the patient and with due care to prevent harm.

The third and fourth meanings, on the other hand, most appropriately require involvement of the patient. The third use of the maxim focuses on the result of a risk-benefit calculation in deciding on a treatment plan. It requires that one choose the treatment plan that carries the most favorable balance between chance of success and risk of harm. Gillon has argued for this meaning and changed the maxim to *primum nocere* and *adjuvare,* or benefit with minimal harm.[5] It must involve patient input because of the different weight individuals will place on certain benefits and certain burdens as well as their individual tolerance for risk. This third sense of the maxim is that which relates most closely to vaccination. In making decisions about vaccinations, patients will weigh the benefits offered by the vaccine in question against the risk of potential harm. It is this sense of the maxim *primum non nocere* that most often leads to conflict between those promoting childhood immunization and parental refusal of permission to carry it out.

Finally, the fourth sense of the maxim is similar to the third, in this case seeking the most favorable result in a benefit-detriment equation. Whereas the third sense of the maxim might seek to avoid harm, the fourth sense recognizes that some treatments will inevitably result in harm. The maxim in these cases demands that we do no harm unless that harm is associated with a benefit that at least compensates for the harm done. Again, the patient's input into the importance of the harm and benefits in question will be necessary for applying the maxim in this sense. In the case of vaccination, those requiring injection will inevitably cause some pain. The fourth application of the maxim *primum non nocere* would require that the benefits of the immunization at least compensate for the discomfort of the injection.

These final two aspects of the maxim become more problematic in children. The principle of respect for autonomy influences the maxim *primum non nocere* by requiring that the values of a mature patient influence the ways in which benefits are measured against risks and burdens. Much of pediatrics involves the care of individuals who have yet to develop the capacity to make those kinds of decisions. Since most vaccination involves children, the third and fourth meanings of *primum non nocere* cannot rely on the decision of the person who stands to benefit and to assume some of the risks of potential harm. Rather, a surrogate decision maker must make that decision for the child.

Parental Refusals and the Best Interests of Children

Health care providers and parents are bound by the duty to seek medical benefit for their children while minimizing harm to them. When faced with the decision to immunize a child, the welfare of the child should remain primary. The proper standard for measuring decisions made on behalf of others ought to be a best interests standard. In many cases, more than one approach to the problem may reasonably appear to be in a child's best interests. In those situations, the identification of a reasonable range of decisions that might benefit the child and the elimination of those that are unequivocally harmful to the child is the best we can do.[6] Those most closely situated to the child, usually their parents, should be free to make choices between those options which could reasonably be interpreted as in a child's best interests.

Those who resist immunizing their children often argue that the risk of immunization exceeds any benefit their child will derive from immunization. Though many will recognize the importance of vaccination to the health of a population, they might argue that the benefit to their child is minimal. There are abundant data to suggest that vaccination of children effectively reduces the incidence of childhood disease, and that when vaccination rates in a community fall, outbreaks of disease frequently occur.[7] However, in a community where immunization rates remain high and disease incidence remains negligible, even an unimmunized child may be unlikely to contract the disease in question.

Of course this argument holds only for certain vaccines. Pertussis, diphtheria, and polio, for example, are contracted after contact with an infected individual. As long as an unimmunized individual has no contact with an infected individual, the unimmunized person will not be at risk of disease. However, diseases such as tetanus and rabies are contracted in other ways—through contact with dirt containing the spores of the tetanus bacterium or through the bite of a rabid animal. Vaccinations against tetanus are given to protect individuals against a risk that does not decrease as vaccination rates rise.

In making decisions about vaccination on behalf of their children, parents must consider several factors that will influence the benefit-risk ratio of receiving the vaccine. These factors include the value placed on any discomfort associated with administration of the vaccine, the probability of having a reaction to the vaccine, the value placed on the initial morbidity associated with those reactions and any resulting permanent disability or sequelae, the probability of contracting the disease if unimmunized and the value placed on the expected morbidity from the disease itself, and the probability of contracting significant complications of the disease and the value placed on those complications. While these probabilities are often known for a given vaccine and illness, the values placed on each of the benefits and risks will vary from individual to individual. In the case of children, the values placed on each risk and benefit by their parents will replace the child's inability to value these factors. Zalkind et al. published a decision analysis model that formalizes this kind of noneconomic risk-benefit calculation for the swine influenza vaccine.[8] Using a similar decision analysis, the same could be done for other vaccines.

The results of such an analysis will vary depending upon the prevalence of disease in the community. The balance between the risks and benefits to a given individual favors vaccination when vaccination rates in the community are low and disease prevalence is high. In most cases, however, as vaccination rates climb and disease prevalence drops, the balance tips the other way.[9,10] While the benefits of a pertussis vaccine program, for example, clearly outweigh the risks at a population level,[11] an unvaccinated child living in a well-vaccinated community derives significant indirect protection from herd immunity.[12] One parent might reasonably conclude that refusing the pertussis vaccine is in the best interests of a child living in a community with a 95 percent immunization rate since they are unlikely to contract pertussis and can be spared any risks associated with the vaccine. Another parent might decide differently given the same set of circumstances. In both cases one can reasonably interpret the decision as in the child's best interests since each determination reflects a reasonable assessment of the value placed on each of the potential benefits and risks associated with the disease and the vaccine. In fact, it has been argued that "any successful vaccination programme will inevitably create a situation, as the disease becomes rare, where the individual parent's choice is at odds with society's needs."[13] With a vaccine like the rabies vaccine, the risk of contracting rabies remains low enough that vaccination is rarely sought. However, after contact with a potentially rabid bat, the risk of contracting almost universally fatal rabies rises significantly, shifting the analysis in favor of receiving the vaccine.

The parents or guardians of a child are bound by a duty to make such decisions based upon what they believe to be in the child's best interest. The role of the physician or health care provider in these situations is to provide the risk and benefit information necessary to make an informed decision. The health care provider must also decide in each case what constitutes a range of reasonable decisions using the best interest of the child as a guide. In some situations, the health care provider may disagree with the parents' assessment of the relative risks and benefits of the vaccine and disease in question and thus on what approach would be best for their child. In general, parental decisions should be accepted unless they clearly fall outside the range of what would be a reasonable decision concerning the child's best interest. In those rare cases where the decision of a parent places the child at substantial risk of serious harm, the health care provider may be obligated to involve state agencies in seeking to provide the necessary vaccination in defiance of the parents' objections. For example, in the situation where a child has sustained a deep and contaminated puncture wound, it might be justified to override the decision of a child's parents to refuse treatment with tetanus vaccination.

Feinberg refers to this sort of coercive action as "presumptively nonblamable paternalism" which "consists of defending relatively helpless or vulnerable people from external dangers, including harm from other people when the protected parties have not voluntarily consented to the risk, and doing this in a manner analogous in its motivation and vigilance to that in which parents protect their children."[14] In these cases, the state acts *in loco parentis*, in the place of the parents. While this role of the state has been recognized as constitutionally valid in the United States, courts have closely examined such actions, showing reluctance to require medical treatment over the objection of parents "except where immediate action is necessary or where the potential for harm is rather serious."[15]

Primum Non Nocere and Community Interests

Thus far, we have looked at the problem of vaccination from the individual patient's perspective, with particular reference to the principle of *primum non nocere* as it applies to the person being vaccinated. However, the principle *primum non nocere* is one that has broader application than the therapeutic relationship. All individuals, not exclusively physicians, have a moral duty to avoid causing harm to others. What makes immunization programs different from most other individual health interventions is that immunization has both a direct health benefit to the individual in terms of immunity to certain diseases and an indirect benefit to other individuals in the community—those who remain unimmunized or nonimmune despite immunization. When discussing the ethical issues surrounding vaccination of children, an analysis would be incomplete without examining the duty of parents to have their children vaccinated in order to prevent harm to others in the community within which they live and from which they derive many other benefits.

The first question that arises concerns whether those who refuse to participate in vaccination programs cause harm to other individuals in the community. Veatch has pointed out that the group of individuals most likely to be harmed by those individuals who refuse to be vaccinated is, ironically, the same group of individuals who have refused vaccination.[16] Those individuals who have already been vaccinated are less likely to benefit from herd immunity since most possess individual immunity. Herd immunity benefits those individuals who remain unvaccinated and those few who remain or become susceptible despite vaccination. Unvaccinated individuals can hardly argue that others have a duty to receive immunization in order that they may safely forgo immunization themselves. What complicates this situation, however, is that most vaccination programs target children, whose parents make the decision on their behalf. Thus, children potentially become involuntary participants in vaccination nonparticipation. Because of their vulnerability and inability to make decisions on their own behalf, children have a plausible claim on their parents to make reasonable efforts to protect them from harm. For the same reason, children may have a claim on other individuals to make reasonable efforts to protect them from harm when their parents have failed to do so. Thus, while Veatch argues that a competent individual choosing to remain unvaccinated has no legitimate claim on others to be vaccinated in order to protect themselves from harm, the situation differs for children. Parents choosing not to immunize their own children increase the potential for harm to other children who remain unvaccinated not because of their own decisions, but because of the decisions of their parents.

Veatch illustrates two other ways in which those who remain unvaccinated potentially harm others.[17] First, immunized individuals are harmed by the cost of medical care for those who choose not to immunize their children and whose children then contract preventable disease. Of course, a less coercive approach than forced vaccination could minimize the harm of increased medical cost. Veatch proposes higher insurance premiums for those individuals remaining unvaccinated.[18] Alternatively, a tax credit provided to those with proof of vaccination would have a similar effect. A second way is that those who remain unimmunized may harm immunized persons relates to the imperfection of vaccines. A small percentage of vaccinated individuals will either remain or become susceptible to disease. These individuals have done everything they can to protect themselves, yet remain at risk. These individuals do benefit from herd immunity and may be harmed by contracting disease from those who remain unvaccinated.

Refusals of vaccination also raise questions of justice. What sets immunization apart from most other aspects of medical practice is that immunization has a public health benefit in addition to its potential benefit to the individual patient. Community health interests are threatened each time the parent of a child residing in that community refuses to participate in the vaccination program. Even when a parent chooses not to vaccinate a child because that is perceived to be in the child's best interest, issues surrounding the fairness of that decision to others in the community arise.

The problem of fairness that arises has been described as the problem of "free-riders" or "freeloaders."[19-21] As discussed above, situations in which vaccination rates are high and disease rates low present a situation where the risks of vaccination may exceed or equal the risks of contracting disease. Parents may rationally decide to refuse vaccination on behalf of their children. These people are, in a sense, free-riders who take advantage of the benefit created by the participation and assumption of risk of vaccination by others while refusing to participate and share equitably in the risks of the program themselves. They reap the benefits of a vaccination program without sharing any of the risks. These individuals act unfairly to others in the community and slight the community by pursuing self-interest ahead of civic responsibility. Even if the community refuses to coerce or punish these free-riders, they remain morally culpable in an important way. A free and liberal society can exist only if its citizens occasionally make self-interest subservient to the interests of the community. A community that offers its members true freedom must place some restraints on individual freedom. An individual's "freedom" to ignore stop signs while driving, pollute the environment, or spread disease does not ultimately serve the good of freedom.[22] At least, free-riders insult the communities to which they belong, elevating their own interests above those who have acted to make it possible for them to safely do so.

Is Coercion Justified?

Having examined the moral implications of vaccination, let us now turn to a final question concerning whether coercion is justifiable in vaccination programs. It is a well-accepted principle that competent adults should not be forced to undergo medical treatment or vaccination simply because it would be in their best interests. As we have discussed above, children may have vaccination provided against the objections of their parents in situations where parental refusal places the child at significant risk of serious harm. In general, however, coercive measures to force unwanted treatment upon an individual are justified only in those cases where others are placed at risk of harm by the individual's decision or action. In *On Liberty* John Stuart Mill argued:

> The only purpose for which power can rightfully be exercised over any member of a civilized community, against his will, is to prevent harm to others. His own good, either physical or moral, is not a sufficient warrant. . . . The only part of the conduct of anyone for which he is amenable to society is that which concerns others. In the part which merely concerns himself, his independence is, of right, absolute. Over himself, over his own body and mind, the individual is sovereign.[23]

Mill's justification for interfering with the freedom of an individual has become known as the "harm principle." In his work to establish a group of "liberty-limiting principles" that enunciate types of considerations that are always morally relevant reasons to support state action, Feinberg has redefined the harm principle as follows: "It is always a good reason in support of penal legislation that it would be effective in preventing (eliminating, reducing) harm to persons other than the actor (the one prohibited from acting) and there is no other means that is equally effective at no greater cost to other values."[24] What is important to note about Feinberg's analysis is that to justify coercion, it must be both effective at preventing the harm in question and no option that would be less intrusive to individual liberty would be equally effective.

Compulsory vaccination laws in the United States have repeatedly been upheld as a reasonable exercise of the state's police power even in the absence of an epidemic or even a single case.[25,26] They have also been found to be constitutional, even in cases where these laws conflict with the religious beliefs of individuals. In the first such case, *Jacobson v. Massachusetts*, the Supreme Court of the United States held that:

> . . . in every well-ordered society charged with the duty of conserving the safety of its members the rights of the individual in respect of his liberty may at times, under the pressure of great dangers, be subjected to such restraint, to be enforced by reasonable regulations as the safety of the general public may demand. . . . the liberty secured by the Constitution of the United States to every person within its jurisdiction does not import an absolute right in each person to be, at all times and in all circumstances, wholly freed from restraint. There are manifold restraints to which every person is necessarily subject for the common good . . . (Liberty) is only freedom from restraint under conditions essential to the equal enjoyment of the same right by others.[27]

It seems clear that when others are placed at substantial risk of serious harm, the range of choices of the individual may be restricted. But more importantly, is the harm associated with unimmunized individuals great enough to make such restrictions desirable? The answer to this question would seem to be yes in times of epidemic disease when an effective vaccine can end the epidemic and protect those individuals who have not yet contracted the disease. In those situations, however, it is clearly in the self-interest of individuals to receive the vaccine both for themselves and their children. In all likelihood, compulsory vaccination would be unnecessary to achieve adequate levels of vaccination when disease prevalence is high. In this situation, a noncompulsory vaccination program would probably bring about a result similar to a compulsory program without infringing on liberties. Indeed, vaccination rates in several countries without compulsory immunization laws suggest that self-interest in combination with effective education and public relations campaigns may be sufficient to achieve protection of most individuals within a population.[28]

What of the situation in which disease prevalence is low and vaccination rates are high? Should those who remain unvaccinated be compelled to participate in the vaccination program? In this situation, only a very small percentage of those already vaccinated derive any benefit from herd immunity or higher vaccination rates. Most are already protected directly from the vaccine. As discussed above, the economic costs that may be passed on from free-riders who contract disease to those who have been vaccinated could be addressed through a tax credit or price break on insurance premiums. The primary beneficiaries of most compulsory programs to push vaccination rates even higher would be those choosing to remain unvaccinated—the free-riders. Since most of these free-riders have no legitimate claim to the benefit derived from herd immunity—having decided not to participate themselves—Veatch argues that compulsory vaccination programs simply to attain herd immunity may be difficult to justify. Rather, "if immunization is so obviously in the interests of citizens that compulsion is being considered simply to produce herd immunity, then it is likely that the evidence is so overwhelming that immunization is in the best interests of the incompetent persons, and paternal discretion ought to be overridden—overridden on paternalistic grounds, not on grounds of social benefits from herd immunity."[29]

The one exception to the above argument might be those vaccine programs, like measles, in which there may be more susceptible individuals in the community from vaccine failure than from refusal to vaccinate. As a result, until a disease like measles is eradicated, very few nonparticipants can be tolerated if disease prevalence is to remain low and protection of individuals with vaccine failure is to be optimal. The case for compulsory vaccination becomes stronger for a vaccine like the measles vaccine because of the importance of herd immunity to those individuals participating in the vaccination program who remain unprotected. Those individuals do have a legitimate claim on others to optimize the effect of herd immunity in order to decrease their risk of disease acquisition.

Some Final Thoughts

Most vaccines carry with them a small, but measurable risk. At a population level that risk of currently accepted vaccines is almost always justified by the benefit of widespread vaccination to the population. With the polio vaccine, for example, the trade-off is that one person will suffer vaccine-induced paralytic disease per million people vaccinated as opposed to some 5,000 people developing paralytic disease per million unvaccinated people. The trade-off appears simple at the population level.

Yet there remains the problem that an occasional individual will bear a significant portion of the cost for the benefit which is provided to the rest of the population by a vaccination program.

Given the unequal sharing of the burdens associated with vaccine programs, it seems that a minimal requirement of those nations with vaccination programs would be to bear the financial burden of vaccine-induced disease and injury by providing adequate compensation and health care to those few affected adversely by vaccine administration.[30,31] It seems fair and reasonable that those who are protected by the vaccination program and who bear no burden as a result be asked to help bear some of the burden of those injured by the program which has led to that benefit.[32] A tax-based system of compensation can easily be justified.

A similar argument can be made concerning the costs of the vaccine program itself. The benefit of the program to the public is significant. Since all within the community, even those refusing to participate through vaccination, gain the benefits of the vaccination program, the costs of the vaccination program should be borne by the public rather than individuals. Charging individuals the cost of vaccines has a negative effect on vaccination rates by offering a financial disincentive to vaccinate. At the same time, it allows free-riders to avoid the financial costs of a program which benefits them. For those reasons, a strong argument can be made to support vaccination programs through a tax-based system into which all citizens contribute.

Jonsen points out that the maxim *primum non nocere* is as much as anything a call to humility for those practicing medicine. Those who practice medicine often focus on the benefit of their craft, while ignoring the harm that often results from what they do in trying to practice beneficently:

> When good persons possess great powers and wield them on behalf of others, they sometimes fail to recognize the harm done as they ply their beneficent craft. The medical profession has such power and its practitioners usually intend to use it well. They must become sensitive to its shadow side.[33]

The shadow side of vaccination appears in the form of uncommon but potentially devastating adverse effects, and those practicing medicine must remain sensitive to the impact these infrequent events have on some children. Likewise, good communities must assure citizens that at a minimum, the financial costs of these unfortunate events will be fully compensated. However, the principle *primum non nocere* applies to all individuals. Refusal to participate in vaccination programs also has its shadow side—the possibility of contracting potentially severe disease and spreading that to others. Those considering nonparticipation as an option must also remain sensitive to the shadow side of their actions.

Notes

1. Committee on Infectious Diseases, American Academy of Pediatrics. 1997 Red Book: Report of the Committee on Infectious Diseases, 24th ed. Peter G (ed). Elk Grove, IL: American Academy of Pediatrics, 1997.

2. Fox JP, Elveback L, Gatewood L, Ackerman E. Herd immunity: basic concept and relevance to public health immunisation practices. Am J Epidemiol 1971;94:179–189.

3. Jonsen AR. Do no harm. Ann Int Med 1978;88:827–832.

4. Ibid.

5. Gillon R. Primum non nocere in paediatrics. In: Burgio GR, Lantos JD (eds). Primum Non Nocere Today: A Symposium on Pediatric Bioethics. Amsterdam: Elsevier, 1994: 29–38.

6. Buchanan AE, Brock DW. Deciding for Others: The Ethics of Surrogate Decision Making. New York: Cambridge University Press, 1990.

7. Gust ID. The pros and cons of immunisation—paper two: the importance of immunisation. Health Care Anal 1995;3:107–111.

8. Zalkind DL, Shachtman RH. A decision analysis approach to the swine influenza vaccination decision for an individual. Med Care 1980;18:59–72.

9. Editorial. Pertussis vaccine. Br Med J 1981;282:1563–1564.

10. Editorial. Vaccination against whooping cough. Lancet 1981;1:1138–1139.

11. Hinman AR, Koplan JP. Pertussis and pertussis vaccine: reanalysis of benefits, risks, and costs. JAMA 1984;251:3109–3113.

12. Fox JP, Elveback L, Gatewood L, Ackerman E. Herd immunity: basic concept and relevance to public health immunisation practices. Am J Epidemiol 1971;94:179–189.

13. Anderson R, May R. The logic of vaccination. New Scientist 1982;96:410–415.

14. Feinberg J. Harm to Self: The Moral Limits of the Criminal Law. New York: Oxford University Press, 1986.

15. Wing KR. The Law and the Public's Health, 3rd ed. Ann Arbor, MI: Health Administration Press, 1990.

16. Veatch RM. The ethics of promoting herd immunity. Fam Community Health 1987;10:44–53.

17. Ibid.

18. Ibid.

19. Ibid.

20. Menzel PT. Paper four: noncompliance: fair or free-riding. Health Care Anal 1995;3:113–115.

21. Ball LK, Evans G, Bostrom A. Risky business: challenges in vaccine risk communication. Pediatrics 1998;101:453–458.

22. Gaylin W, Jennings B. The Perversion of Autonomy: The Proper Uses of Coercion and Constraints in a Liberal Society. New York: Free Press, 1996.

23. Mill JS. On Liberty. Indianapolis, IN: Bobbs-Merrill, 1956.

24. Feinberg J. Harm to Self.

25. McMenamin JP, Tiller WB. Children as patients. In: American College of Legal Medicine. Legal Medicine: Legal Dynamics of Medical Encounters, 2nd ed. St. Louis, MO: Mosby Year Book, 1991:290–291.

26. Dover TE. An evaluation of immunization regulations in light of religious objections and the developing right of privacy. U Dayton Law Rev 1979; 4:401–424.

27. *Jacobson v. Massachusetts*. 197 U.S. 11 (1905).

28. Noah ND. Immunisation before school entry: should there be a law? Br Med J 1987;294:1270–1271.

29. Veatch RM. Ethics of promoting herd immunity.

30. Gust ID. Pros and cons of immunisation.

31. Anderson, May. Logic of vaccination.

32. Gelfand HM. Vaccination: an acceptable risk? Science 1977;195:728–729.

33. Jonsen AR. Do no harm.

18

Rights and Dangers

Bioterrorism and the Ideologies of Public Health

Ronald Bayer and James Colgrove

The history of American public health is punctuated by controversies over the extent to which the state may legitimately impose restrictions on liberty in the name of the common good and over the extent to which protection of the public's welfare has served as a pretext for erosion of fundamental rights. Such conflicts were animated by deep-rooted mistrust of overreaching, by concerns about arbitrary exercises of power, and by the antiauthoritarian ethos that is such a prominent feature of American politics and civic culture. Periods of divisive controversy alternated with times of consensus during which dissident ideologies and underlying tensions largely disappeared from view. Extraordinary events, however, forced into the open assumptions underlying the dominant views of public health and revealed the existence of unresolved tensions, kindling anew debates over matters long thought to be settled. The shattering of the illusion of American continental impregnability by the events of September 11, 2001, and by the subsequent anthrax scare provided the occasion for a debate over the ideologies of public health. A controversy was sparked by proposals to enact a model emergency health powers act that would radically enhance the power of the state to respond to threats to the public health.

Looking Backward

In the nineteenth and early twentieth centuries public health officials who sought to institute mandatory vaccination programs, quarantines, and surveillance repeatedly faced resistance. Control of smallpox through government authority to compel vaccination and isolation of the infected served as a rallying point for groups and individuals motivated not only by antigovernment ideology but by concrete fears of physical harms that sometimes resulted from the procedure. Many state laws during this period were repealed or modified in response to pressure from opponents, especially in the second half of the nineteenth century when antivaccination societies gained strength.[1] In Milwaukee, for example, forceful application of the state's mandatory vaccination law sparked riots among the city's large German immigrant population in the 1890s.[2] Health officers who went into neighborhoods seeking to vaccinate residents and remove sick individuals to quarantine hospitals were greeted by angry mobs throwing rocks. In Massachusetts, a smallpox epidemic in 1901–1902 was the occasion for a court challenge to the state's compulsory vaccination law that ultimately led to a landmark Supreme Court ruling establishing the right of the government to use its "police powers" to control epidemic disease.[3] In its seven to two decision the Court affirmed the right of the people, through their elected representatives, to enact "health laws of every description to protect the common good."[4]

The history of efforts to impose quarantines on those viewed as threats to public health involved the exercise of authority that from the perspective of less threatening moments looks excessive and profoundly unfair.[5] On occasion the association of diseases with disfavored minority groups led to harsh measures supported by large segments of the population. In New York City, for example, arriving immigrants in 1892 could be isolated under squalid conditions to prevent the spread of cholera and typhus. At a moment of massive immigration and concomitant nativist sentiment, health officials encountered little popular opposition to their efforts.[6]

Finally, popular as well as professional opposition characterized early efforts to initiate case reporting by name to public health registries for purposes of disease control. Physicians opposed such requirements as an intrusion on their autonomy and as a violation of the confidentiality of the doctor-patient relationship.[7] Reflecting on controversies that greeted his efforts to mandate the reporting of tuberculosis cases as he moved forward to begin surveillance of sexually transmitted diseases, Herman Biggs, Commissioner of Health in New York, remarked early in the twentieth century, "The 10 year long opposition to the reporting of tuberculosis will doubtless appear a mild breeze compared with the stormy protest against the sanitary surveillance of the venereal diseases."[8] Despite the existence of such opposition, reporting of cases by name to local and state health departments and to special confidential registries ultimately became part of the tradition and practice of public health.[9] The same was true for mandatory vaccination.

The courts almost always deferred to public health authorities who deprived individuals of their liberty in the name of public health. Thus one state high court declared at the beginning of the twentieth century, "It is unquestionable that the legislature can confer police powers upon public officers for the protection of the public health. The maxim *Salus populi supreme lex* is the law of all courts in all countries. The individual right sinks in the necessity to provide for the public good."[10] Perhaps most remarkable, such a plenary grant of authority could still be found to be constitutional in the seventh decade of the twentieth century. In upholding the detention of a person with tuberculosis pursuant to a statute that provided virtually no procedural protections, a California appellate court in 1966 declared, "Health regulations enacted by the state under its police power and providing even drastic measures for the elimination of disease . . . in a general way are not affected by constitutional provisions, either of the state or national government."[11]

The breadth of public health powers that were virtually unchallenged through most of the twentieth century increasingly became subject to scrutiny in the century's last decades. And when that occurred, the roles of mandatory screening and examination, reporting the names of those who were sick or infected to public health registries, and imposition of quarantine once again became the subject of dispute. Development of a robust jurisprudence of privacy[12] and the "due process revolution" that extended rights to prisoners, mental patients, and others under the authority of the state[13] ultimately brought into question assumptions that protected public health from searching constitutional scrutiny. But whereas the groundwork was prepared in the transformations of American politics, law, and culture in the 1960s and 1970s, it was the AIDS epidemic that forced a fundamental rethinking of the dominant ideology of public health.

The controversies that raged during the 1980s, when the HIV epidemic emerged in the United States, reveal the profound effects that political and historical context have had on the enforcement of health. In the epidemic's early years a broad coalition of gay rights activists and civil libertarians were largely successful in their efforts to place the protection of privacy and individual rights at the forefront of the public health agenda.[14] Fierce battles occurred when proposals were made to mandate reporting of people with HIV infection, and it was not until many years later that such reporting became possible. Intense controversy also surrounded efforts to preserve the right of individuals to determine whether they would be tested for the infection. Policies were adopted requiring exacting and specific informed consent for testing, and only in the 1990s did significant public support emerge for relaxing these standards. Finally, every attempt to use the power of quarantine to control those whose behavior placed their sexual partners at risk provoked extensive debate about the counterproductive impact of recourse to coercion.

Paralleling the development of a rights-based perspective on public health, and drawing on some of the same broad cultural changes, was the emergence of a visible antivaccination movement in United States. During the late 1970s and 1980s heterogeneous collections of groups and individuals representing various goals, ideologies, and strategies came together to question the safety and efficacy of vaccines and the ethics of compulsory policies. A common thread of the movement is the argument that public health officials have willfully denied the dangers of immunization, which render any attempt to compel the procedure ethically unjustifiable.[15] An antistatist, antiauthoritarian outlook characterizes many of the groups in the movement. The libertarian Association of American Physicians and Surgeons (2002) thus declared in a position paper, "It's obscene to threaten to seize a child just because his parents refuse medical treatment that is obviously unnecessary and perhaps even dangerous. [We believe] that parents with the advice of their doctors should make decisions about their children's medical care—not government bureaucrats."

Bioterrorism

In the late 1990s the threat of bioterrorism surfaced as a concern of a few public health officials and experts. Alarmed by reports that Iraq had invested in a bioweapons program, the lethal gas attack by a Japanese cult, and information regarding activities of the former Soviet Union, advocates sought to jar America into coming to grips with the danger of and its utter lack of preparedness for a potential attack. That the efforts were spearheaded by D. A. Henderson, who had gained worldwide recognition for his work in the global smallpox-eradication campaign, lent credibility to these efforts.[16] For him, the prospect of the use of biological weapons was "more likely than ever before."[17] In early 1999 President Clinton announced that he was allocating $158 million to the Department of Health and Human Services for research into and preparation for bioterrorism. Additional sums would be requested for the next year.[18]

The mounting concern had its antagonists, especially among those identified with the public health left. Victor Sidel and his colleagues thus wrote in the *American Journal of Public Health,* "Should we be guided by a perspective that focuses on a hypothetical bioterrorism as a main concern while relegating to the background the monumental issues of infectious disease, food borne illness, and chemical accidents, not to mention the daily problems that are inadequately attended? The road to bioterrorism preparedness may be paved with good intentions [but] traveling down that road may be a disastrous course for public health."[19] But such opposition could not stem the growing sense of concern.

On 26–27 April 2001, a meeting to address the public health threat posed by bioterrorism was convened by the Centers for Disease Control and Prevention (CDC), the American Bar Association's Standing Committee on Law and National Security, and the National Strategy Forum. Held outside Chicago, the Cantigny Conference brought together federal, state, and local public health and law enforcement officials, representatives of the Departments of Defense and Justice, as well as university-based researchers. The goal of the meeting, which strikingly did not include representatives of civil rights and liberties organizations, was to consider the extent to which states had the legal capacity to invoke emergency powers in the face of an act of bioterrorism and whether current public health law would be adequate to the challenge posed by such an event. A premise of the meeting was that law was a central component of the public health infrastructure, that there could be no preparedness that did not include the statutory authority that would govern efforts of officials faced with a terrorist-created emergency.

From the outset officials at the CDC underscored the necessity of a legal framework that would govern access to medical and other records, permit the control over private property, allow procurement and rationing of medicines and vaccines, and provide for control over individuals who were thought to pose a risk. Such control would include the possibility of mandatory examinations and implementation of quarantines when deemed necessary to prevent spread of disease. Whereas conference participants appeared to acknowledge that in the face of a bioterrorist attack public health authorities would be able to count on voluntary cooperation of the population, they noted that "statutory mechanisms needed to be in place for dealing with uncooperative people." Although public health officials had experience in the exercise of compulsory powers, the extent to which coercion might be called upon in a bioterrorist event would be much greater.

It was the specific dimensions posed by the threat of bioterrorism that suggested the need to confront the adequacy of public health laws, many of which were enacted in the early twentieth century and had not been updated in decades. Conference participants expressed concern about ways in which some recent modifications in the law were designed to impose due process limits on the exercise of public health powers, and that some privacy protections might serve as impediments to action in the face of an emergency. Thomas Gillespie of the Johns Hopkins Center for Civilian Biodefense Studies, directed by D. A. Henderson, thus noted that it might be necessary to change the health care system, "which currently treats the individual patient with the highest regard and is less concerned with the public good." Most important, given the leadership role he ultimately assumed in drafting the model public health act, Larry Gostin noted that the rights-centered transformation of recent decades had created a situation in which "laws that protect individual rights appear to have superseded those preserving the common good." It was, of course, no small irony that Gostin, director of the Georgetown–Johns Hopkins Center for Law and the Public's Health, had himself been a forceful advocate for civil liberties during the 1980s and 1990s and as such had been instrumental in the very transformation he now viewed with some concern.

Emerging from the Cantigny Conference was a consensus on the powers that would be required by public health officials faced with a bioterrorist event. They mirrored the conventional strategies of infectious disease control that emerged at the end of the nineteenth century and in the first decades of the twentieth century: reporting of cases by medical personnel; mandatory medical examinations; contact investigation; and imposition of isolation and quarantine. In addition, the importance of having authority to seize, confiscate, and make use of private property, including hospitals, was noted.

The Cantigny Conference participants were committed to drafting a model act that would help states clarify and strengthen their existing public health laws. But the time frame for such an undertaking remained unspecified. In part, this was so because an ambitious effort, funded by the Robert Wood Johnson Foundation, to redraft public health laws was already very far along. It took the assaults of September 11 to create the context within which a sense of urgency would take hold.

Ideology, Politics, and the Model State Emergency Health Powers Act

Soon after the events of September 11, Gene Matthews, legal advisor to the CDC, called on Larry Gostin quickly to prepare a model public health emergency act. "It wasn't," said Matthews, "in anyone's interest to have 50 states running off in different directions on this."[20] On October 30, a model act that had been speedily drafted was released to the public. In every way the proposed statute bore the marks of an initiative with powerful and broad-based official backing. A press release by Secretary of Health and Human Services Tommy Thompson noted that the Act was the outgrowth of a "CDC-led process."[21] The CDC's director Jeffrey Koplan commented that adoption of the emergency act would facilitate his agency's efforts. "Many of the current laws don't make sense anymore. . . . This will update the public health laws to fit the world we live in."[22] An official at the National Governors' Association said that the act "goes a long way to helping governors improve their public health infrastructure to respond to today's health emergencies."[23] It is thus not surprising that press reports saw in the proposed act a government initiative. The *Atlanta Constitution* headlined "CDC Pushes Bill Boosting States' Powers."[24] For Gostin and his colleagues the draft, while open to refinement, was "polished and strong,"[25] nearly ready for consideration by state legislatures.[26]

Those who drafted the act were haunted by the specter of a catastrophic threat to the public health, and although the impetus for the proposed legislation was the prospect of bioterrorism, concern extended much more broadly.[27] Indeed the act referred to dangers associated with "emergent and resurgent infectious diseases" as well as "epidemics and pandemic threats." In the face of challenges that posed a "substantial risk of a significant number of human fatalities or incidents of permanent or long term disability," the governor was to be given authority to declare a public health emergency. If the situation warranted, and when prompt action was necessary, such a declaration could be issued without consultation with public health officials. It would also allow the governor to mobilize the state's militia and initiate a range of extraordinary measures that would last for 30 days, at which point it could be renewed. The legislature could intervene to override the executive decision only after 60 days and only by a two-thirds vote of both chambers.

Although its preamble noted the importance of balancing the "common good with individual liberties" and asserted that it was designed to grant authority to prevent and manage emergency health threats without unduly interfering with civil rights and liberties, the act allowed for coercive interventions bearing on privacy, bodily integrity, and liberty backed by the threat of criminal sanction. Health care providers and medical examiners would be required to report to public health authorities within 24 hours the name, date of birth, gender, race, and current address of individuals with conditions that could be related to bioterrorism or other highly fatal or dangerous infectious agents. In a marked departure from convention, pharmacists were to be included among those required to report unusual increases in prescriptions for conditions that could be linked to public health emergencies. Based on such reports, public health officials were to engage in the time-tested process of contact investigation designed to trace the origin and track the potential spread of disease.

Far more striking were the powers enumerated under Article 13 dealing with "control of persons" and the extent to which those powers were to be enforced through the threat of criminal sanction and potential deprivation of liberty. The public health authority was granted the right to "compel" individuals to undergo medical examination and medical testing, and those who refused would be liable for misdemeanors. When authorities were uncertain if individuals who refused to undergo examination or testing had been exposed to an infectious agent or otherwise posed a threat to public health, they could impose isolation or quarantine. When it was determined that public health required either treatment of those who were sick or vaccination of those who were at risk for infection, such interventions could be mandated under threat of a misdemeanor charge. Furthermore, "if by reason of refusal of vaccination or treatment" the individual was thought to pose a danger to public health, he or she might be subject to isolation or quarantine. Health care providers who refused to be party to such interventions would be subject to criminal prosecution.

Recognizing that much had occurred since quarantine laws of an earlier era were enacted, the model legislation sought to balance due process considerations with exigencies imposed by public health emergencies. In general, quarantines and isolation were to be imposed only after courts had issued a written *ex parte* order, based on a showing that probable cause existed that such measures were necessitated by a threat to public health. When urgency dictated immediate action, however, deprivation of liberty could occur without a court order being obtained first. Those quarantined or isolated could request a court hearing and representation by counsel. Such hearings were to be held within 72 hours of the request. The court's determination regarding both initial and continued isolation or quarantine was to be based on presentation of clear and convincing evidence.

In all, the act was a stark expression of the view that grave threats to public health might necessitate abrogation of privacy rights, imposition of medical interventions, and deprivation of freedom itself.

Release of the act was the occasion of considerable media attention, much of which was subtly supportive of the drafters' analyses of public health infrastructural inadequacies and limits of the prevailing legal regime.[28] An editorial in the *New Republic,* for example, concluded, "Here's hoping we won't have to experience a real outbreak before we realize that when it comes to public health, temporarily sacrificing liberty may be the price of staying alive."[29]

That was the perspective shared by sympathetic public health officials and by legislators who moved swiftly in a number of states to introduce legislation that largely mirrored the model act. "In tough times you have to make tough decisions," said an assistant commissioner of public health in Massachusetts.[30] In Minnesota, Thomas Huntley, a Democratic Farm Labor Party representative, announced plans to introduce his public health emergency legislation in January 2002. Noting the existence of quarantine laws the state had relied on in the 1950s, he declared that in the earlier period "the minuscule trade-off in individual liberties was clearly understood in light of the consequences of letting these diseases run rampant. We must be prepared and empowered to take the same course of action if necessary to prevent similar epidemics, particularly since bioterrorists have engaged our country in this kind of warfare."[31] In California, Republican Assemblyman Keith Richman acknowledged that his proposed legislation, which was virtually identical to the model act, would raise questions about civil liberties. But given the risks of smallpox, from which one-third of the infected could die, "we should have a public health law in place that could minimize the situation as much as possible."[32] Finally, in New York, Democratic Assemblyman Robin Schimminger also asserted that civil liberties concerns paled by comparison to what would be necessary in "extraordinary circumstances." "We're dealing with a bona fide public health emergency declared by the governor and confirmed by the legislature in which the hazard to the public is contagious and insidious."[33]

In striking contrast to those who endorsed the model act's provisions, many policy makers and health advocates viewed the proposal as a grave threat rather than as a necessary tool in the struggle against bioterrorism. These critics came from the left as well as the right and shared deep suspicion of the state's authority, even when exercised in the name of public health. Where architects of the act and their allies believed it was possible to delegate extensive authority to officials faced with emergencies, opponents saw only prospects of the abuse of power. Whereas the nightmare that informed the world view of the act's advocates involved tens of thousands of imperiled individuals, the true threat, according to opponents, was arrogation of unlimited executive authority to confront dangers that could instead be managed by measures that were respectful of privacy and individual rights.

Among the broadest challenges was an open letter to the secretary of health and human services by the New England Coalition for Law and Public Health, an ad hoc group of law professors and others concerned with public health policy led by Boston University's George Annas. The coalition asserted that it was not necessary to enhance public health emergency powers. Indeed, what modification was required would entail imposition of constitutional limits on older public health statutes. Whereas the act forcefully asserted the need to engage coercive authority of the state during emergencies, the coalition saw such "undue reliance" on power as a diversion from the central problem: failure adequately to fund public health departments and hospital emergency services or to provide preventive care and treatment to those in need. Recourse to threats and coercion treated the people as if they, rather than pathogens, posed a problem. "In other words this statute limits individual rights without providing individuals with any substantial assurance of protection against bioterrorist attacks or other more ordinary threats to public health."

Finally, the coalition denounced the breadth of statutory language that would permit declaration of a state of emergency when less drastic efforts might suffice. "Individual civil liberties and property rights may be disregarded even when more benign measures might achieve a comparable results."[34] The act was described as a replica of statutes from the early twentieth century, an era of therapeutic limits, "when officials had to rely on quarantining sick people because they have little else at hand."[35] Annas described it as "the old Soviet model of public health (lots of power and no standards for applying it), hardly a 'new' American model."[36]

Like the New England Coalition, groups with special concern about privacy expressed alarm at the way in which the model act treated medical information. The Health Privacy Project at Georgetown University's Law Center noted that the "breathtakingly expansive scope of the definition" of public health emergencies could open the way to name-based reporting of cases of HIV and hepatitis, "a controversial proposition indeed."[37] Furthermore, the act was denounced for the inadequacy of protections afforded medical information on identifiable individuals. Crafted to highlight problematic features of the act's specific provisions, the project's challenge was embedded in a perspective radically distinct from that which animated the work of the drafters. Giving voice to an understanding that had taken hold in the first years of the AIDS epidemic, the critique concluded by asserting that gaps in public health capacity to respond to emergencies could be resolved by "fully" respecting civil liberties and privacy rights. "These ends are not mutually exclusive; rather they are integrally linked."[38]

To the Lambda Legal Defense and Education Fund—a gay and lesbian civil rights organization that had been involved for more than a decade in combating policies such as reporting names of HIV-infected individuals—the act was anathema. With its recourse to compulsory measures, threats of quarantine and criminalization, and reliance on collaboration between public health and law enforcement agencies, it represented a regressive step that could have dire effects on those the AIDS advocacy group had so fiercely sought to protect.[39]

But from whatever vantage point they challenged the act, informing the liberal opposition's position was the unmistakable sense that, wittingly or not, the drafters permitted themselves to bring forth the public health equivalent of policies emanating from John Ashcroft's justice department. As the threat of war and terrorism provided a warrant for cabining civil liberties, the danger of bioterrorism provided justification for yet one more perilous threat to fundamental rights.

But broad and thoroughgoing challenges came not only from those who embraced liberal political values and a progressive social agenda. Conservative libertarians also saw in the act exemplification of an appalling philosophical outlook. It represented "an unprecedented assault on the constitutional rights of the American people [and] on our fundamental principles of limited government and separation of powers."[40] Like critics on the left, groups such as the Association of American Physicians and Surgeons denounced intrusions on privacy that would occur as the result of disease-reporting requirements, imposition of medical interventions and vaccinations, and criminalization of refusals to undergo such treatment. Invocation of a broad power to quarantine was viewed as especially egregious. In short, said the physicians' group, the model act "turns governors into dictators," permitting them to "create a police state by fiat."[41]

Ironically, as liberal civil libertarians responded with dismay to what they took to be Larry Gostin's betrayal of his libertarian past, conservative opponents characterized Gostin as the embodiment of left-wing values. Jennifer King, an official with the American Legislative Exchange Council, portrayed Gostin as a "very strong public health, police state type." Nothing more tellingly revealed his commitments than the work he had done as one of more than 500 consultants assisting the Clintons during the ill-fated effort at health care reform.[42]

Finally, with its authorization of mandatory vaccinations on penalty of criminalization and quarantine, and with its invocation of a much-hated century-old Supreme Court decision upholding imposed immunization, it was inevitable that the act would draw the ire of antivaccination advocates. These groups typically, although not always, shared the antistatist perspectives of the broader conservative libertarian movement. In one such online denunciation,[43] which was especially harsh in its reference to Gostin because of his "long history of trying to brainwash people into sacrificing individuals' rights for society," the act was described as "horrifying." It would impose immunizations on adults and children and would enhance the "powers of public health bureaucrats." The legislation offered the false promise of security in exchange for the freedom to make one's own medical decisions. This was all too predictable given the history of coercive childhood vaccinations. It was time for the "extortion" to stop.

Denunciations from groups that believed that the exercise [of] state authority, even [in] the name of public health, had to be carefully circumscribed, and from those who had a visceral antagonism to state authority, were not unexpected. Perhaps more striking was the response of constituencies that, according to first reports, had enthusiastically participated in the legislative initiative. Indeed, in the weeks after the late-October public release of the act, the very organizations that had been listed as collaborators in its development sought to distance themselves from it. The same official at the National Governors' Association (NGA) who at first described the act as "extremely useful" later was compelled to acknowledge that the NGA had not taken a full position on the act, that a number of states had indicated "we don't need this," and "governors don't like models, they like options."[44] The Association of State and Territorial Health Officials (ASTHO) noted that "at the request of the CDC" it circulated the document for review and comment, and many respondents expressed discomfort with overreliance on criminalization, recourse to mandatory treatment and vaccination, and reliance on quarantines. Most significant, ASTHO noted that the model act would best serve as a "tool" for states as they considered the necessity of new or amended authority; in no way was it to be viewed as a template for a radical revision of extant public health laws. States should "retain the flexibility to adopt all or part of the model act as they deem appropriate for their jurisdictions."[45] A similar stance was adopted by the National Association of County and City Health Officials.[46] Although the National Association of Local Boards of Health did not immediately take a position on the act, its director for governmental relations cautioned about the dangers of thoroughgoing legislative reform. "It has been my experience that the more comprehensive legislation becomes, the greater the effect of the law of unintended consequences. State and legislating jurisdictions within them should be encouraged to adopt as little new law as possible and to focus on amendments of existing statutes only as much as necessary."[47] Finally, the National Council of State Legislatures (NCSL) indicated that it did not typically endorse model acts. An observer sympathetic to the project of reform recounted that the NCSL had "gone ballistic" on being listed as a collaborator on the draft.[48] One account of meetings convened by the council suggested that most attendees saw the model as "bad" legislation. At least two legislators underscored the extent to which it appeared like a "governmental takeover."[49] In lieu of wholesale reform, many groups suggested using the act as a checklist for thinking about the adequacy of extant legislative provisions.

This then was the context in which those who crafted the model act were compelled to undertake the redrafting. It was a process that would seek to preserve core elements of the act while modifying aspects—language and substance—that provoked criticism from those alarmed by the breadth of the statutory formulations and the impact they could have on the rights of those who might become subjects of the act's compulsory dimensions. In undertaking the refinement, drafters could not ignore the fact that even among many who thought legislative reform to meet the challenge of bioterrorism was necessary, there appeared to be no great enthusiasm for the grand recodification foreseen when the act was first released. Thus whatever was done would have to be understood as providing states with a checklist of matters with which they would have to deal. Thus said Maryland's Health Secretary Georges Benjamin, "States should look at [the act] as a menu . . . I think the most important thing is that people not take any model act and simply try to push it through Willy Nilly."[50]

Nevertheless, in light of the fact that the CDC was to be distributing approximately $1 billion to states for emergency preparedness, and that in making its determination the CDC would look for evidence that efforts had been made to provide the legal infrastructure for confronting public health threats, it was inevitable that action at the state level would be forthcoming. Whether CDC funding was viewed as an inducement or a bludgeon depended very much on how one saw the effort to craft a legislative bulwark against bioterrorism.

At the end of December 2001 a new draft was made public. Changes, both cosmetic and substantive, were evident.[51] The amended act reflected the political lessons of the previous 6 weeks. Perhaps most striking was the characterization of the relationship between the legislative proposal and constituencies that had been portrayed as "collaborators" in crafting the earlier effort. Now the act was described as serving to "assist" those very organizations. Indeed the National Association of Attorneys General was simply listed as having provided "input and suggestions." To dispel the illusion that the act represented CDC-endorsed legislation, a disclaimer asserted that the emergency measure did not "represent the official policy, endorsement or views" of the federal agency. Oddly, the disclaimer was extended to the CDC-funded Center for Law and the Public's Health that had itself drafted the model act! In all, a distinct effort was made to avoid the suggestion that states had before them a legislative measure that had the full backing of powerful national public health and law enforcement bodies.

The new draft also underwent significant linguistic transformation. Whereas the earlier version unabashedly employed terms that reflected the necessity of coercive measures, the new draft sought to soften the harsh tone. Thus, for example, the subsection dealing with property—which evoked such concern on the part of those who viewed it as an invitation to unwarranted seizures—was now denominated "management" rather than "control" of property. The subsection dealing with compulsory powers over individuals, which drew the ire of those committed to civil liberties, was no longer termed "control of persons"; now it was called "protection of persons." Finally, the new draft subtly acknowledged that the original version had, by emphasizing the importance of coercive measures, inadequately underscored the centrality of a well-financed and organized public health system. The preamble now declared, "although modernizing public health is an important part of protecting the population during public health emergencies, the public health system itself needs improvement."

More important were substantive changes, all of which sought to prevent exercise of authority from becoming an occasion for abuse of power. First, responding to the alarm evoked by the very breadth of the definition of threats that could occasion the declaration of an emergency, the new draft eliminated references to "epidemic and pandemic diseases" (critics asserted that the flu and AIDS could trigger a declaration). In so doing the drafters sought to demonstrate that their understanding of what constituted an emergency was similar to that of their antagonists, who asserted that there were, of course, situations that might require the exercise of extraordinary public health powers. What had been the sweeping authority of the governor to impose a state of emergency with very limited legislative oversight was now to be subject to the possibility of an override by a simple majority of both legislative houses. Concerns that the October version would have permitted gross violations of privacy was similarly given credence. Mandatory reporting by name remained a central element of the act, but steps were taken to ensure that the data would be protected from unwarranted disclosure and misuse. Criminalization of refusals to undergo treatment and vaccinations by those deemed a potential threat to public health were gone, although those who declined such interventions would still be subject to isolation and quarantine. Gone too were criminal sanctions for physicians and other health care providers who refused to impose treatment or vaccination, although their licensure could be endangered. The capacity to move swiftly to impose isolation and quarantine, so central to the original act, remained untouched. The revised legislative proposal did, however, provide a much more extensive elaboration of due process procedures that would surround such deprivations of liberty.

Some of those who expressed fierce opposition to the October draft acknowledged that the proposed substantive changes had improved the legislation. Core concerns remained, however, revealing a deep philosophical divide. Thus, for example, the Health Privacy Project noted improvements represented by the narrower definition of public health emergencies but continued to voice objections to the way in which the act would violate the privacy of medical information. Bluntly it said, "The necessary changes . . . have not been made."[52] George Annas revealed the gulf that separated those who saw limitations on liberty as central to the response to public health threats and those who were profoundly skeptical of this assumption. "We do not have to trade off civil liberties for public health to effectively respond to a bioterrorist attack."[53] Indeed, he viewed the constitutional premise on which the act was predicated—the 1905 *Jacobson v. Massachusetts* decision—as part of a bygone era. Invoking the lessons of the AIDS epidemic he concluded, "The promotion of human rights can be essential to deal effectively with an epidemic."[54]

The New York Civil Liberties Union, in testimony before a state legislative committee, gave voice to the fundamental opposition that no cosmetic changes or limited adjustments could address.[55] The act was an "anachronism" and failed to "fully anticipate the ways in which [it] would empower the state to violate fundamental rights and liberties." Giving credence to the need to respond to real incidents of bioterrorism, it believed it crucial to recognize the history of abuse by the state. "Government acting in the name of public safety, has demonstrated bad judgment and worse using state police powers in a discriminatory manner to suspend freedoms based upon race or national origin." Given such a perspective it is not surprising that the group challenged even the revised version of the act in every detail: The definition of public health emergency was still too broad; the requirement that names be used for reporting purposes ignored the principle that without demonstration of an overriding interest such a privacy-violating measure was unacceptable; the "protection of persons" clauses presumptively overrode the individual's right to refuse medical treatment; the act failed to incorporate procedural protections already available in some states, including New York. Finally, the limited scope of judicial review on matters of treatment, testing, isolation, and quarantine "constituted a fundamental and 'fatal' flaw in the act."[56]

The arguments of the libertarian right were not very different, although they were informed by a characteristic stridency. The Association of American Physicians and Surgeons denounced the new draft as a "disingenuous effort to mute criticism." Limitations on liberty for ordinary citizens were less severe, but the draft still imperiled clinicians and those who owned medical facilities. "Their property can be commandeered and their skills usurped to perform duties that might well violate their oath to serve patients to the best of their own judgment and ability." In short, the revision was "still a prescription for tyranny."[57] The American Legislative Exchange Council also acknowledged that changes had been made in the October draft but asserted that "the release of a revised draft [did] not mask the original intent of the authors."[58] Finally, Georgia Republican congressional representative Bob Barr described the act as a "fearsome power grab" by the CDC and the nation's governors. Barr drew a parallel between the proposed legislation and the Clinton administration's effort at health care reform. The earlier attempt was a "federal takeover" of the health care industry. Now there was an effort "to hijack not only the health care industry, but also the constitutional freedoms of [Americans]." The entire enterprise was "unprecedented," at least in "nondictatorial regimes."[59]

Although some antivaccine advocates found in the modification an acceptable compromise—quarantine for refusal to undergo immunization rather than criminalization[60]—the most redoubtable voice of the movement continued to denounce the proposal. Terming the CDC-funded drafting effort as one that "treats us like runaway slaves in need of subjugation," Barbara Loe Fisher, head of the National Vaccine Advisory Center, attacked the act's continued use of compulsion as a choice between freedom and vaccination. Linking her struggle to a broad liberty-preserving agenda she declared, "I've said many times during the past decade that if the state can tag, track down and force citizens to be injected with biologicals of unknown toxicity, then there will be no limit on what individual freedoms the state can take away in the name of the greater good tomorrow. Now tomorrow is here."[61]

It was against a backdrop of such fervid attacks and more sober critiques that the work of state legislatures took place. Some states considered legislation based on the revised version, whereas others moved to adopt even more scaled-back versions that would be acceptable to those concerned about overreaching. Thus, for example, in Wisconsin adaptations from the act were characterized as "pretty minor" by a state senator.[62] In Ohio the health department cautiously reconsidered its options given the need to face a legislature "very leery of big government."[63] The California state health department remained skeptical of the need for wholesale legislative action even though a bill closely following the October version of the model act was introduced into the legislature.[64] In Minnesota, the need to accommodate those opposed to the act resulted in a legislative proposal that was "barely adequate," according to the state's epidemiologist, who had been among the proponents of a more expansive version.[65]

But despite such resistance it was clear by March 2002, five months after the model act was first proposed, that significant legislative activity was inspired by the proposal to create a legal infrastructure responsive to the threat of bioterrorism. Indicative of the state of affairs was the enthusiastic involvement of Richard Gottfried, chair of the New York State Assembly's health committee.[66] Long an advocate of both public health and privacy rights, an architect of the state's extensive AIDS confidentiality act, Gottfried assisted the Milbank Memorial Fund in convening two meetings in early 2002 for state legislators and their staff members. At those sessions the concept of creating a legal infrastructure for responding to bioterrorism received an enthusiastic response. As of April 2002 the Center for Law and the Public's Health reported that legislation had been introduced in 32 states based wholly or in part on the model act.[67] In many states, bills were being sponsored by legislators with considerable political influence, in contrast to the first round of bills in the fall of 2001, some of which were introduced by less well-connected lawmakers. Nevertheless, despite such extensive activity, only two states, Utah and South Dakota, had by the spring of 2002 enacted emergency health powers legislation. Only in the case of the former did the model act serve as a template.

Conclusion

Whatever the ultimate legislative outcome, the debate inspired by the MEHPA [Model Emergency Health Powers Act] illuminated the enduring ideological tensions that inform the world of public health. In the 1980s the AIDS epidemic provided the occasion for articulation of a new paradigm of public health. Given biological, epidemiological, and political factors that shaped the public policy discussion, it became possible to assert that no tension existed between public health and civil liberties, that policies that protected the latter would foster the former, and that policies that intruded on rights would subvert the public health. And what was true of AIDS was true for public health more generally. Indeed, the experience of AIDS provided the opportunity to rethink the very foundations of public health with its legacy of compulsory state powers. Even when some elements of the privacy- and rights-based approaches to AIDS were subject to modification in the 1990s as the epidemic was "normalized," the core values that had taken hold remained largely undisturbed.

The effort to articulate a new public health ideology masked a conflict that, however dormant, remained prime for exacerbation under appropriate conditions. At one pole were those who, like health and human rights activist Jonathan Mann, had come to believe that "it may be useful to adopt the maxim that health policies and programs should be considered discriminatory and burdensome on human rights until proven otherwise."[68] Very different was the view that respect for individual rights, however important, could and should be subordinated to the common good when threats to public health emerged. From this perspective the compulsory vaccination decision of the Supreme Court in 1905 rested on sound moral as well as constitutional assumptions.

It was possible, given the nature of HIV as a behaviorally transmitted virus, to avoid confronting tensions between these ideologies of public health because of the strategic importance of engaging those most at risk in the work of prevention. But with a threat that involved virulent communicable viral or bacteriological agents, such strategic constraints would not inform the discussion. It was inevitable, then, that in the shadow of September 11 the conflict over rights and dangers would resurface, shattering for the time being the illusion of a single guiding vision for public health.

Notes

1. Kaufman, Martin. 1967. "The American Anti-Vaccinationists and Their Arguments." *Bulletin of the History of Medicine*. 41.5: 463–478.

2. Leavitt, Judith Walzer. 1982. *The Healthiest City: Milwaukee and the Politics of Health Reform*. Princeton, NJ: Princeton University Press.

3. Albert, Michael R., Kristen G. Ostheimer, and Joel G. Bremen. 2001. "The Last Smallpox Epidemic in Boston and the Vaccination Controversy, 1901–1903." *New England Journal of Medicine*. 344.5: 375–379.

4. *Jacobson v. Commonwealth of Massachusetts*. 1905. 197 U.S. 11.

5. Fox, Daniel. 2002. Interview with Ronald Bayer. 7 March.

6. Markel, Howard. 1997. *Quarantine! East European Jewish Immigrants and the New York City Epidemics of 1892*. Baltimore, MD: Johns Hopkins University Press.

7. Fox, Daniel. 1988. "From TB to AIDS: Value Conflicts in Reporting Disease." *Hastings Center Report*. 16 (December): 11–17.

8. Winslow, C.-E.A. 1929. *The Life of Herman Biggs*. Philadelphia: Lea & Febiger.

9. Thacker, S. B., and R. L. Berkleman. 1988. "Public Health Surveillance in the United States." *Epidemiologic Reviews*. 10: 164–190.

10. Parmet, Wendy. 1985. "AIDS and Quarantine: The Revival of an Archaic Doctrine." *Hofstra Law Review*. 14: 53–90, citing p. 61.

11. In re Halko. 1966. 54 Cal. Report. 661.

12. Karst, K. L. 1980. "The Freedom of Intimate Association." *Yale Law Journal*. 99: 624–692.

13. Tribe, Lawrence. 1978. *American Constitutional Law*. Mineola: New York Foundation Press.

14. Bayer, Ronald. 1988. *Private Acts, Social Consequences: AIDS and the Politics of Public Health*. New York: Basic Books.

15. Freed, G. L., S. L. Katz, and S. J. Clark. 1996. "Safety of Vaccinations. Miss America, the Media, and Public Health." *Journal of the American Medical Association*. 276.23: 1869–1872.

16. Bor, Jonathan. 1999. "Spreading the Word about Bioterrorism." *Baltimore Sun*. 27 December, A1.

17. Henderson, D. A. 2001. "Biopreparedness and Public Health." *American Journal of Public Health*. 91.12: 1917–1918, citing p. 1918.

18. Garrett, Laurie. 1999. "Wake-Up Call on Germ Warfare." *Newsday*. 21 February, A4.

19. Sidel, Victor W., Hillel W. Cohen, and Robert M. Gould. 2001. "Good Intentions and the Road to Bioterrorism Preparedness." *American Journal of Public Health*. 91.5: 716–718, citing p. 717.

20. Matthews, Gene. 2002. Interview with Ronald Bayer. 6 March.

21. U.S. Department of Health and Human Services. 2001. "Statement by HHS Secretary Tommy G. Thompson regarding the Model Emergency Health Powers Act." News releases. October 30.

22. McKenna, M. A. J. 2001. "CDC Pushes Bill Boosting States' Powers." *Atlanta Journal and Constitution*. 30 October, A8.

23. Center for Law and the Public's Health. 2001a. "Model Emergency Health Powers Act in Response to Bioterrorism Written for the CDC and Governors." News release. 30 October.

24. McKenna, M. A. J. 2001. "CDC Pushes Bill Boosting States' Powers." *Atlanta Constitution*. 30 October, A8.

25. Durraj, Susan Muaddi. 2001. "Model Legislation: Balancing Civil Rights and Public Health." *Johns Hopkins Public Health Magazine*. Special Edition, late Fall 2001. Available at http://www.jhsph.edu/Publications/Special/model.htm (accessed 5 February 2002).

26. Center for Law and the Public's Health. 2001a. "Model Emergency Health Powers Act in Response to Bioterrorism Written for the CDC and Governors." News release. 30 October.

27. Center for Law and the Public's Health. 2001b. *The Model State Emergency Health Powers Act (Draft as of October 23, 2001)*. Washington, DC: Center for Law and the Public's Health.

28. Copeland, Larry. 2001. "CDC Proposes Bioterrorism Laws." *USA Today*. 8 November, A3.

29. Brownlee, Shannon. 2001. "Why America Isn't Ready for Bioterrorism." *The New Republic* Online. Available at http://www.thenewrepublic.com/102901/brownlee102901.html (accessed 23 January 2002).

30. Lasalandra, Michael. 2001. "Smallpox Attack Preparedness Plan Would Give Officials Sweeping Powers." *Boston Herald*. 8 November, 16.

31. deFiebre, Conrad. 2001. "More Power Sought to Fight Bioterror." *Star Tribune* (Minneapolis). 6 November, B1.

32. Tansey, Bernadette. 2001. "Health Bill Endangers Civil Rights." *San Francisco Chronicle*. November 25, A1.

33. Ernst, Tom. 2001. "Bill Proposes Quarantine Powers During Crisis." *Buffalo News*. 21 November, B3.

34. New England Coalition for Law and Public Health. 2001. Letter to Health and Human Services Secretary Tommy Thompson. 13 November, citing p. 2.

35. Parmet, Wendy E., and Wendy K. Mariner. 2001. "A Health Act That Jeopardizes Public Health." *Boston Globe*. 1 December, A15.

36. Annas, George. 2001. Letter to James Hodge. 1 November.

37. Health Privacy Project, Institute for Health Care Research and Policy, Georgetown University. 2001. Letter to Lawrence O. Gostin. 7 November, citing 1–2.

38. Health Privacy Project, Institute for Health Care Research and Policy, Georgetown University. 2001. Letter to Lawrence O. Gostin. 7 November, citing 5.

39. Lambda Legal Defense and Education Fund. 2001. Letter to Lawrence O. Gostin. 20 December.

40. Schlafly, Phyllis. 2001. "Where Do Politicians Go in Their Afterlife?" *Toogood Reports*. December 20. http://www.toogoodreports.com/column/general/schlafly/122001.htm (accessed 4 March 2002).

41. Association of American Physicians and Surgeons. 2001. "Model Emergency Health Powers Act (MSEHPA) Turns Governors into Dictators." Association of American Physicians and Surgeons Web site. Available at http://www.aapsonline.org/testimony/emerpower.htm (accessed 4 February 2002).

42. Betsch, Michael. 2001. "Bio-terror Response Plan Would Invade Civil Liberties." CNS News Web site. Available at http://www.cnsnews.com/Nation/Archive/200112/NAT20011211a.html (accessed 15 April 2002).

43. Richardson, Dawn. 2002. Posting to groups.yahoo.com/group/i-v-y/message/5971 (accessed 18 March 2002).

44. Thomasian, John. 2002. Interview with James Colgrove. 8 March.

45. Association of State and Territorial Health Officials. 2001. *Summary of Comments on October 23, 2001, Draft of Model State Emergency Health Powers Act, November 5.* Washington, DC: Association of State and Territorial Health Officials.

46. Brown, Donna. 2002. Personal communication to James Colgrove. 29 January.

47. Pratt, Ted. 2001. Memorandum to Lawrence Gostin, James Hodge, and Richard Goodman. November 8.

48. Fox, Daniel. 2002. Interview with Ronald Bayer. 7 March.

49. Guiden, Mary. 2001. "Lawmakers Not Keen on 'Model' Public Health Law." Available at http://www1.stateline.org/print_story.do;jsessionid =gi6uwx91d1?storyId =212079 (accessed 4 March 2001).

50. Gillis, Justin. 2001. "States Weighing Laws to Fight Bioterrorism." *Washington Post.* 19 November 19, A1.

51. Center for Law and the Public's Health. 2001c. *The Model State Emergency Health Powers Act (Draft as of December 21, 2001).* Washington, DC: Center for Law and the Public's Health.

52. Health Privacy Project, Institute for Health Care Research and Policy, Georgetown University. 2002. *Health Privacy Project Comments on Model State Emergency Health Powers Act, January 18, 2002.* Washington, DC: Institute for Health Care Research and Policy.

53. Annas, George. 2002. "Bioterrorism, Public Health, and Civil Liberties." *New England Journal of Medicine.* 346: 1337–1342.

54. Annas, George. 2002. "Bioterrorism, Public Health, and Civil Liberties." *New England Journal of Medicine.* 346: 1337–1342.

55. New York Civil Liberties Union. 2002. Testimony of Robert Perry on behalf of the New York Civil Liberties Union before the Assembly Standing Committee on Health and the Assembly Standing Committee on Codes Concerning the Model State Emergency Health Powers Act. 14 March.

56. New York Civil Liberties Union. 2002. Testimony of Robert Perry on behalf of the New York Civil Liberties Union before the Assembly Standing Committee on Health and the Assembly Standing Committee on Codes Concerning the Model State Emergency Health Powers Act. 14 March.

57. Association of American Physicians and Surgeons. 2002. "Revised Draft of Model State Emergency Health powers Act (December 21) Still a Prescription for Tyranny." Association of American Physicians and Surgeons Web site. Available at http://www.aapsonline.org/testimony/emerpower2.htm (accessed 4 February 2002).

58. American Legislative Exchange Council. 2002. "ALEC Opposes the Model State Emergency Health Powers Act." American Legislative Exchange Council Web site. Available at http://www.alec.org/viewpage.cfm?phname=5.103 (accessed 4 March 2002).

59. Barr, Bob. 2002. "A Fearsome Power Grab by the CDC and State Governors." Congressman Bob Barr Web site. Available at http://www.hillsource.house.gov/barr/newsdescr.asp?N=20020215170247 (accessed 13 March 2002).

60. Reiss, Lisa. 2002. Testimony on behalf of Connecticut Vaccine Information Alliance before Public Health Committee of Connecticut State Assembly. 19 February.

61. Fisher, Barbara Loe. 2002. "Editorial: Vaccinating America at Gunpoint." National Vaccine Information Center Web site. Available at http://www.909shot.com/smallpoxspecialrpt.htm (accessed 13 March 2002).

62. Rosenweig, Peggy. 2002. Interview with James Colgrove. 15 March.

63. Govern, Jodi. 2002. Interview with James Colgrove. 18 March.

64. Reilly, Kevin. 2002. Interview with James Colgrove. 6 March.

65. Hull, Henry. 2002. Interview with Ronald Bayer. 7 March.

66. Gottfried, Richard. 2002. Interview with Ronald Bayer. 14 March.

67. Hodge, James. 2002. Personal communication to Ronald Bayer.

68. Mann, Jonathan M., Lawrence Gostin, and Sofia Gruskin. 1994. "Health and Human Rights." *Health and Human Rights.* 1: 7–23, citing p. 16.

Further Reading

Gostin, Lawrence O., "Pandemic Influenza: Public Health Preparedness for the Next Global Health Emergency," *Journal of Law, Medicine & Ethics* 32.4: Winter 2004, 565–573.

Gostin, Lawrence O., and Zita Lazzarini, *Human Rights and Public Health in the AIDS Pandemic* (New York: Oxford University Press, 1997).

Moreno, Jonathan D., ed., *In the Wake of Terror: Medicine and Morality in a Time of Crisis.* (Cambridge: MIT Press, 2003).

Oppenheimer, Gerald, Ronald Bayer, and James Colgrove, "Health and Human Rights: Old Wine in New Bottles?" *Journal of Law, Medicine & Ethics* 30.4: Winter 2002, 522–532.

Orenstein, Walter A., and Alan R. Hinman, "The Immunization System in the United States: The Role of School Immunization Laws," *Vaccine* 17 Suppl. 3: 29 October 1999, S19–S24.

PART V

REGULATION AND ENVIRONMENTAL AND OCCUPATIONAL HEALTH

Introduction

Environmental hazards and occupational health threats expose us collectively to the risks of disease, disability, and death. As such, they require collective interventions designed to provide us with protection. In some cases, exposure levels must be reduced. In other circumstances, certain products or production processes may be deemed unacceptably toxic, requiring more radical measures, even bans. In part V, the issues posed by public health regulations of the environment and the workplace are examined.

When does a risk become unacceptable? And when does an unacceptable risk become the subject of regulation? At stake are factual questions, moral considerations, and political factors. In an effort to bring conceptual clarity to this issue, William Lowrance has pointed out that we commonly think of measuring risk as an empirical problem.[1] When we consider safety, however, we have shifted into the normative and political realm because we are making a determination about whether something is acceptable. We must decide who shall bear what burdens. Both the act of regulating and the determination not to regulate thus entail questions of distribution and redistribution. Hence, they raise questions of justice.

Complicating the matter even further is the extent to which the very task of measuring risk may be beset by uncertainties. The National Research Council noted: "The choices encountered in risk assessment rest, to various degrees, on a mixture of scientific fact and consensus, on informed scientific judgment, and on policy determinations (the appropriate degree of conservatism). . . . A desire to err on the side of overprotection of public health by increasing the estimate of risk could lead a risk assessor to choose the most conservative assumptions throughout the process for components on which science does not indicate a preferred choice."[2] And of course, a desire to minimize the costs of regulation would dictate very different assumptions in the face of uncertainty.

Regulation of environmental and occupational hazards, therefore, is not simply a question of how to distribute potential burdens most fairly but how to distribute the burden of uncertainties equitably. Given the stakes involved, it is not surprising that political controversies have whirled around air and water pollution control and global warming. Those who would be required to pay the cost of regulation have tended to emphasize the scope of uncertainty and the need for caution. Those who might suffer the consequences of exposure have tended to dismiss such "scientific" concerns as a pretext for inaction, as masking narrow economic self-interest. As critics of inaction in the face of uncertainty have asserted, "A clinician cannot wait for scientific consensus among experts regarding diagnosis before deciding whether or not to operate on a suspected case of appendicitis. Similarly environmental regulation cannot delay regulating a suspected harmful exposure until scientific consensus exists. In both instances decision-making under uncertainty is necessary."[3]

In his analysis of the apparent conflict between the requirements of scientific rigor and the need to frame policy in the face of data that do not meet those exacting standards, Carl F. Cranor in chapter 19 draws a parallel between the differences in the evidentiary requirements of criminal law—where the rule is that guilt is determined by asking if a charge has been proven beyond a reasonable doubt—and civil law, where the much less demanding preponderance of the evidence standard applies. "Different kinds and amounts of *evidence* may be needed before one asserts for purposes of *understanding* the definitive existence of causal claims versus *deciding* for public health purposes what to do."[4]

Chapter 20, To Foresee and to Forestall, provides a statement of the precautionary principle, which has emerged as a central moral statement and political platform for many environmentalists. Developed as a challenge to those who relied on scientific uncertainty as a justification for retarding the pace of regulation, the principle is forthright: "When an activity raises threats of harm to human health or the environment, precautionary measures should be taken even if some cause and effect relationships are not fully established scientifically." Many questions are posed by the precautionary principle, including the role and limits of science as the foundation for public health action, the role of expert versus lay knowledge, and the risk-benefit ratio of regulation when risk may not materialize as contrasted with the failure to regulate when risk may materialize.[5]

Part V next turns to occupational health and safety, which has many of the same issues. But because the risks in the workplace are borne by selected groups rather than the population at large, some of ethical questions that must be considered take on a different cast. A broad legislative framework, the Occupational Safety and Health Act, provides the legal framework for addressing these matters. The preamble to the act asserts that the secretary of labor must establish standards "which most adequately assure, to the extent feasible, on the basis of the best available evidence, that no employee will suffer material impairment of health or functional capacity even if such employee has regular exposure to the hazard dealt with by such standard for the period of his working life."[6] Each of the operative terms—"adequately assure," "feasible," and "best available evidence"—invites controversy, with the resolution as much a matter of moral considerations as empirical.

In the more than three decades since the passage of the act, the extent to which it has served to guide public health policy has shifted with the political tides. Administrations with greater commitment to protection of the market from regulatory impositions have been reluctant to impose strict regulation. Administrations with stronger ties to labor have moved more aggressively. But at every turn, regulatory moves have been the subject of political controversy.

It is therefore critical to retain an interest in the ethical as contrasted with the legal issues at the heart of occupational health and safety: What does justice require in terms of the scope of worker protection from dangerous exposures? Should toxic exposure standards be designed to protect the average worker or those who, for biological reasons, are the most vulnerable? How should questions of cost-benefit be considered in the setting of health and safety standards? Do workers assume some risk when they enter the workplace? How should prevailing market conditions affect our judgment about whether risks are "freely" assumed? Should workers be free to trade safety and health for higher wages?

These ethical questions are the subject of analysis by Norman Daniels in the selection Doth OSHA Protect Too Much? Of particular note is Daniels's confrontation with the question of how the limited options of the labor market that create "quasi coercive" contexts ought to influence our consideration of regulations that appear to be paternalistic. Confronting that issue opens the way to an engagement with another dimension of the ethics of regulation.

Notes

1. William Lowrance, *Of Acceptable Risk: Science and the Dilemma of Safety* (Los Altos, CA: William Kaufman, 1976).

2. National Research Council, *Risk Assessment in the Federal Government: Managing the Process* (Washington, DC: National Academy Press, 1983), pp. 36–37.

3. James Robins, Philip Landrigan, Thomas Robins, et al., "Decision Making under Uncertainty in the Setting of Environmental Health Regulations," *Journal of Public Health Policy*, September 1985, 322–328.

4. Carl Canor, *Regulating Toxic Substances: A Philosophy of Science and the Law* (New York: Oxford University Press, 1993).

5. Cass Sunstein, *Risk and Reason: Safety, Law and the Environment* (New York: Cambridge University Press, 2002).

6. Cited in Gilbert Omenn, "Values in the Debate over Workplace Safety and Health: The Rancorous Rhetoric about Regulation," in H. Tristram Englehardt and Arthur Caplan (eds.), *Scientific Controversies* (New York: Cambridge University Press, 1987), pp. 437–464.

19

Regulating Toxic Substances

A Philosophy of Science and the Law

Carl F. Cranor

Public Policy Issues

Since the reporting, interpretation, and use of epidemiological data are not normatively neutral, and we could change traditional scientific practices, we should face the use of the 95% rule in these contexts as a normative question, no matter who makes the interpretative decisions. The 95% rule . . . serves as a surrogate or as an exemplar for the use of demanding standards of evidence for regulatory purposes. We have seen how this can adversely affect the health-protective goals of regulation. Thus, the reader should keep in mind plausible generalizations of the 95% rule as examples of how demanding standards of evidence or other scientific practices could frustrate pursuit of legally mandated goals when more sensitive and more flexible interpretations of data would better serve legal aims.

In other institutional contexts we have clearly faced such issues. In the criminal law, for example, avoiding wrongful damage to someone's reputation and well-being is so important that we spend considerable sums of money and deliberately impose difficulties on proving guilt in order to avoid wrongly inflicting harsh treatment and condemnation on the defendant. We could save money and have more unjust outcomes if we thought it worth the human costs, but we do not. Clearly a number of moral and cost considerations have influenced the institution of the criminal law. We have been quite self-conscious in debating the considerations that bear on the design and workings of the criminal law. Somewhat analogous problems arise in environmental health law concerning the interpretation and use of scientific studies; I suggest that similar debates should address these issues.

An additional problem is that the conventional evidentiary practices of science (use of the 95% rule) may well be much more demanding than the evidentiary requirements and aims of the tort and regulatory law. . . .

Thus, the problem is that the evidentiary standards of science as exemplified in the 95% rule may be much more demanding than the legal standards of evidence where the scientific evidence will be used. If this is correct, then, if regulators or courts in tort cases use conventional scientific standards, by default their science will in many cases beg the normative question at issue. Under postmarket regulatory statutes (which predominate in governing the regulation of carcinogens) a commitment to demanding scientific standards may well prevent the discovery of risks and lead to lowered protections for the public. When epidemiologists study relatively rare diseases with small samples, they will be forced to choose between high false-negative rates or high false-positive rates (that would be intolerable for normal scientific work). If they choose to tolerate high false negatives to protect the integrity of their scientific work, they thereby favor nonregulation or less regulation by their choice of evidentiary standard.

Furthermore, given the wider aims of both the regulatory and tort law and the evidentiary standards that typically must be met in the law compared to science, there may not be good reasons in these legal contexts to require risk assessment science to meet the same evidentiary burdens as normal scientific pursuit of the truth for its own sake. Thus, I would urge that for regulatory science, agencies adopt evidentiary standards much closer to those of the legal institutions it is meant to serve. . . .

The following reasons might be offered for retaining the 95% rule even in regulatory and other legal contexts:

1. It is the prevailing tradition.
2. Scientists should be cautious about additions to scientific knowledge so that additional bricks of knowledge are well made and well cemented to the existing scientific structure.
3. The 95% rule provides a useful standard, a benchmark against which all epidemiological studies (and scientific studies more generally) can be compared. If studies were conducted with substantial departures from the 95% rule, they would no longer have a kind of automatic credibility (represented by the 95% rule) and perhaps would have to be scrutinized much more closely.
4. If the aim in an epidemiological study is to establish a causal relationship between a substance and a disease, not using the 95% rule undermines this aim.
5. The 95% rule, when used in certain regulatory contexts, protects the commercial status quo.

None of these arguments provide overriding reasons for always using the 95% rule, and several do not constitute even a prima facie reason for using it.

Reason 1, although true, begs the question whether the rule should be followed in all contexts, especially in regulatory and legal ones. The second reason, although correct for basic research that aims to add to the stock of fundamental knowledge, is less appropriate for regulatory contexts. For regulation epidemiological studies are aimed not at discovering new scientific results, but at trying to discover whether risks to health exist. And sometimes the aim is merely to confirm or deny the carcinogenicity of a substance that is in a chemical class with other substances known to be carcinogenic. Neither case presents a good reason for always adhering to the 95% rule.

The third reason is an important reason of consistency, but only that. Consistency is not an overriding reason for following a certain practice, if the practice otherwise would produce bad results in a particular area. In addition, such studies are not automatically accepted at present—they receive considerable scrutiny. If the 95% rule were abandoned in some regulatory contexts this would add only marginally to the usual controversies. In particular, not using this rule would merely add to the existing complaint by some interest groups seeking to undermine risk assessment that risk assessments are not "scientific."

A related point is that a commitment to scientific standards of evidence may be the only stable reference point in debates that otherwise seem driven by political interests, policy considerations, and a good deal of uncertainty. There is much to this concern. However, it is not clear that a commitment to the 95% rule, which can beg regulatory questions, is the best way to address it. Presenting data in the most objective manner is quite important. But how the data are used, whether to infer a risk of concern or to infer no such risk, is clearly a matter of one's broader moral and political philosophy, or a matter to be settled in the law by the statutory guidance of regulatory law or by the procedures of the tort law. How much of a "clue" to carcinogenicity is provided by studies that fall short of the 95% rule is an important issue to be settled by the evidentiary standards appropriate to the institutional context.

Furthermore, it is a good thing to have questions of health risk decided in large part on normative policy grounds. Some degree of inaccuracy in estimating risks is important, but risk assessment is an inexact "science."[1] As I indicated earlier, perhaps it is much better to treat both the *kind and amount of evidence* needed to estimate a risk and the *acceptability of the risk* in part as social decisions, rather than treating the first as a purely scientific decision and the second as the only policy decision, especially when the scientific part of the decision may beg the normative issues. In addition, several researchers have found that scientists' attitudes toward their research results and toward public policy issues are substantially influenced by their place of employment. Industry scientists are more skeptical that substances pose risks of harm than are academic or government scientists.[2] Given the possibility of normative "slants" to scientists' work, it seems a better approach is to choose openly and deliberatively the normative concepts we want to influence the choice of models in risk assessments and the interpretation of statistical studies. A public, community decision about these matters through the mechanism of a regulatory agency seems the appropriate approach in a democracy.

Fourth, if indeed the aim is to establish a causal relationship between a substance and a disease, then we surely want to understand this. However, whether we should wait until that is definitely established before we decide to take *action* as a matter of regulatory policy is another matter. Different kinds and amounts of *evidence* may be needed before one asserts for purposes of *understanding* the definitive existence of causal claims versus *deciding* for public health purposes what to do. For regulatory purposes one might well accept the results of epidemiological studies not based upon the 95% rule in order better to detect potentially harmful substances. For more fundamental research purposes, for example, discovering whether a whole class of substances–say, the arsenicals—appeared to be carcinogenic, one might want to have at least some of the studies established by the 95% rule.

Finally, although in fact the 95% rule used in evaluating commercially valuable chemical carcinogens may protect these commercial interests, it is for precisely this reason we should reexamine the use of the rule. For small samples and relatively rare diseases, use of the 95% rule in many circumstances may well protect commercial manufacturers and sellers of a substance better than potential victims. In weighing the balance between risks of wrongly regulating commercial substances and wrongly leaving people exposed to potentially carcinogenic substances, the latter seems the more important concern, although this depends upon the facts of the case and one's larger legal and moral philosophy. . . .

In addition to the preceding rebuttals, there are some more positive reasons for modifying the 95% rule for various legal purposes. When sample sizes are small and the background rate of disease is relatively rare (<8/10,000), departures from the 95% rule make it possible for epidemiologists better to detect harmful substances at a certain relative risk. This is especially important for detecting low but possibly substantial relative risks. In regulatory contexts, where a major aim of the enterprise is to predict risks to human health and prevent them, if possible or feasible, departures from the 95% rule may better serve this preventive aim. Similarly, in toxic tort suits where the aim is to compensate victims who have probably been harmed by defendants, a departure from the 95% rule might be appropriate.

This is not to suggest that the 95% rule should be abandoned in all scientific contexts or even that it should be abandoned in all regulatory contexts. Instead scientists and policymakers should be more discriminating in their use of the rule and carefully consider the consequences of its use. In clinical trials of a drug in which the goal is to discover if a drug has therapeutic effects, the 95% rule might be relied upon, for research endeavoring to add to our fundamental knowledge about biochemical and therapeutic mechanisms should not be conducted if chances of incurring false positives are significant. Similarly, when one is conducting epidemiological research to establish knowledge as a foundation for further research, one might well want to retain the 95% rule.

I suggest that on moral and legal grounds it is likely there will be reasons for departing from the 95% rule in at least these contexts:

> in screening substances to try to discover those that pose harms to health;
> in preventive regulatory proceedings where the major concern is the forward-looking prevention of health harm and there is little fundamental research to be gained or upon which to build . . . ;
> in the tort law where the typical standard of proof is not nearly as demanding as the 95% rule, perhaps courts should permit such departures. . . .

For example, it might be useful for preventive health purposes for an agency like EPA [Environmental Protection Agency] or OSHA [Occupational Safety and Health Administration] to commission a number of epidemiological studies with chances of false positives higher than .05 simply to screen for potentially harmful substances. Where there were positive results, the agency could then conduct further tests of one kind or another if additional evidence was needed, or it could randomly conduct some studies that relied upon the 95% rule in order to check for false positives.

There is a generalization to the concerns raised in this section. Any specialist (at least in academic disciplines) is concerned about the validity and defensibility of his or her inferences. We tend to be cautious in drawing inferences in order to avoid mistakes. Frequently we are hyperskeptical in order to protect the field and prevent pursuit of false leads. The 95% rule is an exemplar of a minimal standard for good statistical inferences in scientific inquiries. By analogy with the arguments about epidemiology, to the extent that scientists are reluctant to conclude that suspect substances to not cause disease or death because the inferences cannot be justified on the *best* inference standards for the discipline, a debate whether to regulate or not may be begged in favor of nonregulation. By analogy with the recommendations made previously, scientists should scrutinize other scientific inferences used in risk assessment and other public policy debates to see whether regulatory outcomes are biased by evidentiary practices used in the discipline.

Similarly, the use of strict scientific inferences in regulatory contexts should be addressed as moral or social policy questions. In many cases evidentiary practices in science will beg policy questions, thus they should be examined for this *possibility*.

Conclusion

Several conclusions emerge from the discussions in this chapter. Sufficient uncertainties plague risk assessment procedures based on animal studies, the foundation of agency standard setting, to make risk assessment somewhat different from ordinary core areas of science. Adoption of the ideals of research science in these circumstances may result in false negatives and underregulation. Demanding standards of evidence exemplified by the 95% rule may produce a similar result. An implicit commitment to avoiding false positives may dominate risk assessment instead of some more appropriate balancing of false positives and false negatives relevant to the legal context. And, finally, assessment of the risks posed by carcinogens proceeds much too slowly to evaluate existing chemicals or to keep pace with the introduction of new substances. . . .

Clearly, there will be mistakes, whether we consider estimates of risks to human health based upon animal studies or epidemiological studies. Mistakes are a result of the state of knowledge or of practical and theoretical limitations in the tools available to risk assessors. These mistakes will impose costs on someone. On whom the cost of such mistakes should fall is a normative issue. Thus, we must face the evidentiary questions posed by these different risk assessment procedures as normative matters, much as we have in designing legal procedures so that they promote and do not frustrate the larger institutional goals in which these risk projections are used. But this raises philosophical questions about the institutions involved, about what standards of evidence should be used to guide risk assessments or to establish the causal connections needed in particular institutional settings. . . .

Notes

1. See Cranor, C. (1988). Some public policy problems with the science of carcinogen risk assessment. *Philosophy of Science* 2:467–488.

2. Lynn, F. M. (1987). "OSHA's Carcinogen Standard: Round one on risk assessment models and assumptions." In *The Social and Cultural Construction of Risk*, ed. B. B. Johnson & V. T. Covello. Bingham, MA: D. Reidel, pp. 345–358.

20

To Foresee and to Forestall

Carolyn Raffensperger and
Joel A. Tickner

When Rachel Carson completed her book, *Silent Spring,* she dedicated it to Albert Schweitzer, who said, "Man has lost the capacity to foresee and forestall. . . . He will end up destroying the earth." To foresee and forestall is the basis of the precautionary principle. It is the central theme for environmental and public health rooted in the elemental concepts of "first do no harm" and "an ounce of prevention is worth a pound of cure." In its simplest formulation, the precautionary principle has a dual trigger: If there is a potential for harm from an activity and if there is uncertainty about the magnitude of impacts or causality, then anticipatory action should be taken to avoid harm. Scientific uncertainty about harm is the fulcrum for this principle. Modern-day problems that cover vast expanses of time and space are difficult to assess with existing scientific tools. Accordingly, we can never know with certainty whether a particular activity will cause harm. But we can rely on observation and good sense to foresee and forestall damage.

We have failed to heed Carson and Schweitzer's warning. Industrial development increased rapidly following World War II, with little regard for human health or the environment. Growth was considered akin to prosperity, and some small environmental damage was a small price to pay for the benefits of industrialization. Research and legislation developed during the late 1960s and early 1970s acknowledged that there were substantial adverse impacts associated with unlimited growth. With increasing knowledge about the complexities of ecosystems, the human body, and the impacts of various stressors, we have realized that we actually understand much less than we thought we did about these systems.

During the 1970s and 1980s, tools such as risk assessment and cost-benefit analysis were developed to assist decision makers in making more rational decisions about industrial activities and their impacts. However, their incorporation into decision-making structures was based on the misguided belief that humans could fully understand the impacts of their activities on the environment and establish levels of insult at which the environment or humans could rebound from harm. Too much emphasis was placed on the role of science to model and predict harm in extremely complex ecological and human systems. Risk assessment, which was originally developed for mechanical problems such as bridge construction where the technical process and parameters are well defined and can be analyzed, took on the role of predictor of extremely uncertain and highly variable events. The risk-based approach, now central to environmental and public health decision making in the United States, has in part led to a regulatory structure based on pollution control and remediation rather than fundamental prevention.

The quantitative, risk-based approach to environmental and public health regulation has taken on an importance in government agency operations. It allows agencies to justify and defend their decisions to the courts, businesses, and the public in the guise of objective, unbiased numbers, avoiding mention of the values implicit in decisions affecting public and environmental health. This approach is viewed as the "sound science" approach to decision making, where decisions are made on the basis of what we can quantify, without considering what we do not know or cannot measure. That is lumped under the category of "uncertainty," which can be addressed in a neutral way through additional information and modeling. The risk assessment process, however, is as much policy and politics as it is science. A typical risk assessment relies on at least 50 different assumptions about exposure, dose response, and relationships between animals and humans. The modeling of uncertainty also depends on assumptions. Two risk assessments conducted on the same problem can vary widely in results.

Current environmental and public health decision-making processes, based primarily on the level of risk, suffer from several limitations, which constrain their ability to identify, anticipate, and prevent potential harm to human health and the environment. Decisions to take action to restrict potentially dangerous activities are often taken after science has established a causal association between a substance or activity and a well-defined, singular adverse impact. Proving causality takes both extensive time and resources. During this research period, action to prevent potentially irreversible human and environmental harm is often delayed in the name of uncertainty and the harmful activity continues. For a variety of reasons, it may not even be possible to demonstrate a causal association in complex human/ecological systems.

For example, even basic knowledge about the impacts of the most widely used toxic chemicals is unavailable. Analysis of the impacts of human activities on health and the environment is fraught with uncertainty. This ignorance leads to an important question for decision makers: "How can science establish an 'assimilative capacity' (a predictable level of harm from which an ecosystem can recover) or a 'safe' level when the exact effect, its magnitude, and interconnectedness are unknown?"

Further, regulatory programs often demand the achievement of statistical significance in experimental and observational research. Even though an effect is not significant to a statistician, it still may be significant to the person or community. This "laboratory" model of science places an emphasis on minimizing type I errors (incorrectly concluding that there is an effect when one does not exist) and thus unnecessary regulation at the expense of increasing the potential for type II errors (incorrectly concluding that there is not an effect when there is one), placing humans and the environment in jeopardy. Achieving adequate statistical power (the predictive potential of an experiment) for a study to be considered acceptable is difficult if the number of subjects or effect is small.

Even low-level exposure to stressors may cause adverse impacts. These impacts may be impossible to monitor or control. For example, there is growing evidence that some synthetic chemicals may disrupt the hormone system at very low levels of exposure and not at high doses (an inverted U-shaped dose response), with effects happening when exposure takes place during sensitive periods in the development of a fetus. It is virtually impossible to know what level of exposure will affect a fetus or what impacts that exposure will cause.

Science has not begun to address the wide range of physical and chemical stressors to which humans and ecosystems are exposed since it focuses on single chemicals/stressors in single media. If we are ignorant about the impacts of only single human activities on health and the environment, we are even more ignorant about the cumulative effects of many potentially harmful activities.

Finally, risk assessments and other analyses are very time consuming, contentious, and costly. For example, a single risk assessment on a single chemical might take up to 5 years and cost upward of $5 million. This excludes the cost of the harm that may be caused by the activity under study. Focusing on opportunities to prevent harm (e.g., using the precautionary principle) is a much more cost-effective use of limited resources.

There is a need for decision makers to bridge the gap between uncertain science (and the need for more information) and the political need to take action to prevent harm. As trustees of ecosystem and public health, government agencies have an obligation to prevent harm despite the existence of uncertain impacts. They must consider that there could be large political and economic consequences if they are wrong. The question of what society should do in the face of uncertainty regarding cause and effect relationships is a question of public policy, not science. A decision not to act in the face of uncertainty, to await further scientific evidence, is as much a policy decision as taking preventive action.

History of the Precautionary Principle

The term *precautionary principle* is relatively new to the national and international environmental policy arena, though the concept has its roots in hundreds of years of public health practice. Even early environmental legislation encompassed a precautionary approach to environmental protection. For example, in the legislative history to Sweden's first environment act, the minister of justice noted that environmental policy should lead to actions in the face of uncertainty and shift the burden of proof of safety to those who create risks.

The principle emerged as an explicit basis of policy during the early 1970s in West Germany as *Vorsorgeprinzip* or the "foresight" principle of German water protection law. At the core of early conceptions of this principle in Germany was the belief that society should seek to avoid environmental damage by careful "forward-looking" planning, blocking the flow of potentially harmful activities. The Vorsorgeprinzip has been invoked to justify the implementation of vigorous policies to tackle river contamination, acid rain, global warming, and North Sea pollution. Implementation of the foresight principle has given rise to a globally competitive industry in environmental technology and pollution prevention in Germany.

The precautionary principle was first introduced internationally in 1984 at the First International Convention on Protection of the North Sea, designed to protect the fragile North Sea ecosystem from further degradation due to the input of persistent toxic substances. At the Second North Sea Conference, ministers noted that "in order to protect the North Sea from possibly damaging effects of the most dangerous substances . . . a precautionary approach is addressed which may require action to control inputs of such substances even before a causal link has been established by absolutely clear scientific evidence." Following this conference, the principle was integrated into numerous international conventions and agreements including the Maastricht Treaty, the Barcelona Convention, and the Global Climate Change Convention, among others. The principle guides sustainable development in documents like the 1990 Bergen Ministerial Conference on Sustainable Development and the 1992 United Nations Conference on Environment and Development. It has become a central theme of environmental law and policy in the European Union and many of its member states.

The precautionary principle itself is a relatively new concept to environmental protection in the United States. However, as in many other countries, the general notion of precaution underlies much of the early U.S. environmental and public health legislation. For example, the former Delaney Clause of the Food, Drug, and Cosmetics Act prohibited the incorporation into processed food of any level of a substance that had been found carcinogenic in laboratory animals. The National Environmental Policy Act (NEPA) requires that any project receiving federal funding and that may pose serious harm to the environment undergo an environmental impact statement, demonstrating that there were no safer alternatives. The Clean Water Act (CWA) established strict goals in order to "restore and maintain the chemical, physical, and biological integrity of the Nation's waters." The Endangered Species Act requires the protection of threatened species beyond economic interests. The Occupational Safety and Health Act (OSHA) was designed to "assure so far as possible every working man and woman in the Nation safe and healthful working conditions." The OSHA draft Carcinogen Standard (which was never put into practice) required precautionary actions any time a chemical used in the workplace was suspected of being a carcinogen in animals.

Early court decisions also gave substantial deference to the Environmental Protection Agency (EPA) to take action to prevent harm even before considerable evidence of cause and effect was gathered. For example, in the Reserve Mining Case, the court ruled that "the public's exposure to asbestos created a sufficient health risk to justify taking precautionary and preventive measures to protect the public health." In a case over EPA regulations requiring reductions in lead additives in gasoline, the court noted, "Where a statute is precautionary in nature, the evidence difficult to come by, uncertain or conflicting because it is on the frontiers of scientific knowledge, . . . we will not demand rigorous step-by-step proof of cause and effect."

Much of the early precautionary nature of U.S. environmental and occupational safety and health policy was lost during the 1980s, when the Reagan administration disarmed these protections. In addition, a U.S. Supreme Court case involving occupational health standards for benzene, and the rise in supremacy of quantitative risk assessment and cost-benefit analysis in environmental and occupational health, eroded the early precautionary nature of environmental and public health protections. The protection of health and environment has not fully recovered from these actions.

A strong public backlash to losses in environmental and health protections, coupled with the industrial disasters in Chernobyl and Bhopal, led to a rejuvenation of the grassroots activism in the United States and new calls for the public's right to know and expanded environmental protections. Creating a public right to know led to an understanding that companies were emitting enormous amounts of pollutants into the environment. This, coupled with a realization that pollution-control strategies were not eliminating but rather shifting pollution, led to the passage of the Pollution Prevention Act of 1990, which sets prevention as the highest priority in environmental programs.

Responding to the public's strong pro-environment sentiment, the U.S. government signed the Rio Declaration at the United Nations Conference on Environment and Development in 1992. Section 15 of the declaration calls for states to adopt the precautionary principle. The U.S. Environmental Protection Agency has admitted that it is bound by the Rio Declaration and must identify ways to implement the precautionary principle. In 1996, the U.S. President's Council on Sustainable Development, a multistakeholder presidential board, issued a statement of principles for sustainable development, among them an implicit definition of the precautionary principle: "There are certain beliefs that we as Council members share that underlie all of our agreements. We believe: (number 12) even in the face of scientific uncertainty, society should take reasonable actions to avert risks where the potential harm to human health or the environment is thought to be serious or irreparable."

Perhaps the most noteworthy work on the precautionary principle in the United States has occurred in the Great Lakes region and on the state level. In the Great Lakes, the International Joint Commission (IJC), a 100–year-old binational body established to protect waters along the Canadian-U.S. border, determined that attempts to manage persistent and bioaccumulative pollution in the Great Lakes had failed, and these could not be managed safely. As a result, the commission issued a call to sunset all persistent toxic substances, noting that action is needed to protect health and environment "whether or not unassailable scientific proof of acute or chronic damage is universally accepted." Gordon Durnil, who was appointed by President Bush to head the U.S. delegation to the commission, relates how the IJC reached its conclusions. First he asked the various scientists serving on committees within the IJC to describe what they knew. He received myriad provisos on lack of evidence and absence of significant proof linking chemicals to harm. Next he asked these scientists what they believed. They believed that there was harm linked to these substances, even if they could not prove it.

On the state level, at least 25 states have established some type of pollution prevention legislation. California passed Proposition 65, which requires companies and other establishments to label any products that contain substances that could cause cancer or developmental harm. The Commonwealth of Massachusetts has passed several laws that are precautionary in nature. For example, its wetlands statute requires those building near wetland areas must demonstrate that no harm to wetland integrity will occur. The commonwealth's Rivers Act requires that anyone building within a river buffer zone demonstrate that there is no other option for building. And the Toxics Use Reduction Act requires firms using certain toxic chemicals to identify alternatives to reduce or eliminate their use. Most recently, a bill was introduced in Massachusetts establishing the precautionary principle as a general duty for government agencies and businesses.

Business organizations have also begun to recognize the importance of implementing the precautionary approach as a corporate responsibility and its benefits to business. Both the International Chamber of Commerce and the World Business Council for Sustainable Development have endorsed the precautionary principle as a management tool necessary to achieve sustainable development. There are numerous examples of individual companies and industries (e.g., British Petroleum with regard to global warming) taking precautionary action to avoid environmental and health harm. Author Stephen Schmidheiny explains that business leaders are "used to examining uncertain negative trends, making decisions, and then taking action, adjusting, and incurring costs to prevent damage." They support the precautionary principle not only because it can help them avoid liabilities, but also because of opportunities for innovation, improved corporate image, and product development. . . .

In 1993, the *New York Times* published a series of articles by Keith Schneider that stated that many environmental problems of modern times were exaggerated. This series of articles led to the publication of more articles, books, and the establishment of so-called sound-science organizations. The attack on environmental and occupational health regulation during the 104th Congress incubated a need for the development of proactive measures to fight this attack. Emerging issues, such as global climate change and endocrine disruption, reinforced the demand for new approaches to decision making in the face of uncertainty. Environmental groups, as well as the scientists and lawyers working with them, felt that the precautionary principle represented an important paradigm that addresses the limits of science while promoting action to prevent harm.

Environmentalists recognized that the precautionary principle had achieved some prominence in Europe and in international treaties but not in the United States among other countries. While they understood the underlying basis of the principle, it was unclear what precaution actually meant in practice. There was also no clear structure to integrate the principle into decision making in the way that risk assessment had been integrated over the past 15 years. To bring the precautionary principle to the forefront of environmental and public health decision making in the United States, advocates felt that a meeting was needed to develop a structure and methods for operationalizing the principle. From this need the Wingspread Conference on Implementing the Precautionary Principle was born.

During the weekend of January 23–25, 1998, the Science and Environmental Health Network convened 35 academic scientists, grassroots environmentalists, government researchers, and labor representatives from the United States, Canada, and

Europe to discuss ways to formalize the precautionary principle. The workshop focused on understanding the history and scientific and political contexts under which the principle developed, its basis, and how it could be implemented in toxic chemicals policy, agriculture, and biodiversity. The Wingspread participants issued a consensus statement calling for and defining the precautionary principle. It states: "When an activity raises threats of harm to human health or the environment, precautionary measures should be taken even if some cause and effect relationships are not fully established scientifically."

The Wingspread Statement on the Precautionary Principle represents an important definition for the principle because it amplifies and clarifies both the Rio Declaration and the President's Council's statement. The Wingspread statement starts off with a call to action, because we have already reached our capacity for environmental insults. As defined at Wingspread, the precautionary principle has four components: (1) Preventive action should be taken in advance of scientific proof of causality; (2) the proponent of an activity, rather than the public, should bear the burden of proof of safety; (3) a reasonable range of alternatives, including a no-action alternative (for new activities) should be considered when there may be evidence of harm caused by an activity; and (4) for decision making to be precautionary it must be open, informed, and democratic and must include potentially affected parties.

Since the Wingspread Conference, the precautionary principle has been invoked in places the convenors could not have predicted before January 1998. While toxics have traditionally been the domain for the precautionary principle internationally, in the United States it is gaining its greatest support among sustainable agriculture advocates. In Washington State, people protesting the use of hazardous waste in the manufacture of fertilizers called for decision making to be based on the principle. It has also been identified by advocates as the single most important issue in the enormous grassroots response to the U.S. Department of Agriculture's draft organic agriculture rule. Opponents of genetic engineering have also used the Wingspread Statement in international meetings.

In the United States it is likely that the principle will first be solidified at the local and state levels, given the more conservative nature of federal government policies and the entrenchment of risk assessment. Once successes are made at these levels, pressure can be brought on the federal government to institutionalize the principle. This differs from international experience with the principle, where it starts as a global concept and then works its way down to the local level. Nonetheless, several federal agencies are considering how to incorporate the principle into children's environmental health and other environmental concerns, and the precautionary principle was included in the "description" of endocrine disruption developed under the U.S. EPA's Endocrine Disruptor Screening and Testing Committee. In the summer of 1998, the Indiana Republican Committee adopted the precautionary principle as the basis for its environmental platform. The concept of precaution is beginning to take hold in the United States; however, it will be some years before it reaches the level of prominence held in Europe and other regions of the world.

21

Doth OSHA Protect
Too Much?

Norman Daniels

Fair Equality of Opportunity and Preventive Health Care

A health care system can protect an individual's share of the normal opportunity range both by curing disease when it arises and by reducing the risks of disease and disability. If we are obliged to protect opportunity, we may neglect neither curative nor preventive measures. The fair equality of opportunity account thus has a bearing on the debate about whether the health care systems of the United States and other Western countries overemphasize acute therapeutic services as opposed to preventive and public health measures. There are two general implications of the account for preventive health care: protecting opportunity will require (1) reducing the risk of disease and (2) seeking an equitable distribution of the risk of disease.

The first implication is fairly obvious. It is often more effective to prevent disease and disability than it is to cure them when they occur (or to compensate individuals for loss of function, where cure is not possible). Cost-effectiveness arguments will have some bearing on claims about the appropriate distribution of acute versus preventive measures. But the general point emphasized by the equal opportunity account is that the burdens of disease—even where the disease can be treated, and leaving aside financial burdens—have effects on fair equality of opportunity. This suggests that many types of preventive service and practice which reduce the risk of disease will be given prominence in a system governed by the fair equality of opportunity principle.

The second implication of the account, the importance of equalizing the risk of disease, needs some explanation. Suppose a health care system is heavily weighted toward acute care and that it provides equal access to its services. Thus anyone with severe respiratory ailments—black lung, brown lung, asbestosis, emphysema, and so on—is given adequate comprehensive services as needed. Does the system meet the demands of justice?

The fair equality of opportunity account implies the system is incomplete. If some groups in the population are differentially at risk of getting ill, it is not sufficient merely to attend to their illnesses. Where risk of illness differs systematically in ways that are avoidable, guaranteeing equal opportunity requires that we try to eliminate the differential risks and to prevent the excess illness those experience. Otherwise the burdens and risks of illness will fall differently on different groups, and the risk of impaired opportunity for those groups will remain, despite the efforts to provide acute care. Care is not equivalent to prevention. Some disease will not be detected in time for it to be cured. Some is not curable, even if it is preventable, and treatments will vary in efficacy. We protect equal opportunity best by reducing and equalizing the risk of these conditions arising. The fact that we get an equal chance of being cured once ill—because of equitable access to care—does not compensate us for our unequal chances of becoming ill.

For these reasons, the fair equality of opportunity account places special importance on measures which seek the equitable distribution of the risk of disease. Some public health measures, such as water and waste treatment, have the general effect of reducing risk. But historically, they have also had the effect of equalizing risk between socioeconomic classes and between groups living in different geographical areas. Many other environmental measures, such as recent clean air laws and pesticide regulations, have both general effects on risk reduction and specific effects on the distribution of risks. For example, pollutants emitted from smokestacks have a different effect on people who live downwind from those who live upwind. Gasoline lead emissions have greater effect on urban than rural populations. But other health-protection measures primarily have an effect on the distribution of risks: The regulation of workplace health hazards is perhaps the clearest example. Only some groups of workers are at risk from workplace hazards. The general implication of the fair equality of opportunity account is that stringent regulation in all of these ways must be part of the health care system. . . .

Prevention and OSHA Regulation

In this chapter I will discuss preventive health care measures in an institutional setting, the workplace. In part, I choose this focus because the regulation of workplace risks is clearly mandated by and emphasized by the fair equality of opportunity account, which urges the equalization of the risk of disease. But I also choose this focus because the workplace is a context in which actual regulation and not just education, as in matters of lifestyle choice, has been initiated. This regulation has been the object of great public controversy, largely because it has forced employers to bear the considerable costs of cleaning up workplaces. Without such cleanup, the costs are "externalized"; they are borne by workers, in the form of increased disease and disability, and by society, which pays the resulting increased health costs in the form of higher insurance premiums. The fair equality of opportunity account points toward the need for rather stringent hazard regulation. Its goal is to protect fair equality of opportunity, which implies that the significantly increased risks of disease faced by particular groups of workers are to be avoided to the extent it is possible to do so. Moreover, the fact that there may be significant costs to protecting equal opportunity in this way, or that such stringent protection may not be economically efficient, does not override the requirement of justice in this regard. The priority we give to fair equality of opportunity means that we must be willing to accept some economic losses of this kind.

Though much of the public debate about health hazard regulation has focused on costs, there is another, extremely important issue which also is raised as an objection to stringent regulation, and thus to my account. The objection is that the account comes into conflict with other requirements of justice, namely, the protection of individual liberty. Specifically, it threatens the liberty of workers and employers to contract, through hazard pay, to distribute the benefits and burdens of risk taking to their mutual advantage. Stringent regulation seems unduly paternalistic, perhaps valuing workers' health more highly than workers themselves value it. It is in this context, then, that there arises a sharply defined conflict between equality—in the form of stringent prevention efforts—and liberty—in the form of eliminating consent to risk as a method of distributing the burdens and benefits of risk taking. . . .

The form my discussion will take is to consider a rather restrictive form of health hazard regulation, one that might well be required by the fair equality of opportunity account. The task will be to determine if such restrictive regulation, viewed as an "upper bound" on stringency, can be justified without violating legitimate concerns for the protection of individual liberty. The upper bound to be considered is not hypothetical: It is the *actual* criterion for regulative standards embodied in the Occupational Safety and Health Act of 1970 [which created the Occupational Safety and Health Administration (OSHA)], namely, the "technological feasibility" standard. If this actual standard can be shown to respect individual liberties, then it is plausible to think that the fair equality of opportunity account will be consistent with those components of the general theory of justice which protect individual liberty.

This focus of my discussion needs further explanation because there is an asymmetry between acute and preventive care which is relevant here. A just health care system provides equitable access to medical services which are themselves equitably allocated—but it remains an individual's decision whether to use such services. The social obligation is to protect opportunity by providing the institutions which make individual consumption of these services possible. There is an elaborate doctrine of *informed consent* which intervenes between the framework of services society makes available and individual choices about consumption. Risk taking, including the risks of medical treatment, is generally viewed as a matter which should be left for individual decision: deep strands of liberal political philosophy coalesce to form a protected space within which the individual is to be sovereign in his self-regarding decisions. But in preventive contexts, especially where groups are protected, as in the workplace, the issue of consent arises in a much more complicated form. The central issue in this chapter will be to reconcile the demands of justice—that we provide a just distribution of preventive health services through stringent regulation of exposure to health hazards—with these concerns about individual liberty. . . .

The OSHA "Feasibility" Criterion:
In Search of a Rationale

The Occupational Safety and Health Act of 1970 requires the U.S. Secretary of Labor to set *standards* for dealing with toxic or harmful materials in the workplace. Such standards specify permissible exposure levels and require various practices, like the wearing of air masks, and means, like monitoring devices, for insuring that exposure does not exceed these levels. But when is a standard a good standard? How much protection should a good OSHA standard afford, assuming full compliance and enforcement? A centrally important feature of the 1970 act is the *criterion* it specifies for acceptable standards: A standard should "assure, *to the extent feasible,* on the basis of the best available evidence," that no employee will suffer material impairment of health.[1]

. . . OSHA has taken "feasibility" to mean *technological (or technical) feasibility.* A standard must protect workers to the degree it is technologically feasible to do so. In fact, however, OSHA must make a modest concession to economic considerations: the costs of compliance with the standard should not result in putting a whole industry out of business, though it may drive out marginal producers. In this discussion, I shall ignore this economic concession and shall refer to the criterion as the *strong* or *technological feasibility criterion.* . . . [T]he strong feasibility criterion has teeth. It compels the stringent regulation of hazards and is therefore seen as an essential feature of the OSHA Act by many proponents of public health regulation. . . .

The Feasibility Criterion:
Beyond Market Regulation

One way to see the issues raised by . . . the feasibility criterion is to notice how the criterion moves OSHA beyond the role of mere "market adjuster." Suppose we held the view that the task of government is to intervene in markets where individuals exchange goods only when the markets depart in specifiable ways from the conditions that define ideal or fair market conditions. The goal of such intervention is to adjust conditions in the direction of the ideal. We might then look at the "market" for such commodities as health care protection and willingness to take risks (daring) and ask if the exchanges workers and employers make in this market take place under fair or ideal market conditions. To the extent that they do, we would be assured that the resulting distributions of risks and benefits are both efficient and *fair.* They are fair because the market process which led to these outcomes is fair, and well-known optimality theorems prove they are efficient.

Where ideal market conditions or prerequisites are not met, however, we would authorize interventions to reestablish them or we would impose compensatory mechanisms which mimic their presence. For example, the market model presupposes that exchanges between employers and workers, such as the buying of daring with hazard pay, take place with adequate or full information about the nature of the risks involved. If there is a systematic absence of relevant information, or if access to the information is systematically unequal, then a regulatory intervention is needed to ensure that only informed exchanges take place. Uncertainty would otherwise undermine both efficiency and procedural fairness. Similarly, markets will be efficient and procedurally fair only if the commodities in them are priced at their true social cost. To the extent that many of the costs of health damage to workers are *externalized* and not priced in the health hazard market, since the bill for illness and disability is picked up by society as a whole, the market will be neither efficient nor fair in its outcomes. Such a "free" market would embody a form of freeloading. In it advantageous bargains would be made between workers and employers at the expense of nonconsenting third parties outside the market. To restore the market to ideal conditions would require a mechanism compelling the internalization of the externalized costs.

To the extent that the health hazard "market" in fact fails to provide for *informed* exchanges and fails to price all factors of production *at true social cost,* a major role would be provided for OSHA as a market adjuster. Such a role would have to be agreed to by any who accept the underlying rationale for the fairness and efficiency of ideal markets themselves. In this case, OSHA would have the role of guaranteeing that information is provided to all parties involved in the exchanges—and this task would involve many of the monitoring, research, and notification requirements incorporated in current OSHA standards. Indeed, it might involve more vigorous protection of workers' "rights to know" than we now find in practice. Similarly, OSHA would have the task of making sure the market properly priced the commodities exchanged in it. Of course, there are many possible ways to promote the internalization of externalized costs: Instead of standards defining permissible dose exposures, forcing the costs of cleanup on the company (at least initially), there might be taxes imposed on relevant employers, the revenues from which would be earmarked to defray the externalized costs. Presumably, these taxes would no longer be available to employer and worker as part of the pie that they divide among themselves. But another way of internalizing costs might be to use a *cost-benefit* feasibility criterion in the design of protection standards. Such a criterion would force the internalization of externalized costs only when, and to the point where, further "internalization" was counterproductive from the point of view of third parties.

But now it should be clear just how the stricter, feasibility criterion pushes OSHA well beyond the role of mere market adjuster or regulator. The effect of the standard is to eliminate completely the market in which daring is exchanged for hazard pay, at least for all hazards that it is technologically feasible to eliminate. Ideally, there would be no hazards left to bargain about. But if this is the effect of upholding the technological feasibility criterion, why should we single out this market for such drastic intervention, indeed elimination? Why not allow exchanges within the modified, adjusted market that would result from a weaker OSHA, one which merely provided information and which internalized externalized costs? *We need an argument to show that health protection in this setting is so special that it should not be treated to any degree as a market commodity.* So the shift from a cost-benefit to a techno-logical feasibility criterion is more than a mere question of degree. . . .

The "Specialness" of Health Protection and the Problem of Consent

I have suggested that the technological feasibility criterion seems to commit us to some very strong views about the special importance of health protection. Such strong views might be needed to . . . justify the virtual elimination of a market for risk tak-ing under OSHA regulation. Are there bases for such strong views?

One possible basis involves an appeal to individual rights, specifically a right to bodily integrity and freedom from assault.[2] Just as my bodily integrity is violated by a punch in the nose, so, too, it is threatened by toxins and carcinogens others place in the environment, including the workplace. Just as I have right claim against those who would punch me in the nose, so, too, I have one against those who would batter my lungs, liver, or DNA with hazardous materials at work. Just as I may need the help of police and the courts to protect my rights against assault and battery of my nose, so, too, I may need OSHA to protect me against battery of my DNA.

Whatever the strengths and weaknesses of such a rights-based account in gen-eral, it falls dramatically short of helping us with the problem we are considering, namely, the justification of the technological feasibility criterion. To use the indi-vidual rights model to justify the strong criterion, one would have to supplement it with two features, neither of which is intuitively plausible. First, one would have to assert that the only, or most satisfactory, way to respect these individual rights is to bar exposures to the degree required by the criterion. But it is not clear that these rights fail to be adequately respected by other combinations of measures, for example, by combining a cost-benefit feasibility criterion with special insurance protections against the contingency that health is damaged, or with special liability protections, such as an enhanced Workman's Compensation program, or even with a more lib-eral approach to torts for these cases. Second, one would have to treat the right as nonwaivable.[3] Yet, I can waive my right not to have my nose punched. Indeed, were I a world-class boxer, I might be able to get $10 million for doing so. So, too, it would seem, I should be able to consent to have my DNA assaulted, especially if I feel the compensation I get (with costs internalized) for taking that risk is worth it. Only if it can be shown why my consent and waiver is to be ignored in just the cases OSHA regulates can we resurrect the rights view in support of the technological feasibility criterion. Moreover, what will be doing the philosophical work here is *not the ap-peal to the rights* themselves, but the *supplementary theory* that explains the extent of the right and the limits of consent in these particular contexts.

Support for the special importance of health hazard protection might derive from an argument from fairness which requires that there be equity in the distribution of risks. To see the force of the argument, we must first ask a more general question. When do the risks I impose on another through various activities I engage in give rise to claims for compensation? After all, as Charles Fried[4] points out in his discus-sion of this argument,[5] if I drive to the corner store to buy a newspaper, I impose risks on others all along the route, risks to which they have not explicitly consented. Do they have a right claim against me to refrain from imposing these risks? The answer depends on pointing out that there is reciprocity in the imposition of such risks: My neighbor *normally* imposes them on me, just as I do on him. Since the pursuit of our ordinary, otherwise nonproscribed activities is *roughly reciprocal,* we ought to accept the balance of threats and risks that emerges as the price for collectively living normal, reasonable lives. The "risk pool" that results ought to be consented to, even if it is not usually the object of explicit consent. Tolerating these "normal" reciprocal risks is a fair way for each of us to "use others" to advance our own ends.

But if the argument from fairness justifies the imposition of some unconsented-to risks, it does so only if a central presupposition is met. As Fried notes in his discussion, the risks must be *roughly equally distributed.* If risks to health and safety are unequally distributed, then simple arguments from fairness will count *against* their acceptability to those facing the greatest risks. A paradigm case of such unequal distribution of avoidable risk is the health risk imposed by hazards in the workplace—at least in societies where we do not all rotate our jobs periodically. This argument from fairness implies, then, that workplace hazards are not part of the socially acceptable risk pool, and workers have a claim against their being imposed.

Viewed as a vehicle for justifying the technological feasibility criterion, the argument from fairness founders on the same rocks as the rights-based view. Though workers may have a claim, based on fairness, against having unequal health risks imposed on them, the argument does not specify how they are to be protected or compensated for their loss. Some form of compensation may be all that is needed to meet the fairness argument. More importantly, the claim of such workers is only against risks to which they do not consent. If workers are willing to face the risks in exchange for other benefits (assuming they actually can bargain for benefits and keep them in the long run), the fairness argument becomes irrelevant, or so it would seem. If consent is not a reliable risk-distributing mechanism in these contexts, we will have to know why, and it is *this* explanation, not the fairness argument above, that will be needed to justify the strong feasibility criterion.

Perhaps the argument from fairness fails because it is too general: It pays too little attention to what is *special* about health and therefore about the protection of health. The fair equality of opportunity account is just such an account: It shows why health care needs are of special importance and why they give rise to social obligations to provide needed services. Does it also show why protecting worker health is so important it warrants the strong feasibility criterion?

I think not. The fair equality of opportunity account also falls short of providing a direct and clear rationale for the strong feasibility criterion so central to the OSHA Act. Health may be special or important from the perspective of a theory of justice because of its impact on opportunity, and this importance may give rise to social obligations to protect health. But nothing in this view makes health protection *so* overriding a concern that we may deny individuals the autonomy to take risks that endanger life, liver, and lungs. Consequently, it cannot be just the special importance of health that justifies the strong feasibility criterion Congress imposed. Rather, there may also be something special or peculiar about the context in which these risks to health arise that justifies the imposition of the strong criterion. If so, our search for a justification will compel us to examine what is distinctive about the context.

More Protection Than I Want:
A Libertarian Lament

To focus our problem it may be useful to consider the lament a libertarian worker might make against the technological feasibility criterion. Of course, few actual workers would be likely to argue in this fashion. Indeed, most have sought stringent government regulation.[6] Nevertheless, however unusual or hypothetical the lament, it forces us to face squarely an important moral issue.

Imagine, then, that the lament is voiced by a libertarian moral philosopher, driven by market conditions out of academe into the industrial workforce. Having been forced to flee the safety of academic life, Bob, we shall call him, suddenly discovers his willingness to take risks. Indeed, it is one of his few marketable talents. More accurately, it *would* be marketable except that OSHA's technical feasibility criterion almost eliminates the market for such daring in regulated contexts. Bob can negotiate for hazard pay only with regard to a residue of ineliminable risk. In contrast, an economic feasibility criterion, say one that merely guaranteed the internalization of costs, would leave him a greater range of risks for which he could negotiate hazard pay and would increase the market value of his daring. In fact, the more stringent criterion, with its greater compliance costs, might mean fewer jobs and less job security than would be possible in a market which allowed employers and workers room to negotiate a distribution of burdens more congenial to them.

Bob's complaint, then, is that protection from risks is being valued more highly than he values it, given the relevant information. Bob's lament is that his liberty to exchange daring for dollars or greater job security is unnecessarily restricted. What is worse, the restriction is completely out of keeping with our other practices regarding autonomy and the regulation of risks. People take risks with their health, and are allowed to do so, in other contexts, in work, in play, and in everyday living. Why, then, these stringent restrictions in selected work settings?

Consider, for example, the inconsistency between stringent OSHA standards and the autonomy granted in other work contexts. Many workers, ranging from specialists, like stunt drivers and test pilots, to policemen, firemen, and ironworkers, face great risks in their work. They are permitted to negotiate hazard pay for the full range of these risks, and no government agency intervenes to insist that risks be eliminated to the extent technologically feasible. . . .

Second, many lifestyle choices bring with them risks to health of greater magnitude than risks from many workplace health hazards. Yet people are not prohibited from smoking, drinking excessive alcohol, failing to exercise, or eating too much fatty meat. Nor are they prohibited from hang gliding, scuba diving, driving without seat belts (in the United States), or sun bathing. Indeed, the very workers we refuse to allow to face even modest exposure to carcinogens in the workplace we still allow to drive to work with cigarette in mouth and seat belt unhooked (even if we require automakers to install the belts). . . .

Autonomy, Paternalism, and Risky Lifestyle Choices

So far I have rejected the suggestion that the special importance of health protection alone provides an adequate rationale for OSHA's strong feasibility criterion. That defense seemed unduly paternalistic in view of the risk taking we otherwise permit both in work and play. Consequently, either we must find those distinctive features of OSHA-regulated *risks* or *contexts* which justify the strong or we must abandon this strategy for defending it. We may derive some clues from our inquiry from a brief look at the related problem of risk taking in lifestyle choices.

Though most of us would agree that promoting health lifestyles is an important social goal, we are also justifiably hesitant about permitting too much social intrusion into individual decision making about lifestyles. We seek to promote autonomy in the definition and pursuit of our conceptions of the good life. Of course, we accept some social constraints, such as those justice imposes on our construction and pursuit of individual conceptions of the "good." Yet, we resist the suggestion that there is only one acceptable conception of the good, or that self-regarding features of these conceptions must all agree on basic points, for example, in the importance placed on avoiding risks to health. We have no conception of the good life that embodies just one degree of risk-aversion. Nevertheless, even a view that holds the individual to be the best architect of his ends and judge of his interests rests on important assumptions about the *information* available to the agent, the *competency* of the agent to make these decisions rationally, and the *voluntariness* of the decisions he makes. It is because these assumptions are not always met that we require a theory of justifiable paternalism.

One attractive version of such a theory invokes the notion of a social contract.[7] Individuals who value their autonomy must nevertheless realize that sometimes their competency to make rational decisions is temporarily or permanently undermined. They may then engage in self-destructive behavior which runs counter to their "true" interests. Their "true" interests are defined counterfactually as the interests they would claim were they competent, informed, and acting voluntarily. It would be rational for such individuals to insure themselves against such harmful outcomes by authorizing others to act on their behalf, even contrary to their expressed wishes, when specifiable failures of competency make rational choice impossible. But it is critical to this theory that the conditions under which paternalism is permitted are well defined and involve failures of decision-making competency, which I here take to include threats to the voluntariness of the decisions.

Notice that this rationale for paternalism imposes constraints on both the *grounds* for interventions and the *kinds* of intervention it justifies. Specifically, decisions which others regard as self-destructive, including decisions that threaten health, do not constitute conclusive grounds for intervention. Only if these decisions are the result of independently defined and detected failures of competency is paternalistic intervention justified. The theory leaves room, then, for informed patients to refuse life-saving medical treatment and for rational suicide. Moreover, interventions should act first to restore, where possible, the diminished decision-making abilities. Only if restoration is impossible is a more direct intervention in the long-term determination of goals and acts permitted.

Clearly this rationale for paternalism has implications for the kinds of coercion or regulation we may use to intervene in lifestyle choices that affect health. Specifically, health-threatening behaviors—smoking or not wearing seat belts—are not themselves evidence of diminished capacity for rational decision making. Many of these behaviors, after all, are associated with natural effects—the relaxation of smoking—that are also desirable and whose payoffs individuals may weigh differently. To intervene in these behaviors would require independent evidence that the behavior is the result of diminished capacity to make decisions or is in some specifiable way not voluntary. Moreover, where there is such evidence, the intervention must be restricted, where possible, to restoring the decision-making capacity; it should not involve permanent prohibition of the behavior. Of course, people may have diminished competency to judge the rationality of these behaviors if they lack relevant information about them.[8] But then the preferred intervention is the provision of the information in an effective manner. Only if it is impossible to assure that information will be accessible can we impose more stringent restrictions on outcomes. For example, stringent safety standards imposed by the Consumer Product Safety Commission can be justified on the assumption that we could never guarantee that risk taking by consumers would be adequately informed (e.g., the consumer or user may not be the purchaser). Such standards insure us against making the uninformed decisions we consumers are likely to make.

We can obtain another clue for our inquiry, one that bears on the voluntariness of decision making, by looking briefly at a nonpaternalistic argument in favor of intervening in health-threatening lifestyle choices. Indeed, the very factors which weigh against paternalistic intervention to promote healthy lifestyles, especially the lack of evidence for diminished competency, might incline us to turn to this argument from equity or fairness. Unhealthy lifestyles impose a burden on the portion of society that chooses healthy lifestyles, the burden of sharing the costs of the excess illness induced by unhealthy lifestyle choices. For example, if insurance schemes do not pool risks by reference to lifestyle choices, then people with healthy lifestyles have grounds for complaint. The insurance premiums are not actuarially fair to them, for they involve a cross-subsidy to the risk takers. There is a parallel here to the point made earlier with regard to hazard pay in contexts where costs are not internalized. "Free" choices by high risk takers freeload on the risk-averse. It might then be argued that the burden should be redistributed, say in the form of a differential insurance premium or through special taxes on smoking, hang gliding, and so on.

Nevertheless, many people are reluctant to accept this argument from "fairness" for redistributing the costs of risky behaviors.[9] One central worry is that many of the lifestyle choices are not so clearly *voluntary,* or are not ones for which we feel comfortable ascribing full responsibility, even if there is no way to claim diminished decision-making competency. Many factors, such as induced "false consciousness" through cigarette advertising, exposure to special peer pressures as a teenager beginning to smoke, or the influence of a cultural background which emphasizes the macho image of heavy smoking or drinking, raise questions about the fairness of redistributive measures themselves.[10] Such measures seem to treat people as more responsible for these decisions than they really are.

If these are indeed ways in which *voluntariness,* and thereby responsibility, is systematically diminished, a distinct argument for protective, paternalistic regulation might be justified, even though the redistributive argument fails. At least the intrusive factors that diminish voluntariness should be attacked. However, the rather minimal step of informing people about the risks of smoking by warnings on cigarette packs and in commercials falls well short of addressing the issue of diminished voluntariness. We are caught apparently by conflicting considerations in our public policy concerning lifestyle choices. The worry that certain sanctions would be unjustifiably paternalistic stops us in one direction. The worry that redistributive measures would be punishing those not fully responsible stops us in the other direction. These are not inconsistent worries, though there is a slight air of paradox. We compromise by taking minimal steps toward making sure relevant information is present.

Our discussion of paternalism and lifestyle choices suggests a strategy for trying to defend OSHA's strong feasibility criterion. In general we ought to preserve autonomy: This was the point behind the libertarian lament. But we are not bound to preserve the illusion of autonomy. If unregulated worker "choices" about risk taking must fail, or generally do fail, to be *informed, competent,* or *truly voluntary,* then we are not compromising autonomy by intervening. Rather, we are merely avoiding the illusion of autonomy and insuring ourselves against the harms that would result from living with the illusion. Our task, then, reduces to seeing whether choices unregulated by strong OSHA standards would fail to be autonomous in these specifiable ways.

Information and Competency

We may be able to motivate two lines of argument in favor of stringent OSHA regulations by noting some contrasts often drawn between *the kinds of risk* faced, by chemical workers, for example, and other risks we do not regulate as stringently. Risks from toxins or carcinogens are not *visible* in the same way that the risks to a fireman of building collapse or smoke inhalation are.[11] The latter risks are apparent in the work situations in which they arise—no special knowledge or information is needed to make one aware of them. They are familiar. They are dramatic and direct in their action on us. We know exactly what it is to encounter the risk in a particular situation; moreover, each time the fire is put out, we are aware of having survived the risk. That is, their action is immediate. In contrast, the risks from exposure to hazardous materials may be incremental, operating over a very long term. This of course is the case with many of the familiar instances: cotton dust, coal dust, asbestos. Walking out of the mill or mine each day does not mean the danger has been avoided for at least that encounter. To be sure, we can reformulate both types of risks into frequencies or probabilities of disability or death. But it is arguable that the common coin of this reformulation does not remove the difference in the *graspability* of the risks facing the fireman, stunt driver, or hang glider as compared to that facing the textile worker.

This difference in the "graspability" of the risks also suggests a second contrast. The more visible, familiar, direct kinds of risk seem to be apparent to anyone. The invisible, unfamiliar, indirect risks become apparent only when there is access to considerable epidemiological information. But such information is difficult to obtain and is more accessible to employers than workers. So connected to the difference in the graspability of the risks is a potential inequality in access to information about them.

These two differences give rise to distinct arguments about the importance of stringent OSHA regulation of the sort required by the strong feasibility requirement. The first argument expands on the difference in the graspability of these risks and claims that there is diminished competency to make rational decisions about the less graspable risks. Indeed, our risk-taking competence developed primarily around the more visible, direct kinds of cases, so we have some reason to rely on our normal competency in these contexts; but we have no comparable reassurance about competency in the other instances. Since the information about these other risks must be couched statistically, and generally it is in the form of a low risk of a serious outcome, we have even more reason to worry about individual competency. A recent body of psychological literature has shown that we are notoriously unreliable and inconsistent "rational deliberators" about just the kind of risk-taking decisions imposed on us by the invisible, long-term risks.[12] Consequently, to rely on individual decision making in a hazard pay market for these risks would be to rely on a competency we have definite reason to think is diminished. Moreover, merely supplying more statistical information may not compensate for the deficit in graspability and thus lead to improved competency. The "autonomy" a hazard pay market for these risks involves is thus illusory, and regulation eliminating such illusory choice making is not a threat to autonomy.

The problem with this argument is that it seems to prove too much. The same sort of invisible, indirect, "low-graspability" risks are part of the fabric of our everyday lifestyle choices. Thus the decisions to accept the risks of smoking, or not exercising, or eating too much fatty meat—all seem to involve decisions very much like the risk taking involved in exposure to cotton dust or benzene. If we want to challenge competency in one domain, consistency requires we do so in the other, unless there are still other countervailing differences. Our problem then, is that this argument fails to meet the conditions of adequacy on a successful rationale imposed by the libertarian lament. Though we have found a difference between OSHA-regulated risks and some other risks in which we allow autonomy, the difference does not generalize to cover the relevant cases.

The second argument draws on the potential for inequality in access to information about the risks. In effect, it says that even the best efforts of a regulatory agency which concentrated on making information accessible to all parties to hazard pay agreements will fall short of giving reasonable assurance that decisions are adequately informed. But if no such assurance about the adequacy of information is achievable merely through regulation, then we have no assurance that autonomy will be real and not illusory in agreements between workers and employers. This argument is thus similar to a rationale often given for stringent safety regulation of consumer products. The argument there turns on the fundamental inequality in information between the manufacturer and retailer, on the one hand, and the consumer on the other. There seems to be no way to make sure that a consumer is informed when he makes his purchase; moreover, purchasers of products are not always their users, so there is even more room for failures of information, which thus leads to the imposition of unconsented-to risks. The result is that products must be held to some measurable safety standard, and we cannot rely on the mechanism of consent to distribute the benefits and burdens of risk taking.

The difficulty with this argument is that it again fails to steer the proper course among the obstacles illuminated by the libertarian lament. Why should not the same argument about information apply to consumers of cigarettes, alcohol, cholesterol, and so on? Indeed, it seems more likely that we could take steps to insure equality of access to information in the relatively determinate employer-employee relationship than that we could in the highly diffuse relationship between cigarette manufacturer and consumer. In this regard, the former relationship more closely resembles the doctor-patient relationship than does the latter. And even though there is inequality in power or authority, as well as in access to information, in the doctor-patient relationship, we rely on an ideal of informed, competent, voluntary consent to make sure that autonomy is preserved, at the same time we allow risk taking by individuals. Of course, the analogy is not exact: Inequality in power may be greater in the employee-employer relationship than in the doctor-patient one, and there is no traditional ethic governing the "agency" relationship in the former, as there is in the latter. Still, there seems to be more potential for correcting problems in access to information between workers and employers than there does between smokers and cigarette manufacturers. So if it is information, or the lack of it, that is at the heart of the rationale for OSHA's strong feasibility criterion, we have not cleanly met the libertarian challenge.

Intrinsic and Extrinsic Rewards of Risk Taking

There is another relevant set of differences between the risks faced by workers handling toxins and carcinogens and other risks we do not regulate so stringently. In general, the risks OSHA is supposed to regulate stringently lack three desirable effects which can be associated with various less stringently or unregulated risks. First, workplace toxins and carcinogens are not associated with natural effects that are themselves desirable, as cigarettes are the satisfaction smokers experience. Second, exposure to workplace toxins and carcinogens is not directly connected to consequences of obvious moral significance, like the protection of life and property by firemen and policemen. These direct moral consequences mean that a certain prestige attaches to the risky work, and some people are attracted to the work by a "calling" to perform this sort of social service. In contrast, the beneficial, safety effects of asbestos on brake linings are so indirect that the social significance of the risk taking is negligible; few are likely to feel a calling to be asbestos workers.[13] Third, some risk taking is psychologically gratifying because of the kind of skill, talent, or immediate bravery—and training—it requires. Special prestige may be attached to those who visibly accept such challenges, and various forms of "macho" camaraderie may arise to give psychological support to those who persevere in facing these risks. But the handling of workplace toxins and other hazardous materials usually does not involve special skills or talents or such visible daring. It may involve only the breathing of cotton dust or benzene fumes—unpleasant, insignificant, and undramatic parts of one's daily work routine. And where a "macho" attitude arises, it is more likely to be viewed by others as a pathetic and morbid form of false consciousness.

All three of these differences make it easier to see why people might want, for reasons based on their underlying desires, to take those risks associated with desirable consequences. Accordingly, it is more difficult to intrude paternalistically where people taking risks actually value the direct consequences associated with them. Since the handling of workplace toxins or carcinogens is unconnected to any such desirable consequences, it might seem easier to justify intervention: The risk taker cannot really want to do what he is doing, it seems. The very taking of the risks appears to be evidence in these cases for incompetent or irrational decision making.

But the problem with this argument is that risk taking with carcinogens or other hazardous materials can be associated with *extrinsic* rewards, even if it is not naturally or socially connected to directly desirable consequences. A system of hazard pay establishes just such extrinsic rewards, and these rewards are motivating and connect to underlying conceptions of the good or individual utility functions. The only way to save the argument for paternalism here would be to show that these extrinsic rewards are suspect in a way not true of the more direct, desirable consequences associated with other risks. And whatever the grounds for such suspicion about extrinsic rewards, the argument must leave room for the fact that extrinsic rewards are also attached to risk taking in cases where the intrinsic rewards are demonstrably greater—for example, the high pay of Hollywood stuntmen.

One line of argument to show that the extrinsic rewards are suspect is to suggest that they may be particularly sensitive to factors that affect the *voluntariness* of the risk-taking decisions. For example, the extrinsic rewards might be thought enticing only because the range of available alternatives makes them so. Where risk taking is associated with certain intrinsic rewards, we can imagine particular personality types attracted to them. Such individuals plausibly can be viewed as choosing the risky job because it reflects a definite preference; it is deliberate in a relevant way. Where the rewards of risk taking are all extrinsic, however, e.g., in the form of hazard pay or increased job security in the short run, then we are led to think the risks are accepted only because there is no more attractive alternative available. Moreover, such a restricted choice is *typical* for a broad class of workers. And if the lack of alternatives is the result of a coercive exclusion from alternatives, or even an unfair or unjust denial of alternatives, then we have reason to be suspicious about the voluntariness of the risk-taking decisions.

A number of observations may motivate such an argument. The class of workers which handles the hazardous materials OSHA regulates tends to have fewer skills and less training than other parts of the workforce. In many places, the affected industries are dominant employers. In any case, the affected jobs comprise a significant portion of the available industrial employment in an economy which has high levels of unemployment. These observations suggest that the mobility of workers likely to be faced with the choice of handling hazardous materials is restricted. The bitterness and despair of workers who have fought against risks in the workplace—

which is evident in the struggles of coal miners and textile mill workers—is further evidence of such constraints on alternatives.

In what follows, I shall consider two lines of argument that develop these worries about the voluntariness of the choices workers make when they trade daring in handling hazardous materials for hazard pay. Both lines of argument provide somewhat different rationales for OSHA's strong feasibility criterion. Moreover, they capture a concern frequently expressed in the literature, that the existence of a hazard pay market for these risks does not imply that the risk taking is really voluntary. The inference from market exchange to voluntary exchange is faulty.[14]

Coercion

Is it *coercive* to propose that a worker take hazard pay for accepting certain technologically reducible risks in handling carcinogens or breathing dust? It is tempting to look for an argument that shows coercion would be present in any such hazard pay market or the one we are likely to encounter. Such a result would clearly imply the kind of diminished voluntariness needed to justify the paternalism involved in OSHA's strong feasibility criterion. In contrast, arguments that depend on showing that the range of choices open to workers is unfairly or unjustly restricted are likely to be weaker in either of two ways. Even assuming their premise, that choices are unfairly or unjustly restricted, we still get only a controversial inference to diminished voluntariness in choices about risk taking. Moreover, the premise itself is likely to be controversial, for different theories of distributive justice will produce different judgments about the fairness of the range of choice. So, whereas coercion might be viewed as a *prima facie* wrong by anyone, controversy about justice will undermine confidence in the soundness (validity aside) of arguments in which we infer diminished voluntariness from restricted ranges of choice.

Nevertheless, I think it is difficult to establish any straightforward claims about coercion in the relevant cases for our argument. The reason is that the concept of coercion is itself complex and controversial in ways that make its application to the health hazard context complex and controversial. Indeed, we lack a persuasive, dominant philosophical analysis to which we may appeal in such applications. . . .

Voluntariness and Justice

I shall now sketch an argument which, I believe, both provides a plausible rationale for OSHA's strong feasibility criterion and successfully steers its way around the obstacles erected by the libertarian lament. The argument has a resemblance to arguments which justify paternalism under certain conditions, but the argument straddles a fence between an argument from justifiable paternalism and an argument from justice. The reason it must sit on this fence derives from the considerations in the last section, where we saw the difficulty of making clear-cut, uncontroversial attributions of coercion to cases of the sort we are considering. Despite the argument's plausibility, it is not without its problems, which I note in the next section.

To state the argument I will introduce a bit of terminology which will help us capture the underlying intuition. Let us call a proposal *quasi-coercive* if it imposes or depends on a restriction of someone's alternatives in a way that is *unfair* or unjust; that is, a just or fair social arrangement would involve a range of options for the individual both broader than and strongly preferred to the range in the proposal situation. Some quasi-coercive offers will turn out to be straightforwardly coercive ones: It will depend on *how* the unfair or unjust restriction of options emerged. For example, if the person making the proposal or other relevant persons acted outside their rights, Nozick[15] suggests, we will have a case of coercion. But, contrary to Nozick's view, systematic injustice in social arrangements does not always derive from explicit acts of individuals who go beyond their rights. These forms of injustice may lead to proposals which count here as quasi-coercive.

The intuition underlying calling unfair or unjust restrictions of options "quasi-coercive" is that they involve a diminished freedom of action of the same sort which is glaring in the central cases of coercion. A central difference may be the mechanism through which freedom of action is diminished. We do not have the direct and invasive intrusion into the "choice-space" of the individual which is present in the central cases of coercion, for example, when the mugger exceeds his rights by pointing a gun at my head. Instead, we have an indirect, yet pervasive, erosion of that space as a result of unjust or unfair social practices and institutions. The two share the feature that the restriction is *socially caused*. It is not the kind of restriction that results merely from misfortune; it is an act or institution of man, not God or nature, that produces it. Moreover, there are just, feasible alternatives.

Notice an important fact: Like the slave in Nozick's example, people who standardly suffer from an unfair or unjust restriction of their options may welcome a quasi-coercive proposal. That is, from their perspective, it may represent an offer and not a threat. Locally considered, the proposal may advance their interests. Moreover, its quasi-coerciveness may even seem invisible. Not everyone living under an unjust arrangement may be aware of its injustice. Some may even deny its injustice, say through "false consciousness." Indeed, against the background of a familiar and psychologically accepted range of options, however unfair or unjust it is, jumping at the new "opportunity" embodied in such a proposal, say by trading daring in handling carcinogens for hazard pay, may seem the essence of autonomous action. After all, no one is holding a cocked pistol to my head or threatening prison if I do not take the offer. The quasi-coerciveness of unjust arrangements works in a more subtle, but still restrictive, fashion.

There is another way in which the quasi-coerciveness of some proposals may be hidden: It may be only potential, not actual. That is, if we imagine institutionalizing such proposals, then their effect *over time* will be to produce, or to contribute to, actual quasi-coerciveness, even if initially, and viewed locally, there seems to be nothing worrisome about them, and they seem to be the essence of autonomous exchange.[16] There is just such a worry about a hazard pay market for certain kinds of risk when the market is aimed at workers with a severely restricted range of options. Such proposals might seem unquestionably fair at one time: They are the local manifestation of a process of market exchange which seems procedurally fair under certain circumstances. But such markets will tend to greater inequality over time, especially where there is substantial inequality in bargaining power because workers have highly restricted alternatives. Workers who might at one point be able to sell their daring at a relatively high price—as do, say, movie stuntmen—will find that it is worth little or nothing over time. Risk taking then becomes a condition of getting a job at all, a price only one with an unfair or unjust range of options—one who is quasi-coerced—would accept. . . .

The argument of OSHA's strong feasibility criterion can now be sketched as follows: (1) Hazard pay proposals for technologically reducible risks in the contexts OSHA regulated are quasi-coercive or would tend to be over time. (2) Eliminating such proposals (and the market for them) protects workers from harmful consequences, viz. the destruction of their health at a price that only someone under quasi-coercion would accept. (3) Though hazard pay proposals of the sort involved here may be offers welcomed by certain workers, the autonomy embodied in accepting them is only illusory, for quasi-coercion undermines true autonomy in much the same way coercion does. (4) Just as people would reasonably contract to permit paternalistic interventions which protect them against the harmful decisions they would make when they are not, or cannot be, adequately informed, competent, or free to make autonomous ones, so, too, they would reasonably contract to protect themselves against quasi-coerced decisions of the sort involved here. Thus, (5) OSHA's strong feasibility criterion can be viewed as a social insurance policy against quasi-coercive proposals to trade health for other benefits.

I shall restrict my defense of this sketch to comments on several of its controversial features. One issue of considerable concern is that the argument not prove too much: We do not want to trip over the obstacles illuminated in the libertarian lament. Specifically, the claim about quasi-coerciveness, or potential quasi-coerciveness, assuming we can apply it to OSHA contexts, should not extend readily to hazard pay proposals involving some other kinds of risky work, where we endorse no such stringent regulation. Does the argument cover the right cases?

Earlier . . . I noted that the risks we are most concerned with, the handling of toxins, carcinogens, and other hazardous materials, are not risks which are likely to be chosen for their intrinsic desirability, for the satisfaction that might derive from facing danger or using special skills to survive, or for their instrumental connection to highly desirable consequences, for example, saving lives. Rather, the motivation to take these risks derives entirely from the extrinsic rewards associated with them, rewards like hazard pay or steady employment in areas of limited employment opportunity. Partly as a result of this difference, the choice to be a fireman or stunt driver is *exceptional,* reflecting a high degree of self-selection: Such choices could readily have been forgone for many other kinds of work. In contrast, the choice to be a miner, mill worker, or industrial worker facing health hazards subject to OSHA's strong criterion is *typical.* For a large class of workers, these are the primary forms of available employment. Indeed, these are the typical options, or the sole or most attractive ones, facing a class of workers with a significantly restricted range of options. The restrictions on workers' options are the result of various factors: their limited educational opportunity, their array of marketable skills and talents, accidents of geographical location, or their limited economic resources for financing job mobility.

Moreover, this narrowness of the range of options open to the typical worker is compounded by another factor. The riskiness of exceptional jobs (stunt driver, fireman) can be viewed as stable over time: The worker knows more or less what he is getting into over a standard period of employment. But in "typical" jobs, changes in manufacturing processes can expose workers to risks not anticipated at the inception of an employment period. To impose the burden of dodging these risks on the worker, given possible losses in benefits, pensions, family disruption, is to overestimate his effective options, to assume he has job mobility where it does not exist.

What this point about exceptional versus typical choices means, then, is that hazard pay proposals in one setting, made to one group of workers, may be, or will tend to be, quasi-coercive without all hazard pay proposals being so. The difference will depend on judgments about the range of alternatives open to one group, rather than the other, and on the reasons for the restricted options. Thus the argument does not force us to treat dissimilar groups similarly.

Moreover, nothing in this argument for strong OSHA regulation implies we ought to intervene similarly in lifestyle choices affecting health, even though by doing so we might prevent comparable harms. Like the stunt driver's choices, these lifestyle choices are also not generally or potentially quasi-coerced. Earlier I expressed some worries about the voluntariness of certain lifestyle choices, noting, for example, the effect of strong subcultural influences. But these threats to autonomy are different from quasi-coercion, and arguments based on these more diffuse kinds of influence are not likely to justify comparable interventions. Indeed, they are just the sorts of influence we are fearful of undermining if we respect diversity.

The argument sketched here for the OSHA criterion thus appears to avoid the worries of the libertarian lament. It turns out that only the appropriate hazard pay proposals are quasi-coercive, or potentially so. It is important to remember that the argument does not require that we think the range of options open to regulated workers is already unjustly or unfairly restricted. It is sufficient that we believe the restricted range of options such workers enjoy, though fair or just now, would tip in the direction of injustice and unfairness over the long run. Moreover, we should be concerned that the "tipping" might be hard to detect, and therefore that the quasi-coerciveness would remain hidden and invisible to many participants in the hazard pay market. Consequently, we should be reluctant to rely on our perceptions of fairness once faced with such situations. Just as some incompetent or uninformed individuals may not be in the best position to detect their diminished capacity for making autonomous decisions, so, too, we should not wait till we are quasi-coerced to protect ourselves against diminished autonomy. Rather, it is prudent to impose prior, protective constraints on the framework of markets built on exchanges between workers and employers. These constraints are designed to ensure that market changes remain within the requirements of justice or fairness.

An important objection to this argument sketch is connected to a point made earlier, that the argument straddles a fence. The appropriate reaction to complaints about an injustice, or potential injustice, in the distribution of social goods should be to alter the fundamental institutional arrangements which lead to the unjust distribution. Yet our argument leads us merely to intervene narrowly to block one sort of consequence of such (potential) injustice—the harm that might result from quasi-coerced decisions. This intervention seems to add insult to injury, if the premise about quasi-coercion is correct. We leave all the factors intact which create, or tend to create, the unjust, quasi-coercive setting. Instead, we intervene to stop a vulnerable class of individuals from exercising its own discretion. This paternalism seems vexing because it leaves intact the background conditions which seem to make the intervention necessary. The objection, then, is that worries about injustice should not lead to narrow constraints on autonomy. If the objection is correct, step 4 of the argument sketch is dubious.

I should like to make three points in response to this objection. First, the autonomy that is restricted here is only an illusion if the claim about quasi-coercion is correct. To be sure, the interventions may remain offensive to those who want to accept the offers involved, but if the discussion in earlier sections is correct, we have reason to think the voluntariness of quasi-coerced decisions is diminished in morally significant ways. Second, contrary to the premise of the objection, arguments from justice often involve restrictions on free exchanges among individuals: The restrictions take the general form of restricting some free exchanges to preserve the fairness of others. Does a market which permits quasi-coerced exchanges respect liberty more than one that restricts some exchanges in order to make all exchanges free from quasi-coercion? I would suggest not, but the answer would take us afield into some central questions in the general theory of justice.

My third point is that the modification of distributive institutions involved in OSHA regulations does have an effect on distributive justice, at least if arguments I have made elsewhere about the nature of health care as a social good are at all plausible. No doubt, the importance of health might be argued for in various ways, all of which might justify viewing the trading of health for too low a price as unfair. But on my own view, health is of direct relevance to worries about justice because it contributes directly to the distribution of opportunity in society. Compromising health through quasi-coerced hazard pay bargains thus compromises the ability to maintain fair equality of opportunity in a society. The restricted opportunity range of poor or worst-off classes of workers would act, in hazard pay markets, to further undermine fair equality of opportunity. Earlier, I argued that claims about the special importance of health or health care will not show *by themselves* why we should not rely on consent to distribute risks to health: Health is not *so* important we refuse to let people compromise it in various contexts. The argument sketch for the strong OSHA criterion shows, however, why certain hazard pay proposals would depend on a highly questionable form of consent, consent under quasi-coercion, and that is the crux of the rationale offered here.

Worries and Conclusions

There is a deeply troubling consequence of the argument offered in the last section, one that is important to bring out in the open. The rationale I offered turned on concern about the actual or potential quasi-coerciveness of certain hazard pay proposals. The quasi-coerciveness of the proposals depended on the fact that the class of workers facing such proposals has, or is likely to have, unfairly or unjustly restricted alternatives. But what if we could agree that the distribution of income and opportunity were really fair or just, and that the distribution would not be tipped toward unfairness over time through the operation of a market for such risk taking. Suppose, that is, that we lived in a just social arrangement, one that were stable over time. If the rationale for OSHA's strong criterion depends on the claim about quasi-coerciveness, then there would be no need for the strong OSHA feasibility criterion. Perhaps the class of workers receiving these hazard pay proposals might still face a range of options more restricted than more fortunate groups of workers or professionals, but the inequalities here are no threat to justice (we are supposing). In such circumstances, we would still have a role for OSHA: guaranteeing that adequate information is present for informed decision making about risk taking, and guaranteeing that costs are internalized, so that hazard pay bargains do not freeload on other parties. But the strong OSHA criterion now lacks a rationale.

Some proponents of the strong OSHA criterion might readily agree to this restriction on its applicability: For them, the rationale I have offered would seem to capture their underlying moral view. But some proponents of strong regulation might feel uneasy about the restriction; indeed, I feel uneasy about it myself. It is not clear to me just what follows from this sort of unfocused uneasiness. It could be that there are other components to a rationale which are not captured in this argument from justice. Yet, it is not obvious at all what they are. On the other hand, the problem may lie with this methodology for testing a philosophical argument. Intuitions or considered moral judgments about the rightness of a practice, like stringent OSHA regulations, arise in a particular social setting, one which has many forms of injustice or threats of injustice. It is notoriously difficult to clean up and make the principles underlying these intuitions explicit merely by forming counterfactual test situations in which to deploy them. To be sure, this is standard philosophical method, but its results are often less clear than what we take them to be.[17] Nevertheless, if one cannot show why one is dissatisfied with the kind of "test" of the rationale this hypothetical case involves, then the dissatisfaction will linger to infect the rationale itself. This result should worry proponents of strong OSHA regulation, who must offer an alternative, or more complete, rationale than the one sketched here.

The rationale I have offered, despite these deeper worries that there are still *other* components needed for a complete account, does carry weight wherever we have reason to worry about quasi-coerciveness in our own society. That is, we *do* get a plausible argument for the OSHA criterion as long as we have reason to worry about the fairness or justice of the distribution of options available to the workers most likely to receive the hazard pay proposals in question. But, of course, just such worries are themselves controversial. And differences in moral judgment here depend not only on different estimates of empirical facts, but on different underlying conceptions of what is just or fair. So my rationale also has the strength of locating clearly a source of controversy about the acceptability of the OSHA criterion itself. My rationale will be controversial just where moral controversy about regulation is sharpest in our society. The rationale cannot by itself resolve this dispute. Still, it may help make it clearer what might be needed to do so, given the source of conflict.

Does OSHA protect too much? The answer depends on other moral judgments we make about the justice and fairness of choices open to workers in certain hazard pay markets. My belief is that such stringent regulation is appropriate in our society, and this conclusion has definite implications for the acceptability of the fair equality of opportunity account. Specifically, it shows us how to define the *limits* on the fair equality of opportunity account set by liberty-regarding principles of justice. Stringent regulations of the sort OSHA *in theory* is mandated to provide will be required by my account of just health care wherever there is reason to think consent is an inappropriate mechanism for the distribution of risk since the consent is quasi-coerced or may become so over time. Where we can assume quasi-coercion will not arise, the fair equality of opportunity account will only justify less-stringent forms of health hazard regulation.

This conclusion about how to reconcile the demand for equality central to the fair equality of opportunity approach with a concern for liberty may not generalize directly to other contexts. I already noted that less-stringent preventive measures may be in order in the case of lifestyle choices since these are not in general quasi-coerced. The stringent preventive measures the fair equality of opportunity account endorses in other preventive contexts, e.g., environmental protection, may not face the same libertarian objections. The risks in these contexts are in general not ones we consent to. But one can imagine increased efforts to put decisions about issues of the stringency of environmental protection to public referenda, seeking thereby some form of consent to risk. The recent effort by the U.S. Environmental Protection Agency to seek a community vote on how stringently arsenic emissions should be regulated at a Tacoma, Washington, smelter can be viewed as an effort to obtain consent to risk. I am not sure how to extend the account I have given, based on the notion of quasi-coercion, to these contexts. Still, I think the approach I adopt illustrates the kind of analysis we need if we are to reconcile demands for equality with distribution mechanisms that rely on consent to risk. I have addressed the issue in one well-defined, illustrative context, but I cannot explore all of its variations.

Notes

1. OSHA Act of 1970, Pub. L. No. 91–596, 84 Stat. 1590, codified at 27 USS pp. 651–678 (1976).

2. Gewirth, A. 1980. Human rights and the prevention of cancer. *American Philosophical Quarterly* 17:117–125.

3. Mark McCarthy makes these and other objections. McCarthy, M. 1981–1982. A review of some normative and conceptual issues in occupational safety and health. *Boston College Environmental Affairs Law Review* 9:4:773–814.

4. Fried, C. 1969. *An Anatomy of Values.* Cambridge, MA: Harvard University Press.

5. See also Nozick, R. 1974. *Anarchy, State, and Utopia.* New York: Basic Books, Chapter 4; and Rabinowitz, J. 1977. Emergent problems and optimal solutions. *Arizona Law Review* 9:1:61–158.

6. Berman, D. 1978. *Death on the Job.* New York: Monthly Review Press.

7. Dworkin, G. 1972. Paternalism. *The Monist* 56(January 1972):64–84.

8. Brandt, R. 1979. *A Theory of the Good and the Right.* Oxford University Press, citing 110ff.

9. Wikler, D. 1978. Persuasion and coercion for health: issues in governmental efforts to change life style. *Milbank Memorial Fund Quarterly: Health and Society* 56:303–338, citing 317ff.

10. Guttmacher, S. 1979. Whole in body, mind and spirit: holistic health and the limits of medicine. *Hastings Center Report* 9:2:15–21.

11. See Ashford, N. 1976. *Crisis in the Workplace: Occupational Disease and Injury,* chap. 7. Cambridge, MA: MIT Press.

12. See Kahneman, D., and Tversky, A. 1981. The framing of decisions and the psychology of choice. *Science* 211:453–458.

13. McCarthy, M. 1981–1982. A review of some normative and conceptual issues in occupational safety and health. *Boston College Environmental Affairs Law Review* 9:4:773–814, citing pp. 779–780.

14. McCarthy, M. 1981–1982. A review of some normative and conceptual issues in occupational safety and health. *Boston College Environmental Affairs Law Review* 9:4:773–814, citing p. 780; Ashford, N. 1976. *Crisis in the Workplace: Occupational Disease and Injury,* chap. 7. Cambridge, MA: MIT Press, citing pp. 333–336.

15. Nozick, R. 1969. Coercion. In S. Morgenbesser, P. Suppes, and M. White (eds.), *Philosophy, Science, and Method*, pp. 440–472. New York: St. Martin's Press.

16. Cf. Rawls, J. 1977. The basic structure as subject. *American Philosophical Quarterly* 14:2:159–165; Nozick, R. 1974. *Anarchy, State, and Utopia.* New York: Basic Books, pp. 204–213.

17. See Daniels, N. 1979. Wide reflective equilibrium and theory acceptance in ethics. *Journal of Philosophy* 76:5:256–282.

Further Reading

Applegate, J., "The Precautionary Preference: An American Perspective on the Precautionary Principle," *Human and Ecological Risk Assessment* 6(3): 2002, 413–443.

Bayer, Ronald, "Coal, Lead, Asbestos, and HIV," *Journal of Occupational Medicine* 35(9): September 1993, 897–901.

Bayer, Ronald, "Workers' Liberty, Workers' Welfare: The Supreme Court Speaks on the Rights of Disabled Employees," *American Journal of Public Health* 93(4): April 2003, 540–544.

Daniels, Cynthia R., "From Protecting the Woman to Privileging the Fetus: The Case of Johnson Controls," in Cynthia R. Daniels, *At Women's Expense: State Power and the Politics of Fetal Rights* (pp. 57–95). (Cambridge, MA: Harvard University Press, 1993).

Hardin, Garrett, "The Tragedy of the Commons," *Science* 162(3859): 13 December 1968, 1243–1248.

Sunstein, Cass R., *Risk and Reason* (Cambridge: Cambridge University Press, 2002).

PART VI

GENETICS AND PUBLIC HEALTH

Introduction

At the end of the 1990s, it was alleged that advances in genetics would revolutionize medicine and health care. Some now think that this claim may have been exaggerated, at least in the prevention of common diseases.[1] Nevertheless, it seems clear that the international Human Genome Project, which completed the sequencing of the human genome in 2003, has already had and will continue to have profound effects on both medicine and public health. Already, genomic approaches have been used to assess prognosis and guide therapy in the treatment of breast cancer, to predict the risk of heart attacks, to determine drug resistance, to design new drug therapies, and to improve our understanding of the role of specific genes in the causation of common conditions such as obesity.[2] In part VI, we explore the role of genetics in public health.

Not all genetic uses of information are new. Screening for genetic disease, the topic of chapter 22 by Scott Burris and Lawrence O. Gostin, has a relatively long history. For example, the screening of newborns to identify metabolic disorders, such as phenylketonuria (PKU), started in the 1960s. Today, every state screens the blood phenylalanine level of all babies a few days after birth. Although the disorder is rare, affecting only one in 10,000 to 20,000 births, the benefits to those in whom the disease is detected are very great, as the severe mental retardation caused by the condition can be prevented with a very restrictive diet.

Another kind of screening is done to identify carriers, that is, those who will not develop a disease but who could pass it to their offspring. In the 1970s, carrier screening programs were instituted to test adults in specific at-risk populations for recessive genetic diseases such as Tay-Sachs, sickle cell anemia, and the thalassemias. A third type of genetic screening, instituted in the 1980s, soon became a routine part of

351

prenatal care: the screening of pregnant women at risk for having babies with genetic or chromosomal abnormalities, such as Down syndrome or spina bifida. Today, many pregnant women who do not have risk factors, such as age, ethnicity, or family history, choose genetic testing to avoid the risk of delivering an affected child.

As we learn more about the genetic contribution to disease, the number of genetic tests will rapidly increase. This raises a number of questions for public health practice. What are the criteria for determining when population screening is warranted? Which tests should be offered and to whom? Should testing be voluntary or mandatory? Emphasizing the differences between medicine and public health, Burris and Gostin offer three principles by which to judge the ethical acceptability of a screening program from a public health perspective. These three principles derive from (1) public health's focus on populations, rather than individuals, (2) the fact of limited resources, and (3) the importance of justice to the mission of public health.

According to Burris and Gostin, whereas *medical genetics* "concerns the clinical decision made by a doctor to use genetic technology for the benefit of his or her patient," *public health genetics* is "the systematic application of human genetic technologies to identify, prevent, or ameliorate genetic conditions in whole populations." The distinction is key because a genetic test that may provide benefit to an individual may not improve the health of the whole population or even specific groups within a population. For example, it may make sense to test a woman with a family history of breast cancer for the BRCA1 gene because women who have the BRCA1 mutation have a 50 to 85 percent risk of developing breast cancer by age 70. (By comparison, the risk for any American woman of developing breast cancer in her lifetime is about 1 in 8.) Moreover, testing may be beneficial for the woman, who may be able to protect herself by having more frequent mammograms or may even choose prophylactic surgery. However, this logic does not extend to screening all women for BRCA1 or even a subgroup such as Ashkenazi Jewish women. (Over 2 percent of Ashkenazi Jews carry mutations in BRCA1 or BRCA2 that confer increased risks of breast, ovarian, and prostate cancer.) This is because only 5 to 10 percent of breast cancer is due to genetic, as opposed to environmental, factors. A large-scale screening program would not have the kind of benefits needed to justify it from a public health perspective and might have significant risks of stigmatization and discrimination.

An example of a well-meaning but ultimately disastrous screening program involved sickle cell in the 1960s and 1970s. Several states mandated screening African Americans for the disease. This had two unfortunate effects. The first was an increase in acts of discrimination by government, insurers, and employers against persons afflicted with the disease, as well as against persons who were merely carriers of the traits.[3] The second was a tendency to regard sickle cell as a "black disease." In fact, sickle cell is not limited to people with ancestors from Africa, but also has an appreciably high prevalence in Mediterranean regions. All states now screen all newborns, regardless of race or ethnicity, for sickle cell disease, in part because of the difficulty in determining the race of newborns. Part of the rationale for universal screening is that early diagnosis and treatment, particularly penicillin prophylaxis, can dramatically reduce mortality.

Burris and Gostin also stress the importance of social justice in determining the acceptability of population screening. They note that the limitation of resources makes public health "as inherently political—i.e., concerned with the allocation of resources in society—as it is technological—concerned with the deployment of professional knowledge of illness." Choices about where to allocate resources reflect—and sometimes reinforce—existing distributions of wealth and influence. Thus, Burris and Gostin point out that decisions about how to spend health care dollars cannot be simply a matter of benefiting the greatest number of people: "Spending money to address the leading killers of the population as a whole may exclude expenditures on the leading killers of subgroups in the population." Because vulnerability to disease and injury is at least in part a result of inequitable social institutions, justice requires that health care dollars are spent to redress inequities. "To the extent that disease is a social product, public health ought to act as a conscience."

Public health is political in another, more regrettable, sense, as well. Sometimes screening programs are instituted as the result of political pressure rather than being based on scientific evidence. The example of PKU screening is instructive. Although it has clear benefits, it also has some dangers, including the risk of false positives, that is, incorrectly identifying some babies as having PKU when they were not in fact at risk for mental retardation. Moreover, since the severely restrictive PKU diet can itself cause brain damage, instituting a mass screening program caused some children who would have been of normal intelligence to become retarded. Norman Fost argues that the rush to institute mass PKU screening was the product of a "PKU lobby" composed of well-meaning and passionate advocates for the retarded. "The normal scientific caution that accompanies new tests and treatments was brushed aside, and critics were either dismissed as obstacles in the campaign or their skepticism was suppressed."[4]

Some would argue that disease not only is a social product but also, to some extent, a social construction. That is, what we perceive as a disease or disabling condition depends on the society in which it occurs. For example, hereditary deafness was fairly common on Martha's Vineyard, which meant that even hearing members of the community learned to sign. Deafness in that society was not perceived as a disability but rather as a fairly insignificant difference among people. From this perspective, the problems people with disabilities face stem not from the disability itself, but from the failure of society to provide the accommodations they need. According to Adrienne Asch, a proponent of disability rights who has been blind since infancy, a public health approach should not be focused on genetic testing or screening to prevent the births of children who will have disabilities but rather on changing social arrangements so that all children, whatever their abilities, can reach their full potential.[5]

The idea that disease is a social product—a notion essential to a public health perspective—seems at odds with the idea that genes play a significant role in disease since the genes one has are a matter of biology, not social forces. Many in public health are decidedly wary of research that emphasizes the genetic role in disease and health. They worry about the "geneticization" of disease: the overemphasis on genetic factors to the exclusion of social causes. At the same time, it is becoming increasingly clear that there is a genetic component to most diseases, including cancer, mental illness, and susceptibility to infection. The challenge is to understand the complex interaction between genetic and environmental causes of disease. A recognition of these components can be part of public health research and practice. Moreover, human genetics and public health sciences share certain essential perspectives: a focus on populations, interest in variation, and recognition of the importance of social context.[6] "In the end, public health sciences are the tools for understanding gene-environment interactions at the core of nearly all human diseases."[7]

This brings us to the second selection, by Richard R. Sharp and J. Carl Barrett, which discusses the Environmental Genome Project (EGP). Begun in 1998 by the National Institute of Environmental Health Sciences, it was intended to identify and study a number of common genetic variants that appear to play an important role in environmentally associated diseases. The hope was that a better understanding of genetic influences on environmental response would lead to more accurate estimates of the prospects of disease, as well as early intervention programs aimed at individuals and populations at increased risk. While the EGP has the potential to improve human health by improving our understanding of gene-environment interactions, it raises a number of complex social, moral, and legal issues, including the protection of human subjects, the privacy of genetic information, and the possibility of discriminatory uses of the data generated by the project.

A discussion of the role of genetics in health can move quickly to a discussion of race since race is partly a matter of genetic variation. How, if ever, should race be used in public health practice and research? The answer given by Ellen Wright Clayton in the third selection is, "Very carefully." She begins by discussing the complexities of racial identity, which is shaped in part by genes, but also by social, historical, cultural, and political factors. This means that there is no one-to-one correspondence between genetic variation and race, which makes using race as a predictor for health outcomes problematic. In addition, there are social dangers in categorizing people by race, as the long, sad history of racism and eugenics makes clear. Should public health officials and researchers simply ignore correlations between race and susceptibility to disease? Clayton maintains that, in general, using race in public health practice and research creates more intractable problems than ignoring race. For example, all states now test all newborns for sickle cell disease rather than targeting screening at African American newborns, in part because it is difficult to determine with precision a baby's ethnicity at birth, in part because sickle cell disease is not exclusively an African American disease.

In the last selection, Pamela Sankar and others warn against an overemphasis on genetics. They do not deny that genetics has enhanced our understanding of disease processes in individuals. But they are skeptical that genomic medicine will do much to accomplish the public health goal of alleviating pervasive health disparities that fall along racial, as well as economic, lines. Moreover, an overemphasis on genetics could have several undesirable results: diverting attention from social class and environmental contributions to health disparities and reinforcing racial stereotyping.

Notes

1. Holtzman, N. A., and Marteau, T. M., "Will Genetics Revolutionize Medicine?" *New England Journal of Medicine* 343: 2000, 141–144.

2. Guttmacher, A. E., and Collins, F. S., "Welcome to the Genomic Era," *New England Journal of Medicine* 349(10): 2003, 996–998.

3. Markel, H., "The Stigma of Disease: Implications of Genetic Screening," *American Journal of Medicine* 93: 1992, 209–215.

4. Fost, N., "Ethical Implications of Screening Asymptomatic Individuals," *FASEB Journal* 6: 1992, 2813–2817.

5. Asch, A. "Prenatal Diagnosis and Selective Abortion: A Challenge to Practice and Policy." *American Journal of Public Health* 89(11): 1999, 1649–1657.

6. Omenn, G., "The Crucial Role of the Public Health Sciences in the Postgenomic Era," *Genetics in Medicine* 4(suppl): 2002, 21S–26S.

7. Gwinn, M., and Khoury, M. J., "Research Priorities for Public Health Sciences in the Postgenomic Era," *Genetics in Medicine* 4(6): 2002, 410–411.

22

Genetic Screening from a Public Health Perspective

Three "Ethical" Principles

Scott Burris and
Lawrence O. Gostin

Introduction

The disciplines of medicine and public health are different in their goals and practices,[1] and this difference is centrally important in the context of human genetics. Medical genetics concerns the clinical decision made by a doctor to use genetic technology for the benefit of his or her patient. Public health genetics, on the other hand, may be defined as the systematic application of human genetic technologies to identify, prevent, or ameliorate genetic conditions in whole populations. Genetic testing, then, involves the decision to test an individual patient, while genetic screening involves a decision to systematically test a discrete population.[2]

The ethical and policy implications are quite different depending on whether genetics is applied in the medical or the public health context. From a public health perspective, the benefits of testing are assessed against different criteria, and the line between providing care to the individual patient and providing it to the population represents a dramatic investment of scarce resources, both political and economic. Medical ethics, which can guide the clinical decisions of health care providers, do not adequately address the distributional issues and health-health trade-offs[3] that arise in public health decision making. In this chapter, we discuss the emerging idea of *public health ethics* and set out three principles, rooted in public health, for deciding whether a genetic test should be deployed in a program of population screening.[4]

Public Health Ethics

The language of medical ethics "has been developed in a context of individual relationships, and is well adapted to the nature, practice, settings, and expectations of medical care."[5] It does not provide a vocabulary and analytical framework for addressing the fundamental social causes of disease that must be addressed to provide "the conditions in which people can be healthy"[6] nor the deep social divisions that a recognition of the social roots of disease reveals.[7] An ethics for public health remains, to be written, and such a task is beyond our reach in this chapter. We can, however, make a small contribution in the form of a definition of public health that captures the essential moral choices that public health requires.

We define *public health* as *the process of maximizing, within the bounds of possibility set by the resources allocated, the level and distribution of satisfactory health in a population.* This definition stresses several foundational points. First, public health is devoted to the health of populations, not individuals. Geoffrey Rose has brilliantly described the practical implications of this difference for disease prevention, including the "prevention paradox" that the measures that will most improve the health of a population may also have negligible benefits for particular individuals, and vice versa.[8] Second, public health operates in a world of choices in the allocation of limited resources. The great sanitarian Herman Biggs famously remarked that "public health is purchasable," but because there will always be limits on how much we are willing to buy, public health will always turn on allocational decisions. Thus public health is as inherently political—i.e., concerned with the allocation of resources in society—as it is technological—concerned with the deployment of professional knowledge of illness. Finally, while the principle of maximization suggests that measures should be compared for their costs and benefits, imposing a strong utilitarian element to the analysis, it is not necessary to see an ethics of public health as a purely utilitarian exercise. It has its consequentialist side to be sure, but our definition offers the possibility of a deontological claim based on the intrinsic value of a fair distribution of reasonable health and equitable access to the conditions in which it is possible to achieve it.[9]

The Public Health Interest in Genetic Screening: Three Principles

In the absence of a developed ethics of public health, we offer three principles[10] that follow from a definition emphasizing the population, the struggle for resources, and the importance of an equitable distribution of health.

Principle 1: Screening Should Enhance the Health of the Population

Much of the impetus for using genetic testing has and will continue to come from the health care sector, so it is well to keep in mind that public health and health care aspire to complementary but meaningfully different ends. Public health aims to improve the health of the group, as measured by aggregate outcomes. Medicine aims to improve the health of the individual, as measured largely by improvements in quality of life and the individual's satisfaction with her own outcome. Any number of differences follow from this basic distinction, among which are: population health depends more on the causes of incidence of disease in populations than the causes of illness in individuals, and, from the population standpoint, it is the distribution of cases, rather than the accidental fate of any particular person, that matters. Individual risk factors, which seem to explain why certain people get sick, do not tend to explain why certain ills are prevalent in certain populations. Thus genetic differences may help explain why people exposed to the same environmental cofactors differ in their health, but the environmental factors provide the chief explanation of health differences between populations living in different environments. Because health risks that are constituted in a population are different than those expressed in individuals, even a very powerful individual risk factor may not constitute a public health priority if the prevalence of the marker is low, or if there exists no cost-effective intervention from a population-based perspective.[11] The discovery of the relationship between the BRCA1 trait and breast cancer provides an illustration of a genetic technology that may have beneficial application for an individual but perhaps not for whole populations. As Lerman and Croyle observe, "much of breast cancer is not caused by inherited susceptibility at all, but results from somatic events that produce genetic changes in a woman's breast cells during her lifetime. Moreover, the majority of women who develop breast cancer have no known major risk factors."[12] Even if we can fully prevent breast cancer among women with the BRCA1 trait, breast cancer will continue to be a significant burden on the health of the population.

To find a genetic screening measure "ethical" in the public health sense, then, we need to determine that it has a reasonable probability of leading to information that can be used to reduce the incidence of genetic illness or mortality in the society as a whole or in a significant population facing a special threat. If it does not, the measure, however useful to individuals, ought not be an important public health priority and may not be worthy of significant public sector resources.

A genetic intervention that benefits individual patients may actually be harmful from a population perspective. Health and disease being to a considerable extent socially constructed,[13] a new technology providing new forms of information about health and disease can have dramatic effects on how these concepts are understood in society. A widespread belief that health is "in the genes" could further attenuate popular understanding of behavioral and environmental factors influencing health, making it harder to win support for and compliance with public health interventions. Nor can we blithely ignore the risks that the genetic information so desirable to individuals may support the revival of eugenic ideas and policies in new guises.[14] Susan Wolf has warned of the rise of what she calls "geneticism," which, "like racism and sexism, . . . is a long-standing and deeply entrenched system for disadvantaging some and advantaging others" based on their genetic traits.[15]

*Principle 2: The Measure Should Be an Efficient
and Just Use of Resources*

While it is ethically problematic for many doctors, rationing in public health is a "moral imperative . . . in the face of scarce resources."[16] Ideally, each public health dollar will be spent to achieve the greatest marginal increase in the level and distribution of well-being in the population. Although the problems of comparing incommensurate values quickly bursts any illusions about the objectivity or mechanical quality of this analysis, this principle is nevertheless a useful reminder to build water pipes and sewers before cholera wards and to bear in mind the relative costs and benefits of oral rehydration kits and heart transplants. The high cost of health care accentuates the resource problem. Often doctors can do things for individual patients that are clearly miraculous, yet which not only do not add measurably to the level and distribution of good health in the population, and whose cost may drive out non-medical forms of prevention.[17]

Screening programs often illustrate the significance of marginal cost in public health planning. There is an impulse in medicine to routinize the use of a test or treatment that seems to work for the individual, an impulse that is often quicker off the mark than the validation of the measure's efficacy on a large scale.[18] Making a useful test routine sometimes carries with it in turn the impulse to make it "mandatory." Yet, apart from the difficulties of enforcing compliance, which we will discuss next, the move to routine or mandatory testing makes a more fundamentally faulty assumption: that the cost-benefit ratio of reaching hard-to-find or resistant targets is comparable to that of reaching the compliant and eager. Indeed, where a test offers useful relative risk information or even therapeutic options to the patient, one might most logically start with the assumption that the majority of people at risk will accept the test without any intervention from public health authorities at all.

Both the efficiency and fairness of a public health intervention should be evaluated in more than just monetary terms. It must be recognized that genetic conditions will be experienced by individuals within a web of social relations.[19] We frequently discuss the social implications of having a disfavored trait in terms of stigma, but there is far more to the social risk of a genetic illness or predisposition to genetic illness than the psychosocial experience of a "spoiled identity."[20] Social risk in health may be defined as "the danger that an individual will be socially or economically penalized should she become identified with an expensive, disfavored or feared medical condition."[21] So defined, social risk has two distinct components, each of which imposes its own costs on a health measure: (1) "the threat," i.e., attitudes and behavior that cause or threaten social harm; and (2) "the perception of risk," i.e., the attitudes and beliefs about the threat among those who are in some way tied to the trait or disease. Social risk in these terms is a complex phenomenon, or, better, a constellation of phenomena, that will vary with the type of condition, other traits of the person who has it (such as socioeconomic status, race, gender), and the culture of the relationships in which the trait arises.

Again the experience of HIV is instructive: People at risk of HIV have resisted testing for social reasons, it seems, not because of some clear-cut fears about privacy and discrimination as such, but rather a complicated mix of anxieties tied to racism, homophobia, and alienation from authority. The same may be said for genetic carrier traits, genetic markers (predispositions to disease), and genetic illness. A person's genetic composition has an intimate character that says a great deal about her individuality, her family, and her ethnic community. This deep personal meaning suggests that individual behavior may change when faced with decisions to acquire and use genetic information. Social risk, then, includes fears about societal perception of *self:* What discrete or complex illness do I have or might I acquire in the future? What personality characteristics may be revealed, ranging from shyness or risk taking to aggression or criminal propensities? Social risk may also involve concerns about family: What does this genetic characteristic mean for my parent, sibling, or child? Finally, social risk may involve concerns about my community: What does the incidence of this genetic characteristic (e.g., Tay-Sachs or sickle cell) mean for my religious or ethnic group?

The notion that legal protection can palliate perceptions of social risk is especially problematic, given that for many people social risk comes from the law, or that their experiences with the legal system have not been positive.[22] True justice requires that the perspective of the test subject, in all its complexity, be included in the analyses of the costs and benefits of the measure.

The morality of public health's utilitarianism is rooted in the imperative to improve the distribution as well as the level of health. Were there truly a mechanical formula for achieving the greatest good for the greatest number, ethics would be largely self-executing, for the marginal gains of measures helping a large number of needy would almost always be greater than the benefits of helping the fortunate few.[23] In fact, however, nothing could be more complicated and controversial than deciding who is needy and should get what help. In a politicized world of scarcity, there is a constant danger that health expenditures will reflect existing distributions of wealth and influence. Ill-health follows and reflects social disadvantage; social differences create different health problems.[24] Spending money to address the leading killers of the population as a whole may exclude expenditures on the leading killers of subgroups in the population. Though cancer is the leading cause of death in the population as a whole, spending to find its genetic causes must be seen in light of such facts as the proportion of cancers affected by genetics, the harm of accidents, and the toll of violence on young black men.[25] We believe that a just health policy requires recognition of the pernicious synergies of socioeconomic disadvantage and of the problematic nature of existing social entitlements. To the extent that disease is a social product, public health ought to act as a conscience.[26]

Principle 3: The Measure Should Be as Acceptable as Possible to Its Targets

This principle has roots in both practicality and morality. Public health depends largely on voluntary compliance with its guidelines. This is equally true of "voluntary" advice, like wearing a bicycle helmet, and of "mandatory" rules, like wearing seat belts. Resistance can raise costs enormously, the more as prevalence of the condition rises. It has proven possible, with a fair amount of money and talent, to impose directly observed therapy on a few hundred recalcitrant TB patients in a few major cities;[27] it is unlikely ever to have been feasible to isolate and monitor the sex lives of tens of thousands of people with HIV. Even most "mandatory" measures are either largely voluntary in effect (e.g., premarital screening) or are so broadly acceptable that they are not resisted (like PKU [phenylketonuria] screening of newborns). The success of a public health intervention, and its cost, therefore depend significantly on the degree to which its targets perceive it to be more beneficial than costly.

Resistance to health measures is rarely as irrational as it might seem to the paternalistic professional observer. A measure that leads to immediate and short-term health benefits for targeted individuals is obviously more desirable than one that does not; there is the difference between screening for ALS [amyotrophic lateral sclerosis] and screening for PKU. Monetary or other incentives may increase the benefits of compliance, as is sometimes done with DOT [directly observed therapy]. The costs of compliance are often in something like inverse proportion to the treatability of the condition: The less we can do for a trait, the more social costs screening is likely to entail. Being marked as having a dangerous, untreatable condition may be costly in psychological terms and may expose the subject to social risk. These sorts of costs may be addressed to some extent through counseling and the legal protection of social status, but this is difficult and problematic in its own way.[28] In moral terms, this principle emphasizes the fairness of allocating both the benefits and burdens of a disease that threatens public health on the public generally, rather than primarily on the shoulders of those who have the illness.

In the HIV epidemic, resistance to public health rules has taken on a perhaps unprecedented but now widely followed political dimension. Legal and advocacy organizations, capable of generating grassroots action and of effectively lobbying and litigating, have demonstrated their capacity to influence the development of public health policy.[29] In many respects this has proven a boon to public health, facilitating the social negotiation necessary to design broadly acceptable measures. It has also, however, added even more complexity to the rich symbolic politics of health and disease. Thus a final caution under the heading of the principle of acceptability is that measures may not always be judged for their intrinsic merits, or even their objective likelihood of causing harm to the target population. HIV reporting in the United States typifies a measure that has in many places been strongly opposed by advocates, despite the excellent record of health departments in protecting the confidentiality of their records.[30] In this instance, the fear of what government might someday do with an "AIDS list" outweighs health departments' excellent track record.[31] The same, of course, can be said about genetics, where the public has strong beliefs, and some irrational fears, about the application of genetic technologies to human populations. The principle of acceptability thus becomes a good heuristic for analyzing and responding to a health measure's social meaning.

Discussion

Putting aside the assumption that widespread collection of genetic data is both desirable and inevitable sets a very different genetic agenda for public health law. As a preliminary matter, we are required to ask, what are the criteria that need to be satisfied to justify a particular genetic intervention in public health terms, and to what extent have they been satisfied? It is well beyond the purpose of this chapter to apply the principles we offer to any particular genetic screening initiative. Nevertheless, a general overview of genetic screening shows the need for caution in designing large-scale screening programs in the name of improving the public's health. Genetic illness is an important threat to public health. Historically, genetic disease has been seen as both a major source of ill-health and premature mortality, and as largely intractable.[32] With its significant impact on both the population as a whole and on distinct subpopulations, genetic illness is obviously an important challenge to public health.[33]

Some level of pure research would surely be a wise and just use of resources for population health, provided always that information about the impact of genetic factors on health is integrated into a broader examination of the determinants of health.[34] There is good historical evidence that the facts of the germ theory had a greater impact on the decline in mortality in the United States in the past century than did the medical interventions derived from them.[35] Research may help identify important cofactors for illness in the environment or help provide behavioral guidance. Likewise, epidemiological research, including formal surveillance, is justified precisely because of the difficulty of assessing the potential of genetic knowledge on public health.[36] Public health data collection is a prerequisite for according genetic illness greater public health priority.

The value of screening individuals in medical care depends from a public health point of view on factors like the extent and severity of the condition in the population, the cost of detecting it, and the availability of some intervention to cure or prevent the expression of the condition. In those relatively few instances in which the identification of a genetic trait leads to effective, life-sustaining therapy at a reasonable cost—PKU for instance—screening evidently has real public health value. And, of course, as more is known about human genetics, science is likely to offer more effective means to prevent and treat genetic illness. More controversial but comparably effective at the population level is prenatal screening to which the preventive response is contraception or abortion, raising the specter of eugenics. CVS [chorionic villus sampling] and amniocentesis, for instance, have led to a substantial reduction in the prevalence of Down syndrome at birth, but possibly at the cost of further stigmatizing those children who are born with the condition. To the extent one regards preventing the birth of children with Down syndrome to be desirable, there are now racial and ethnic differences in prevalence that may reflect unequal access to prenatal diagnostic services.[37] As the complexity and cost of the response increases— as might happen in the area of prenatal surgery—the eugenic issues, the public health cost-benefit ratio, and the problem of access, all increase.

The most problematic use of genetic screening, from both the medical and the public health standpoint, is where there is little or nothing to be done to prevent an illness or intergenerational transmission of illness. Genetic screening is also problematic where the genetic factor is but one contributor to a higher relative risk of an illness that depends also on unknown individual or environmental cofactors. The psychological value of knowing about something one cannot alter may be positive or negative for the individual,[38] and likewise may make for a net increase or decrease in the sum total of public well-being. Stigma and stress add to the social costs of screening for risk factors, as does an increase in the prevalence of that most modern of ills, being "at risk." In the case of illnesses that have behavioral cofactors, there has been some support for the proposition that personalized relative risk information can enhance the chances of behavior change, but the impact may be slight and short term, and in any event must be placed in the context of the difficulties of behavior change overall.[39] In a larger sense, genetic screening threatens to be a readily commodifiable, culturally powerful approach to dealing with disease that will further complicate the discovery and alteration of the pathogenic elements of the ecology. Clarke argues that "the focus on genetic factors may distract attention from 'the real challenge of the future which appears to be the behavioral and social issues of risk reduction.'"[40]

Although the potential costs of genetic screening are high, they are not uniformly distributed across all uses of the technology. Genetic databases collected by the government, or under its auspices, for research purposes can be reliably protected, even in a largely electronic records environment, because there is no need to allow access for medical care or payment purposes. Such programs could move as much as possible to blinded collection or storage and can maintain rigid barriers to access without significantly burdening bona fide research.

The acceptability of genetic screening is also likely to be very diverse, reflecting the variety of social and medical impact genetic information can have, and the varying degrees to which various populations have access to those benefits and confidence in legal protection of social status. There is likely to be a fair amount of resistance on the general ground of state intrusion into privacy, including spillover from efforts to gather and use genetic information for identification and law-enforcement purposes.[41] Markers of serious future or inheritable diseases are likely to be socially risky to some degree, particularly to the extent they are used by insurers and employers to avoid health care costs. As genetic factors have more and more influence on individual social status, we can expect more principled resistance to screening. The popularity of prenatal screening, for example, is giving rise to concerns about the perceived value of disabled lives.[42] More broadly, much will depend upon the degree to which the benefits of genetic knowledge are distributed in the population: If genetic technology leads to improvements in health care, its practical value will depend upon the population's actual access to the care; if it identifies environmental pathologies, its value will depend on the degree to which society is prepared to alter how it produces, distributes, and consumes.[43]

Conclusion

The use of genetic screening for public health purposes will tend to be most effective when it serves a clear population goal, has a healthy ratio of overall economic and social benefits to costs, entails a just use of resources, and is acceptable to the populations it targets. We recognize that the public health agenda is never written by fully autonomous, fully informed rational actors on a clean slate.[44] Yet precisely because public health policy is so heavily influenced by social and political factors, it is important to seize the opportunity for reflection before the time for action arrives and to at least aspire to rationality in the heat of action.

Notes

1. Jonathan M. Mann, "Medicine and public health, ethics and human rights" *Hastings Center Report* May–June 1997, at 6.

2. Centers for Disease Control and Prevention. *Translating Advances in Human Genetics into Public Health Action: A Strategic Plan* (1997).

3. Cass R. Sunstein, "Health-health tradeoffs" 63 *University of Chicago Law Review* 1533 (1996).

4. Scott Burris and Lawrence O. Gostin, "Genetic screening from a public health perspective: some lessons from the HIV experience" in *Genetic Secrets: Protecting Privacy and Confidentiality in the Genetic Era* (New Haven, CT: Yale University Press) 137, 139 (Mark Rothstein ed. 1997).

5. Mann, at 8.

6. Institute of Medicine, National Academy of Sciences, *The Future of Public Health* (Washington, DC: National Academy Press), 38–40 (1988).

7. Scott Burris, "The invisibility of public health: population-level measures in a politics of market individualism" 87 *American Journal of Public Health* 1607 (1997).

8. Geoffrey Rose, "Sick individuals and sick populations" 14 *International Journal of Epidemiology* 32 (1985).

9. C. L. Soskolne, "Rationalizing professional conduct: ethics in disease control." 19 *Public Health Review* 311–321 (1991–92).

10. In this we follow the model of Brandt and colleagues. *See* Allan M. Brandt, Paul D. Cleary, and Lawrence O. Gostin, "Routine hospital testing for HIV: health policy considerations" in *AIDS and the Health Care System* (New Haven, CT: Yale University Press) (Lawrence O. Gostin ed. 1990).

11. For discussions of the differences between medicine and public health goals, upon which we have relied, see generally Rose; Mann; Bernard Lo, "Ethical dilemmas in HIV infection: what have we learned?" 20 *Law, Medicine & Health Care* 92 (1992); Mary Northridge, "Public health methods: attributable risk as a link between causality and public health action" 85 *American Journal of Public Health* 1202 (1995); Ralph L. Keeney, "Decisions about life-threatening risks" 331 *New England Journal of Medicine* 193 (1994).

12. Caryn Lerman and Robert Croyle, "Psychological issues in genetic testing for breast cancer susceptibility" 154 *Archives of Internal Medicine* 609 (1994).

13. Allan Brandt, *No Magic Bullet: A Social History of Venereal Disease in the United States Since 1880* (New York: Oxford University Press, 1987).

14. David H. Stone and Susie Stewart, "Screening and the new genetics; a public health perspective on the ethical debate" 18 *Journal of Public Health and Medicine* 3 (1996); P. Harper, "Genetics and public health" 304 *British Medical Journal* 721 (1992).

15. Susan Wolf, "Beyond 'genetic discrimination': toward the broader harm of geneticism" 23 *Journal of Law, Medicine, and Ethics* 345, 349 (1995).

16. Richard H. Morrow and John H. Bryant, "Health policy approaches to measuring

and valuing human life: conceptual and ethical issues" 85 *American Journal of Public Health* 1356 (1995).

17. See, e.g., Robert M. Kliegman, "Neonatal technology, perinatal survival, social consequences, and the perinatal paradox" 85 *American Journal of Public Health* 909 (1995).

18. For a recent example, see Dermot MacDonald, "Cerebral palsy and intrapartum fetal monitoring" 334 *New England Journal of Medicine* 659 (1996); Karin B. Nelson, et al., "Uncertain value of electronic fetal monitoring in predicting cerebral palsy" 334 *New England Journal of Medicine* 613 (1996).

19. Jerome Bruner, *Acts of Meaning* (1990).

20. Erving Goffman, *Stigma: Notes on the Management of Spoiled Identity* (Harmondsworth, U.K.: Penguin, 1963).

21. Scott Burris, "Law and the social risk of health care: lessons from HIV testing" 61 *Albany Law Review* 831 (1998).

22. Scott Burris, "Driving the epidemic underground? A new look at law and the social risk of HIV testing" 12 *AIDS and Public Policy Journal* 66 (1997).

23. *See, e.g.,*Morrow and Bryant.

24. *See, e.g.,* Paul Sorlies, Eric Backlund, and Jacob Keller, "U.S. mortality by economic, demographic, and social characteristics: the National Longitudinal Mortality Study" 85 *American Journal of Public Health* 949 (1995); David Blane, editorial: "Social determinants of health—socioeconomic status, social class, and ethnicity" 85 *American Journal of Public Health* 903 (1995); Thomas A. LaVeist, "Segregation, poverty, and empowerment: health consequences for African Americans" 71 *Milbank Quarterly* 41 (1993); George D. Smith and Matthias Egger, "Socioeconomic Differences in Mortality in Britain and the United States" 82 *American Journal of Public Health* 1979 (1992).

25. J. M. McGinnis and William Foege, "Actual causes of death in the United States" 270 *Journal of the American Medical Association* 2207 (1993).

26. See Mervyn Susser, "Health as a human right: an epidemiologist's perspective on public health" 83 *American Journal of Public Health* 416 (1993).

27. *See, e.g.,* Thomas R. Frieden, Paula I. Fujiwara, Rita Washiko, and Margaret A. Hamburg, "Tuberculosis in New York—turning the tide" 333 *New England Journal of Medicine* 229 (1995).

28. Burris.

29. *See, e.g.,* Ronald Bayer, *Private Acts, Social Consequences: AIDS and the Politics of Public Health* (New York: Free Press, 1989); Robert M. Wachter, *The Fragile Coalition: Scientists, Activists and AIDS* (New York: St. Martin's Press, 1991).

30. Lawrence O. Gostin, John W. Ward, and A. Cornelius Baker, "National HIV case reporting for the United States: a defining moment in the history of the epidemic" 337 *New England Journal of Medicine* 1162–1167 (1997).

31. For data on the fears of gay men with regard to data collection, see Karolynn Siegel, Martin P. Levine, Charles Brooks, and Rochelle Kern, "The motives of gay men for taking or not taking the HIV antibody test" 36 *Social Problems* 368 (1989).

32. *See* Thomas McKeown, *The Role of Medicine: Dream, Mirage, or Nemesis* (London: Nuffield Provincial Hospitals Trust, 1980).

33. *See, e.g.,* Centers for Disease Control and Prevention, *Surveillance for and Comparison of Birth Defect Prevalences in Two Geographic Areas—United States, 1983–1988,* 42 MMWR SS-1 (1993); Centers for Disease Control and Prevention: *Surveillance for*

Anencephaly and Spina Bifida and the Impact of Prenatal Diagnosis—United States, 1985–1994, 44 MMWR SS-4 (1995).

34. See Angus Clarke, "Population screening for genetic susceptibility to disease" 311 *British Medical Journal* 35 (1995).

35. See Samuel H. Preston and Michael R. Haines, *Fatal Years: Child Mortality in Late Nineteenth-Century America* (Princeton, NJ: Princeton University Press, 1991).

36. James W. Hanson, "Birth defects surveillance and the future of public health" 110 *Public Health Reports* 698 (1995).

37. CDC, *Down Syndrome Prevalence at Birth – United States 1983–1990,* 43 MMWR 617 (1994).

38. See Sandi Wiggins, et al., "The psychological consequences of predictive testing for Huntington's disease" 327 *New England Journal of Medicine* 1401 (1992); Lerman and Croyle; Paul R. Marantz, "Blaming the victim: the negative consequence of preventive medicine" 80 *American Journal of Public Health* 1186 (1993).

39. See generally Rose.

40. Clarke (quoting R. R. Williams, "Nature, Nurture and Family Predisposition" 318 *New England Journal of Medicine* 769 (1988)).

41. Lawrence O. Gostin, "Genetic privacy" 23 *Journal of Law, Medicine and Ethics* 320–330 (1995).

42. See Lois Shepherd, "Protecting parents' freedom to have children with genetic differences" 1995 *University of Illinois Law Review* 761.

43. Bruce G. Link and Jo Phelan, "Social conditions as fundamental causes of disease" 1995 [extra issue] *Journal of Health and Social Behavior* 80.

44. Geoffrey Vickers, "What sets the goals of public health?" in *Health and the Community: Readings in the Philosophy and Sciences of Public Health* (A. H. Katz and J. S. Felton, eds., New York: Free Press, 1965).

23

The Environmental Genome Project

Ethical, Legal, and Social Implications

Richard R. Sharp and J. Carl Barrett

The National Institute of Environmental Health Sciences recently launched a new research initiative known as the Environmental Genome Project (EGP).[1-3] The EGP will examine how genetic variation affects response to environmental exposures. Initially, the project will identify polymorphic variation in genes that appear to play an important role in environmentally associated diseases. Having identified these genetic polymorphisms, researchers then will examine their functional implications more carefully.[4] These functional studies will be multidisciplinary in approach, incorporating research methodologies from biochemistry, epidemiology, genetics, pharmacology, and toxicology.[5]

Proponents of the EGP hope that the information learned will be instrumental in improving public health.[6] A better understanding of genetic influences on environmental response could lead to more accurate estimates of disease risks and provide a basis for disease prevention and early intervention programs directed at individuals and populations at increased risk.[7] Identifying functionally significant polymorphisms also could shed light on disease pathways and suggest targets for therapeutic intervention.[8,9]

As with all research, these potential benefits must be weighed against possible risks. Following the precedent developed in connection with the Human Genome Project,[10,11] there are plans to support research on the ethical, legal, and social implications of the EGP.[12] By examining these issues, we may be able to anticipate problems before they arise and develop policies that maximize the benefits of the EGP while minimizing its risks.[13]

In this paper, we highlight several ethical, legal, and social issues raised by the EGP. These issues are presented in the order that they likely will present themselves to researchers, beginning with the protection of research participants and concluding with potential long-term implications of environmental genomic research. Our goal in providing this overview is to draw attention to future research needs and encourage others to join us in thinking about these difficult and complex issues.

Current Issues: Protecting Research Participants

The most immediate ethical, legal, and social issues raised by the EGP relate to the protection of individual research participants.[14–16] Genetic studies often present special challenges in protecting human subjects because genetic research frequently poses psychosocial risks that may be difficult to anticipate and convey to prospective participants.[17] These risks can include possible discrimination or stigmatization, disrupted relationships between family members, and adverse effects on a participant's self-image.[18]

The presentation of research-related risks to participants is especially troublesome in connection with the EGP because of the many uncertainties surrounding the study of genetic hypersensitivities to environmental exposures. Studies of gene-environment interactions often do not allow for precise quantification of the respective genetic and environmental contributions to disease.[19] As a result, research findings may be difficult for researchers and participants to interpret. A study may identify a genetic polymorphism that appears to play a role in environmental response, but the extent to which its effects are mediated by environmental factors often will remain unclear. Without more information on an individual's genome and past environmental exposures, the detection of such a polymorphism is of uncertain value in predicting future disease. These uncertainties complicate the process of informed consent, particularly the communication of potential risks and benefits to prospective participants.[20] The inability to quantify the precise extent to which a particular polymorphism increases disease risks also makes it difficult to determine whether research results should be disclosed to participants, and if so, in what manner.[21]

If study results are conveyed to participants, still other complications present themselves.[22] In many genetic studies, specially trained genetic counselors discuss findings with participants. This approach helps minimize potential psychosocial risks. Although genetic counselors could be used to convey results obtained in connection with the EGP, the current shortage of these professionals likely would make this a practical impossibility. Moreover, if many laypersons overestimate the predictive value of genetic information,[23] it may be difficult to present findings on genetic hypersensitivities to environmental exposures in a manner that avoids placing too much emphasis on genetic contributions to disease. It is more likely that information on increased susceptibility to environmentally associated diseases will be viewed fatalistically, prompting some to infer that because they have a genetic predisposition to a disease, they will eventually develop that condition. Such misunderstandings are a concern in presenting study results to individual participants, as well as in presenting research findings more generally.

Other immediate ethical, legal, and social issues relate to the breadth of the consent obtained in connection with EGP studies.[24] Associations between individual alleles and particular environmental exposures are difficult to identify. As a result, researchers are interested in designing studies that look at possible associations between many different allelic variants and many different exposures concurrently. Although such studies increase the likelihood of identifying functionally significant polymorphisms, they complicate the consent process. As more genes and exposures are considered simultaneously, it becomes increasingly difficult to anticipate the potential risks and benefits of the research.[25,26] Hence, it also becomes more difficult to ensure that individual participants are fully informed about the possible risks and benefits of their participation. At the extreme, the worry is that individual consent becomes a blanket permission for genetic research in general.[27] These broad permissions are considered morally problematic because it is unclear how participants could be fully informed about such a wide range of potential research uses.[28]

A related concern is that current policies governing informed consent could place inappropriate restrictions on research in environmental genomics.[29] Although the present standards for informed consent in genetic research may be appropriate for studies of highly predictive alleles, they may be overly demanding for studies of genetic hypersensitivities to environmental exposures, particularly because such studies generally present more limited risks to individual participants. Thus, the challenge facing the EGP is to establish consent procedures that allow individuals to make genuinely informed choices about their participation in studies that examine many different alleles and multiple exposures concurrently. The permissions granted by participants should be broad enough to permit diverse research interests, yet specific enough to allow individual participants to assess the possible risks and benefits of their participation.

Emerging Issues: Protecting Socially Identifiable Groups

Many of the ethical, legal, and social issues surrounding the EGP are familiar to experienced researchers and institutional review boards. Although the EGP complicates these familiar areas of concern, studies of genetic influences on environmental response also introduce other less familiar ethical and social considerations. These concerns will become more prominent as research in environmental genomics expands and information on common genetic hypersensitivities becomes more widely available.

One such issue is the protection of socially identifiable groups, including racial and ethnic populations. Some allelic variants are more common in certain populations and less common in others. As specific genetic polymorphisms are associated with increased susceptibility to environmental exposures, it is likely that some genetic hypersensitivities will be associated with particular social groups.[30] The association of genetic hypersensitivities with race or ethnicity could threaten the employment and insurance opportunities available to entire groups of individuals, not just those who choose to participate in research.[31,32] Members of these populations also could encounter broader forms of discrimination and stigmatization, for example, in child custody disputes or adoption efforts.[33,34] In this regard, the association of Ashkenazi Jews with BRCA1 mutations (and increased risk of breast cancer) is suggestive of the type of risks presented by studies of genetic influences on environmental response.[35,36]

In response to these research-related risks, some have proposed that members of study populations be involved directly in the review of proposed research.[37,38] Involving community representatives early in the design of research protocols could help identify potential risks that otherwise could go unnoticed.[39] This approach has been controversial, and the effectiveness of these supplemental protections has been questioned.[40,41] Additional discussion and empirical research are needed to determine how best to incorporate the perspectives of study populations in the review of genetic research.[42]

Long-Term Issues: Shifting Social Priorities and Responsibility for Health

Although it is difficult to speculate on the long-term consequences of any area of research, there are a number of broad social considerations suggested by the EGP. One such concern is that research on genetic influences on environmental response could affect how we view an individual's responsibility for his or her overall health. It seems reasonable to suggest that individuals with known genetic hypersensitivities to particular exposures are responsible for avoiding those adverse exposures. Individuals who know that they are particularly susceptible to the toxins found in cigarette smoke, for example, should quit smoking. What is less clear, however, is how far this moral obligation extends.

For instance, suppose an individual has a known hypersensitivity to an environmental exposure that is very common and difficult to avoid—exposure to low levels of direct sunlight, for example. An individual may be able to avoid such adverse exposures, but only by taking extraordinary measures. Although preventive interventions are available, it is unclear how we should view those individuals who fail to take such extraordinary measures to lower their risk of disease. Insurers, for example, may claim that individuals who do not minimize their exposure to these agents are responsible for any subsequent illness because they knowingly placed themselves at risk. Employers asked to pay for health costs through workers' compensation may refuse based on the idea that it was the individual who knowingly took a job that placed him or her at increased risk. In contrast, individuals with heightened genetic sensitivities may seek protection under the Americans with Disabilities Act or state legislation protecting against genetic discrimination.[43] Currently, it is unclear how to resolve such disputes or the extent to which information on genetic hypersensitivities might be inappropriately used to avoid responsibility for illness. In part, these disputes concern possible discriminatory uses of genetic information, but the more fundamental issue is how information on genetic risks will alter our views on personal responsibility for one's health.[12]

Other examples suggest further complications to the notion of personal responsibility. Suppose gene-modification techniques become more effective than they are at present. When certain genetic polymorphisms help protect against adverse exposures, individuals may wish to alter their genetic makeup to increase their tolerance to these exposures. Given the scarcity of medical resources, such applications of gene-manipulation techniques are unlikely to become commonplace. However, because these genetic enhancements could be purchased by wealthy individuals, their availability would contribute to existing health disparities between the rich and the poor. Genetically enhanced millionaires could live recklessly, engaging in unhealthy behaviors, whereas the poor would be held to a higher standard of accountability for their health.

Related to these considerations regarding medical responsibility are concerns about the effect the EGP and projects like it may have on how we view at-risk, but currently asymptomatic, individuals. As with other known genetic susceptibilities to disease, some individuals who are at increased risk of developing environmentally associated diseases will view themselves, and will be viewed by others, as ill—even though they may not be exhibiting any symptoms of the disease and may never develop the illness in question.[44] If associations between particular polymorphisms and specific diseases prove difficult to quantify, the EGP could foster such fatalistic attitudes by making it difficult to specify the precise extent to which an individual is at increased risk.

Other long-term considerations relate to increased emphasis on the genetic causes of disease. This trend, which has been described as the geneticization of disease,[45] could foster the belief that social problems are primarily the result of genetic causes. This reduction of social problems to biological problems could change how we think about social priorities. For example, employers may be viewed as less responsible for improving workplace conditions, with the focus of disease causation shifting from the hazardous workplace to the predisposed worker. Similarly, research funding may be diverted away from preventive strategies for improving public health, moving instead to approaches stressing genetic influences on disease.[46]

Areas for Future Research

It is expected that as the EGP develops, a wide range of ethical, legal, and social issues will emerge as important areas for additional consideration. There is already extensive literature examining the social implications of genetic research, much of which is directly relevant to the EGP. All too frequently, however, policy recommendations focus on rare alleles that are highly predictive of disease. It is unclear whether these moral and legal perspectives are appropriate guides when the alleles under investigation are much more common and less predictive of future disease.[47,48]

In many ways, the EGP is representative of a new type of genetic research program, with its emphasis on the incorporation of detailed genomic information into our understanding of disease susceptibility and individual response to environmental exposure. Thus, it is not surprising that the social implications of the project have not been adequately discussed in the existing bioethics literature. As the field of environmental genomics develops, researchers, legislators, and policymakers will need to consider the extent to which traditional bioethical perspectives apply to this new area of research. Thoughtful discussions of the ethical, legal, and social implications of environmental genomic research are critical to the overall success of projects like the EGP. We hope that this paper plays a role in fostering those discussions.

For additional information on the ethical, legal, and social implications of the EGP, visit the project's Web site.[49]

References

1. Albers JW. "Understanding gene-environment interactions" [Letter]. *Environmental Health Perspectives* 105:578–580 (1997).

2. Kaiser J. "Environment institute lays plans for gene hunt." *Science* 278:569–570 (1997).

3. Shalat SL, Hong J-Y, Gallo M. "The Environmental Genome Project." *Epidemiology* 9:211–212 (1998).

4. Guengerich FP. "The Environmental Genome Project: functional analysis of polymorphisms" [Letter]. *Environmental Health Perspectives* 106:A365–A368 (1998).

5. Brown PO, Hartwell L. "Genomics and human disease—variations on variation." *Nature Genetics* 18:91–93 (1998).

6. Wilson S. "Response: Environmental Genome Project" [Letter]. *Environmental Health Perspectives* 106:A368–A369 (1998).

7. Khoury M. "Genetic epidemiology and the future of disease prevention and public health." *Epidemiology Review* 19:175–180 (1997).

8. Collins F. "Shattuck lecture: medical and societal consequences of the Human Genome Project." *New England Journal of Medicine* 341:28–36 (1999).

9. Chakravarti A. "It's raining SNPs—hallelujah?" *Nature Genetics* 19:216–217 (1998).

10. Marshall E. "The genome program's conscience." *Science* 274:488–490 (1996).

11. Meslin EM, Thomson EJ, Boyer JT. "The ethical, legal, and social implications research program at the National Human Genome Research Institute." *Kennedy Institute of Ethics Journal* 7:291–298 (1997).

12. Sharp RR, Barrett JC. "The Environmental Genome Project and bioethics." *Kennedy Institute of Ethics Journal* 9:199–212 (1999).

13. Loffredo CA, Silbergeld EK, Parascandola M. "The Environmental Genome Project: suggestions and concerns" [Letter]. *Environmental Health Perspectives* 106:A368 (1998).

14. Schulte PA, Lomax GP, Ward EM, Colligan MJ. "Ethical issues in the use of genetic markers in occupational epidemiologic research." *Journal of Occupational and Environmental Medicine* 41:639–646 (1999).

15. Brandt-Rauf PW, Brandt-Rauf SI. "Biomarkers—scientific advances and societal implications." In Mark Rothstein, ed. *Genetic Secrets: Protecting Privacy and Confidentiality in the Genetic Era.* New Haven, CT: Yale University Press, 1997;184–196.

16. Grandjean P, Sorsa M. "Ethical aspects of genetic predisposition to environmentally-related disease." *Science of the Total Environment* 184:37–43 (1996).

17. National Institutes of Health Office of Protection from Research Risks. *Protecting Human Research Subjects: Institutional Review Board Guidebook.* Washington, DC: U.S. Government Printing Office, 1993.

18. Andrews LB, Fullarton JE, Holtzman NA, Motulsky AG, eds. *Assessing Genetic Risks: Implications for Health and Social Policy.* Washington, DC: National Academy Press, 1994.

19. Schulte PA, Perera FP. "Validation." In Paul Schulte, ed. *Molecular Epidemiology: Principles and Practices.* New York: Academic Press, 1993;79–107.

20. Schulte PA, Hunter D, Rothman N. "Ethical and social issues in the use of biomarkers in epidemiological research." *International Agency for Research on Cancer (IARC) Science Publication* 142:313–318 (1997).

21. Reilly P, Boshar MF, Holtzman SH. "Ethical issues in genetic research: disclosure and informed consent." *Nature Genetics* 15:16–20 (1997).

22. Schulte PA, Singal M. "Ethical issues in the interaction with subjects and disclosure of results." In Steven Coughlin and Tom Beauchamp, eds. *Ethics and Epidemiology.* New York: Oxford University Press, 1996;178–196.

23. Nelkin D, Lindee M. *The DNA Mystique: The Gene as a Cultural Icon.* New York: W. H. Freeman, 1995.

24. Hunter D, Caporaso N. "Informed consent in epidemiologic studies involving genetic markers." *Epidemiology* 8:596–599 (1997).

25. Clayton EW, Steinberg KK, Khoury MJ, Thomson E, Andrews L, Kahn MJE, Kopelman LM, Weiss JO. "Informed consent for genetic research on stored tissue samples." *Journal of the American Medical Association* 274:1786–1792 (1995).

26. Knoppers BM, Laberge C. "DNA sampling and informed consent." *Canadian Medical Association Journal* 140:1023–1028 (1989).

27. Kopelman LM. "Informed consent and anonymous tissue samples: the case of HIV seroprevalence studies." *Journal of Medicine and Philosophy* 19:525–552 (1994).

28. ASHG report. "Statement on informed consent for genetic research." The American Society of Human Genetics. *American Journal of Human Genetics* 59:471–474 (1996).

29. Wilcox AJ, Taylor JA, Sharp RR, London SJ. "Genetic determinism and the overprotection of human subjects." *Nature Genetics* 21:362 (1999).

30. Shriver M. "Ethnic variation as a key to the biology of human disease." *Annals of Internal Medicine* 127:401–403 (1997).

31. King PA. "Race, justice, and research." In Jeffrey Kahn, Anna Mastroianni, and Jeremy Sugarman, eds. *Beyond Consent: Seeking Justice in Research.* New York: Oxford University Press, 1998;88–110.

32. Caplan AL. "Handle with care: race, class, and genetics." In Timothy Murphy and Marc Lappe, eds. *Justice and the Human Genome Project.* Berkeley, CA: University of California Press, 1994;30–45.

33. Rothstein MA, ed. *Genetic Secrets: Protecting Privacy and Confidentiality in the Genetic Era.* New Haven, CT: Yale University Press, 1997.

34. Wolf SM. "Beyond 'genetic discrimination': toward the broader harm of geneticism." *Journal of Law, Medicine, & Ethics* 23:345–353 (1995).

35. Stolberg SG. "Concern among Jews is heightened as scientists deepen gene studies." *New York Times,* 22 April 1998;A24.

36. Struewing JP, Hartge P, Wacholder S, Baker SM, Berlin M, McAdams M, Timmerman MM, Brody LC, Tucker MA. "The risk of cancer associated with specific mutations of BRCA1 and BRCA2 among Ashkenazi Jews." *New England Journal of Medicine* 336:1401–1408 (1997).

37. Foster MW, Sharp RR, Freeman WL, Chino M, Bernsten D, Carter TH. "The role

of community review in evaluating the risks of human genetic variation research." *American Journal of Human Genetics* 64:1719–1727 (1999).

38. Greely HT. "The control of genetic research: involving the 'groups between.'" *Houston Law Review* 33:1397–1430 (1997).

39. Weijer C. "Protecting communities in research: philosophical and pragmatic challenges." *Cambridge Quarterly Healthcare Ethics* 8:501–513 (1999).

40. Juengst ET. "Groups as gatekeepers to genomic research: conceptually confusing, morally hazardous, and practically useless." *Kennedy Institute of Ethics Journal* 8:183–200 (1998).

41. Reilly PR. "Rethinking risks to human subjects in genetic research." *American Journal of Human Genetics* 63:682–685 (1998).

42. National Human Genome Research Institute, National Institute on Deafness and Other Communication Disorders, National Institute of Environmental Health Sciences, National Institute of General Medical Sciences. "Studies of the ethical, legal and social implications of research into human genetic variation. RFA HG-99–002." In: *NIH Guide for Grants and Contracts.* Bethesda, MD: National Institutes of Health, 29 April 1999.

43. Reilly PR. "Laws to regulate the use of genetic information." In Mark Rothstein, ed. *Genetic Secrets: Protecting Privacy and Confidentiality in the Genetic Era.* New Haven, CT: Yale University Press, 1997;369–391.

44. Weir RF, Lawrence SC, Fales E, eds. *Genes and Human Self-Knowledge.* Iowa City, IA: University of Iowa Press, 1994.

45. Lippman A. "Prenatal genetic testing and screening: constructing needs and reinforcing inequities." *American Journal of Law and Medicine* 17:15–50 (1991).

46. Edlin GJ. "Inappropriate use of genetic terminology in medical research: a public health issue." *Perspectives in Biology and Medicine* 31:47–56 (1987).

47. Juengst ET. "The ethics of prediction: genetic risk and the physician-patient relationship." *Journal of Genome Science and Technology* 1:21–36 (1995).

48. Parker LS. "Ethical concerns in the research and treatment of complex disease." *Trends in Genetics* 11:520–523 (1995).

49. Environmental Genome Project. Available at: http://www.niehs.nih.gov/envgenom/home.htm. Accessed 23 December 1999.

24

The Complex Relationships of Genetics, Groups, and Health

What It Means for Public Health

Ellen Wright Clayton

Genetics offers real opportunities for public health actors. Increased understanding of genetics will illuminate some of the factors that affect disease and, in many cases, will lead to more effective treatments. The recognition that phenylketonuria was caused by a metabolic defect that led to the accumulation of toxic levels of phenylalanine, an elevation that could largely be averted by adopting a low-phenylalanine diet, is an early example. Some cases of what was thought to be sudden infant death syndrome, a diagnosis used when no etiology is known, now appear to have been caused by metabolic defects in fatty acid oxidation[1] and sodium channel defects.[2] One of the tasks that has already been undertaken by the public health sector is to ensure that genomic information is incorporated into clinical care when the robustness of findings and their clinical utility have been well defined.

The focus of this paper is on the problems that arise when public health entities move beyond making sure that genetic tests are used appropriately to intervening directly into people's lives on the basis of genetic information to improve health.[3] Examples outside genetics illustrate some of the issues presented when one thinks about health in terms of providing services to populations. Many public health interventions, such as provision of clean water and efficient sewer systems, are directed at the entire population. Even such general interventions can be controversial, as the ongoing debate about fluoridation of public water supplies demonstrates.[4]

Matters immediately become more complex when public health activities, whether surveillance or therapeutic intervention, are directed at a segment of the population. Here, let us consider a hypothetical effort to identify among a particular, perhaps disfavored, subpopulation an infectious, but not particularly contagious, disease for which effective therapy exists. The group being tested may welcome the intervention, particularly if the risk of untreated disease is great and the therapy effective and not too onerous. Risks, however, attend targeted programs no matter how strong the potential medical benefits are. The group may feel "singled out" in ways that affect both how they feel about themselves and how others regard them. Depending on numerous factors, such as the nature of the disease that is sought to be identified or prevented, how the disease is contracted, and the nature of the targeted group, the program may cause the group to become stigmatized or increase already existing stigma. Public health activities can affect members of the group as individuals as well, subjecting them to surveillance or testing, whether voluntary or mandatory, that otherwise would not occur, which they may see as invasions of their privacy.

Targeted public health interventions pose particular risks to group members who are not actually at risk or affected but who find themselves suddenly officially labeled by governmental actions. One need only think back to the stigma experienced by Haitians when that group was identified as a high-risk group for HIV/AIDS. The difficulty of targeted approaches is that almost all population-based strategies include some, and sometimes even a large number of, people who are not at risk. This raises the question of whether the costs of such labeling are "worth it." The answer, of course, requires consideration of many factors, such as the level of threat to affected individuals and the extent to which it can be ameliorated. More important for this discussion are the degree to which the population being targeted is already disfavored, the extent to which the targeting strategy actually captures those at risk, and whether less overinclusive strategies exist or can be devised and at what cost. Approaches that use classifications, such as race and ethnicity, that have historically been used discriminatorily, that sweep too broadly,[5] or that can ascertain only a small part of the population at risk[6] are particularly difficult to justify.

In the discussion that follows, I will analyze the extent to which patterns of genetic variation correlate with categories historically used to define populations, particularly race, as well as the ways in which genetics has been invoked to justify differential treatment. I will conclude that the biological correlation between genetics and populations is poor, particularly for race, which is a highly complex social construct, that both using and failing to use racial designations in genetic testing and research have diverse and even at times contradictory consequences, and that as a result public health practice and research should include a multipurpose process of community consultation as well as ongoing public education.

Defining Groups

The prospect of greater knowledge of genetics and the recognition that targeted public health activities can have mixed social effects bring new urgency to the question of how groups are defined. The problem is complex. Although some people view themselves as belonging to a single group, most are members of several, some based perhaps on occupation, some on race, others on religious affiliation, others on shared heritage, and still others on recreational or aesthetic preferences. Which ones of these group identities are most important to the individual may vary over time, and the attributions that are most important to the person may not be the most important in the eyes of third parties. For purposes of public health interventions, it may matter a great deal whether a person is a coal miner, a health care worker, or a motorcycle rider, even though that person may define himself primarily in relation to his family or religious beliefs.

All groups of attribution are defined at least in part by social factors—by their history, by their activities, by their shared beliefs, to name only a few. This is obvious in the examples above—the cultural meaning of being a biker both to the biker and to others is entirely the result of social experience and understandings. Notably, the understandings may vary depending on the viewer's perspective and may be based on information that is not entirely accurate. Not all bikers are youthful outlaws; many are responsible, middle-aged people with jobs and families.

Social factors are also involved in defining populations, even for groups that have an element of genetic relatedness. The Old Order Amish share more alleles than usual as a result of their practice of marrying within their own community. As a result, they have an unusually high incidence of a number of metabolic disorders, which has made them the subject of much genetic research.[7] Nonetheless, the Amish are not identified "solely" or even primarily by the genes they have in common, a characteristic that rarely enters the public discourse, but rather by their shared beliefs and cultural practices.

It is worth reflecting on the Old Order Amish for a moment to make the point that being an identifiable group need not necessarily lead to widespread public stigmatization[8] or to punitive state intervention. Indeed, this group has often received preferential treatment, such as exemption from routine public health interventions, including newborn screening[9] and immunizations,[10] even at some risk to their own communities and to others. The Amish have been afforded special protection by no less than the U.S. Supreme Court, which held in *Wisconsin v. Yoder*[11] that this community was entitled under the U.S. Constitution to remove its children from public school prior to high school, citing its long religious history and success in child rearing. It is possible, therefore, to be "different" and even viewed as "odd" without being systematically disfavored.

Society has not always been so willing to acknowledge the social factors that contribute to group identity nor to be so tolerant of differences. History is replete with efforts to "reduce" groups to their genes, usually for the purpose of justifying discrimination against them. This was a major theme of the eugenics movement in the first part of the last century, leading among other things to the imposition of limits on immigration from populations that were thought to be genetically inferior.[12] Similar rhetoric about the Jews contributed to the political atmosphere that led to the Holocaust.[13]

Genetics and Race

In the United States, nowhere is this tendency to genetic reductionism clearer than in the context of race. Antimiscegenation laws were adopted to prevent the sullying or contamination of the white race by interbreeding with minority populations.[14] These statutes ultimately were struck down because they violated the Equal Protection

Clause of the U.S. Constitution, which severely limits the government's power to make distinctions on the basis of race, not because these laws in fact had no biological justification.[15] (By contrast, the Supreme Court ruled that the involuntary sterilization law in *Skinner v. Oklahoma* violated the Equal Protection Clause specifically *because* the legislative line drawn in that case had no plausible biological basis.[16]) Today, white supremacists argue that racial differences are primarily genetic, specifically minimizing the role of cultural influence, and assert that blacks are inherently inferior to whites.[17] Even scientists as well known as James Watson have been known to attach substantial importance to genetic differences between races.[18]

Responding to this distressing history of reducing race to genetics, some commentators have asserted that there are no genes for race[19] or that race has no biological meaning.[20] These statements, however, ultimately are not very helpful, primarily because they fly in the face of common experience—even young children learn and can identify racial categories. While it is true that no single gene can be tested to determine what race a person is, many of the characteristics typically used to define race—skin and hair color and hair texture to name only a few—are largely or solely determined by genetic variation. People usually identify a person's race on the basis of what they see, and what they see for this purpose is largely the product of genes. Similarly, population geneticists have demonstrated that they can with a high degree of accuracy discern a person's race by examining genetic variation at a relatively small number of well-chosen loci,[21] which will doubtless be of enormous forensic interest.

But acknowledging that genes have something to do with race does not mean that genetic difference is the sole basis of race. History, cultural beliefs, political practice, and a host of other factors have an enormous impact on how race is defined both within and outside different racial groups. Lee and her collaborators recently summarized the dramatic variability with which the U.S. Census Bureau has defined and collected information about race.[22] Jews were once labeled as nonwhite. Anyone with even one drop of African blood was at one time counted as black. Race was initially assigned by the census takers, but now is a matter of self-assignment. People are still required to choose one race to assign themselves to even when they see themselves as multiracial. Heated debate surrounded the creation of racial categories for the latest census. Even from the government's perspective, there is no settled definition of race.

Moreover, some government policies, commonly held assumptions, and turns of speech obscure group definitions that may be quite important to the populations themselves. The term *Asian* as it is used in the United States can subsume many groups, some of which see themselves as quite distinct from each other. It also seems strange to use such a sweeping term to encompass such a large portion of the world's population, implying that all people in Asia are the same.

One reason for the confusion about defining race is that there are no inherent lines to be drawn, as the historical debate about who is black reveals. Another reason is that the way race is viewed turns in part on its social meaning and impact, consequences that change over time and with social location. The consequences of being black in America changed with the abolition of slavery and the enactment of the Fourteenth Amendment at the end of the Civil War, and changed again with the Civil

Rights movement and legislation in the 1960s and 1970s. But no matter how great the changes or how malleable its definition, race remains, and in all likelihood will remain, a central factor in social organization.

The Complex Relationships among Genetics, Race, and Health

Recognizing that race is an incredibly complex construct of biology, history, and culture that has enormous social importance must lead us to ask what aspects of race account for its impact on health disparities, for we know that race is highly correlated with health outcomes. African Americans, for example, are more likely than whites to suffer from such common diseases as diabetes mellitus, hypertension, and certain forms of cancer. But these differences can occur for any number of factors, environmental, genetic, and most often complex interactions of the two. Research reveals that differential access to health care is important but is not solely responsible for the variation in observed outcomes.[23] Much work suggests that cultural differences between health care providers and patients, where culture is understood broadly as ranging from beliefs about the etiology and treatment of disease to dietary patterns to language, are important in determining health outcomes.[24] One can hypothesize mechanisms by which these effects occur. Physicians and patients, for example, have difficulty communicating under the best of circumstances.[25] The opportunities for misunderstanding can increase dramatically if the physician and patient have different worldviews and expectations. Such social barriers can also affect that patient's willingness and even ability to adhere to recommended interventions. The social, historical, and cultural differences are not the result of genetic variation, but they may well interact to affect health outcomes.

Genetic variations doubtless play a role as well. Disease-associated alleles vary in their frequency among populations, but they rarely segregate cleanly along racial lines. Variants associated with cystic fibrosis are found most frequently in populations that arose in northern Europe, but they occur in virtually all populations that have been studied to date. Sickle cell disease is found most often in populations that arose in Africa but occurs in many other groups as well. These two examples represent extremes in the correlations observed between genetic disorders and race. Most of the common diseases and the genetic variations that contribute to them are found in significant numbers in all populations. James Wilson and his colleagues recently demonstrated that even though people with different drug-metabolizing alleles do handle drugs in significantly different ways, "commonly used ethnic labels are both insufficient and inaccurate representations" of the different gene patterns.[26] The observation, therefore, that some racial groups respond differently but in predictable ways to certain drugs—that hypertension in blacks is less well controlled by β-blockers and ACE [angiotensin-converting enzyme] inhibitors and is better managed with calcium channel blockers than in whites[27]—need not necessarily be the end of the inquiry about how best to direct therapy.

Nor is the connection between genes and health outcomes necessarily direct. The genetic variations that cause the morphologic features that we use to assign race can trigger a whole host of social responses that affect health status. Racial identity, which is shaped in part by genes, in a racialized society can be a relevant variable. It will be necessary, therefore, to look *through* race to ascertain the *genetic* factors that affect drug response and disease susceptibility. But it will also be necessary to ascertain those social and cultural factors that contribute to the differences observed.

The result of the patterns of variation observed in DNA and of the complex nature and impact of race is that genetic variation, race, and health outcomes do not "map" directly or transparently onto each other. One might conceptualize the relationship as overlapping circles in a Venn diagram, in which the degrees of overlap and the boundaries are not known. Viewed in another way, genetic variation may contribute in a relatively straightforward way to many of the physical characteristics by which people typically assign race. The relationship of such variation to health outcomes, by contrast, is likely to be much more complex, with the genetically influenced physical characteristics triggering all the social constructs of race and their sequelae, while other variations affect disease states more directly.

Genetics, Race, and Public Health

The incomplete concordance of race, genetics, and health has complex and even contradictory implications for public health practice and for research. Although most of the difficulties arise from race-targeted interventions, as will be demonstrated below, ignoring race and the differences among populations presents its own difficulties. Testing is sometimes offered to populations who have a very low incidence of disease or for which the specificity of the test is unknown. It is currently estimated, for example, that Asian Americans have a 1 in 32,000 risk of having a child with cystic fibrosis (CF) with each pregnancy, about 10 percent of the risk faced by Caucasians. No data exist about what percentage of carriers among Asian Americans are detected by current tests or about the reproductive risk such couples face if only one partner is found to be a carrier.[28] In other words, CF carrier testing can provide definitive reproductive risk information to Asian Americans only in the extremely rare event that both partners have detectable mutations. Nonetheless, it was recently recommended that CF carrier testing be offered to all pregnant couples and couples contemplating pregnancy, regardless of their race or ethnicity.[29] The decision was motivated at least in part by the desire not to single out ethnic or racial groups or to deny anyone information they might find valuable.

This proposal on first glance might seem unobjectionable since all that is recommended is that the tests be *offered,* not that they be *performed.* Indeed, the American College of Obstetrics and Gynecologists and the American College of Medical Genetics recommended that lower risk groups be provided written information about testing, with the opportunity for further counseling and testing, if desired. The unstated assumption is that once informed, Asian Americans will decide not to be tested or at least will know what they are (and, more realistically, are not) getting. It is likely, however, that many Asian Americans will be tested, in part because it is easier for the clinician simply to do a test, particularly when it involves drawing one more tube of blood or doing a cheek swab, than it is to counsel about what the test is for and the factors that weigh for and against testing and to document a refusal of testing in a way that protects the clinician in the event of an adverse outcome.

Carol Browner and Nancy Press's study of maternal serum alphafetoprotein (MSAFP) screening in California demonstrates an example of the "it is easier just to do it" phenomenon.[30] In California, all providers who deliver obstetric care are required by law to offer MSAFP screening (now triple screening) to all pregnant women. The primary purpose of screening is to detect fetuses with neural tube defects. Although the state simply requires that the test be offered and even provides written information for the clinician to offer patients, these investigators found that many providers simply tested the women without much discussion. Many women with abnormal levels only found out that they had been tested or the purpose of the test when they went for the follow-up ultrasound which had been ordered to determine if the fetus was affected.

One might attempt to distinguish this study on the grounds that offering MSAFP screening is required by law in California, but most clinicians feel every bit as bound by the recommended standard of care, particularly in a health care environment characterized by brief patient encounters and in a legal system that can impose huge damages for failing to detect a "bad baby." Clinicians understand that the downside risk of doing an unwanted test, the offering of which is recommended as part of the standard of care, is far less than the downside risk of failing to detect a problem that the test would have revealed, and on occasion, some doubtless let this understanding override their ethical commitment to patient self-determination. It seems reasonable, therefore, to expect that at least some Asian American women will be tested for CF carrier status and will receive uninterpretable—or worse, but inevitable with all medical interventions, false-positive—results. The better policy in this instance would have been to recommend that information about CF carrier testing *not* be given to Asian Americans at this time because the test would so rarely be informative.

In general, however, using race in public health practice and in research creates more complex and intractable problems than ignoring race. Targeting interventions on the basis of race is a prime example. All states now screen newborns for hemoglobinopathies, of which sickle cell disease is the best known. A number of states chose at various times to screen only some subset of infants, some testing only black infants, others only nonwhite infants.[31] This practice was justified on the basis of cost-efficacy, reasoning that it would cost less to detect each affected child if only high-risk populations were screened.[32] Problems, not surprisingly, followed. Some went to the actual conduct of the screening program. Affected children who were not screened, of course, were missed. Questions arose about how to determine race: Does one test if the mother is black? If the mother *says* she is black? What about the father's race? What if the baby "looks black"? What about the fact that some black babies have light skin at birth? Ascertainment was sufficiently difficult to lead some states to move to universal screening.[33] Looking at newborn screening for hemoglobinopathies more generally, it soon became clear that some affected children, even when appropriately identified, did not receive appropriate care for their disease, particularly penicillin prophylaxis, which was the justification for screening in the first place.[34] All of this played out in light of the history of the ill-advised sickle cell screening programs of the 1970s and the broader history of discrimination against blacks in this country.[35]

Similar issues have been confronted by Ashkenazi Jews, who share a high number of alleles as a result of founder effects and centuries of being forced into segregated areas. For years, carrier testing and prenatal diagnosis have been offered in this group for a variety of disorders, such as Tay-Sachs and Canavan disease, largely without incident. Problems arose more recently, however, with the identification of mutations in cancer-predisposing genes that were particularly prevalent in this group. These include 185delAG and 5382insC in BRCA1, 6174delT in BRCA2, and I1307K in the APC genes.[36] These variants quickly became identified as "Jewish genes" in the media, raising concerns among the Jewish community that they would be stigmatized as being especially unhealthy.[37] These worries were aggravated by centuries of often-vitriolic attacks on Jews as well as more recent general fears about genetic discrimination. Ironically, these particular alleles were discovered *because* members of this group were willing to participate in research, probably hoping that new knowledge would lead to better interventions or perhaps believing that promoting research simply was a good thing to do.

Much effort went into acknowledging and assuaging this community's concerns,[38] but the lesson that taking part in research can be harmful remained. What exactly were some of the unintended harms of this research on cancer susceptibility genes? One was the association of these alleles with a particular, highly visible social group, which some have viewed over millennia with varying degrees of disfavor. Those who seek to try to belittle Jews could attempt to use this as another weapon, regardless of the fact that *all* people carry deleterious mutations. Other harms arose as a consequence of long-standing but misguided notions referred to earlier of genetic essentialism, of viewing people as their genes and ignoring all other aspects of their lives and histories, and of genetic determinism, of believing that there is a one-to-one correlation between having a mutation and becoming ill. That much of the debate about using genetic information in determining access to health insurance has centered around breast cancer merely increased the focus on these new alleles.

Other groups that have been invited to participate in genetics research have expressed similar concerns, particularly around the tendency to conflate genes with race and the fear that knowledge about genetic risk will be used to stigmatize the group at large. Some Native Americans avoid this research on the grounds that studying tissue violates their religious beliefs or that the findings will challenge their basic beliefs about their origins.[39] Others cite the fear that looking for genetic contributions to diseases such as diabetes mellitus and alcoholism will shift the focus away from the social factors, such as diet, poverty, and stress, that influence these disorders.[40]

Various indigenous peoples throughout the world worry that their genes will be stolen and exploited commercially without any benefit to themselves or their community.[41] Many groups cite the history to abuses in research, such as the syphilis study that was conducted in Tuskegee. In a recent series of focus groups conducted in Nashville about creating a database of DNA and medical records, we found that every group, regardless of race or socioeconomic class, raised the specter that their DNA would be cloned.[42] Some of the worries, then, focus on individual harms, others on harms to the group. Some have a high degree of immediacy, others like cloning seem farfetched and demonstrate the tremendous need for public education about what investigators can and cannot do. Mistrust remains an ever-present theme.

Including Populations in Public Health Research and Practice

Identifying the possibility of group harms, pervasive misconceptions, and the reality of mistrust calls for a variety of responses. At a minimum, investigators and public health practitioners need to be mindful of these issues as they design protocols, as they develop public health interventions, and as they describe their activities and results. That it makes little sense to generalize findings in one small community to the entire United States given the enormous diversity of cultural practices and environments that characterize this country, for example, is a lesson that continually bears repeating. Genetic variation is only part of the picture. Similarly, one cannot make sweeping statements about all Caucasians by looking at a group in Finland or Iceland or Iran or about all Asians by studying only a small population in Japan.

Questions also arise about how fully to involve subject individuals and populations in decision making. That institutional review boards (IRBs) are directed to consider the risks only to subjects and are specifically forbidden to consider the "long-range effects of applying knowledge gained in the research (for example, the possible effects of the research on public policy)"[43]—directives that essentially preclude consideration of group harms—in assessing the risks and benefits of protocols to decide whether the investigators should be allowed to proceed increases the urgency of this inquiry. As a result of IRBs' official inability to consider group harms in weighing the protocol itself, they increasingly insist that information about such harms be included in consent forms. Sometimes the investigator or the group collecting samples for genetic analysis includes such language.[44]

The most complex issues surround the role of the group(s) that may be affected by the research.[45] Leaders of Native American tribes, for example, relying on their sovereign powers, often decide whether their members will be permitted to participate in certain types of research. IRBs for these nations, where they exist, serve a similar function. The reluctance of some of these tribes is so deep-seated that many investigators have decided not to approach even those tribes that might be willing to take part. The most recent revision of the Council for International Organizations of Medical Sciences (CIOMS) guidelines recognizes the role of local governance, stating:

> In some cultures or groups, a researcher may enter a community to conduct research or approach prospective subjects for their individual consent only after obtaining permission from a community leader, a council of elders, or other designated authority. Such customs must be respected.[46]

But one can ask whether respecting the decisions of local leaders, even if legal, is always appropriate as an ethical matter. Should the leaders of such groups be permitted to veto certain types of research? What if the research was addressing the health needs of a disfavored section of the population? At the other end of the spectrum, the political leaders of Iceland decided to sell access to that country's medical and genealogical records to deCODE Genetics, a genomics company in Reykjavik, with a provision that citizens who were opposed could opt out.[47] Should there be some counterweight to the tyranny of the majority or the powerful, as exists in the Bill of Rights in the U.S. Constitution? The answer depends at least in part on matters of political theory—how one defines the legitimacy of government and how much deference ought to be owed by one form of government to another. Even the drafters of the CIOMS guidelines were not always as deferential as the preceding quotation would suggest. They insisted, for example, that *all* research subjects, including women, give individual informed consent to research participation,[48] a position that directly challenges legal rules and cultural practices in much of the world.

Ensuring community involvement is more difficult for the many groups or populations that have no politically credible or even identifiable leadership. Who are the spokespeople for the Ashkenazi Jews who could legitimately decide whether a certain project should go forward? From whom would one seek permission to do research on African Americans?

Driven in part by concerns about the propriety and possibility of group consent, some commentators now advocate a process of group engagement, either in lieu of obtaining the permission of the group's leaders or as an adjunct thereto. As currently conceived in the haplotype map project, an international effort to create a new map of the human genome, the purpose of such a process is not to seek consensus but to elicit all the community's concerns; not to enter into a one-time binding agreement with powerful members of the group giving the investigators authority to proceed but to establish an ongoing partnership in which the participant population has some say in the project and its outcome. The process will proceed in several steps, beginning with understanding the social structure of the group, ascertaining the concerns existing at various levels within the group, bringing together individuals from various parts of the group to develop solutions to the concerns identified, and then assessing the robustness of these solutions by presenting them at more general meetings. It is clearly impossible to identify prior to engagement the full array of concerns that might emerge, but one obvious question is how the group might wish to be described in the resulting map. More work is still required to determine to what extent the process of consultation would actually give power to the group to stop or reshape research projects and how individuals' interests would be protected in the process. The elaboration of this proposal will doubtless be enriched by and informative for the strategies already existing for developing community support for public health interventions.

Thinking about genetics, somewhat ironically, brings questions about the role of community consent and consultation more clearly into focus because, as we have already seen, genetic variation and community, population, and even race do not correlate very well. One might well ask why a community should be able to veto a certain type of genetic research since genetic disorders are rarely limited to a single group, and all the members of a particular community are rarely affected. Viewed from this perspective, it seems difficult to understand how a group could assert that it even "has" its own genes, much less control or ownership over them.

A partial justification for dealing with communities about issues of genetics practice and research comes from the political and social ways in which the relationship between genes and race or ethnicity is understood in society. As diligently as public health actors may point out the limitations of genetic essentialism and determinism, they must contend with long-standing tensions between groups, which have often included attempts to demonstrate that one is "inherently" better or worse than others. "Inherently," in the public discourse of the twenty-first century, translates readily into "genetically." So long as such tensions remain and so long as the contributions of genes and environment to outcomes are not fully understood, community consultation will provide several important benefits: (1) to understand the group's concerns and to develop responses; (2) to help investigators focus on the consequences of their research for the subjects; and (3) to capitalize upon the teachable moment of research to educate the group about genetics, perhaps mobilizing them to participate in a more informed manner in political debates about the appropriate use of genetic information.

This article was supported in part by funds from the National Human Genome Research Institute, 1 R01 HG01974–01. I would like to thank Jay Clayton, Carol Freund, Morris Foster, and Jean McEwen for their helpful comments on earlier drafts.

Notes

1. R. Boles et al., "Retrospective Biochemical Screening of Fatty Acid Oxidation Disorders in Postmortem Livers of 418 Cases of Sudden Death in the First Year of Life," *Journal of Pediatrics,* 132 (1998): 924–933. But see S. Wang et al., "Is the G985A Allelic Variant of Medium-Chain Acyl-CoA Dehydrogenase a Risk Factor for Sudden Infant Death Syndrome? A Pooled Analysis," *Pediatrics,* 105, no. 5 (2000): 1175–1176.

2. M. J. Ackerman et al., "Postmortem Molecular Analysis of SCN5A Defects in Sudden Infant Death Syndrome," *Journal of the American Medical Association,* 286 (2001): 2264–2269.

3. The Institute of Medicine's Committee for the Study of the Future of Public Health concluded that the core missions of public health are "assessment, policy development, and assurance." Committee for the Study of the Future of Public Health, Institute of Medicine, *The Future of Public Health* (Washington, DC: National Academy Press, 1988): at 7.

4. See, e.g., PEN Fluoridation Leadership Team at http://1wwwpenweb.org/fluoride (accessed 15 April 2002).

5. An example might be deciding to screen all blacks for HIV/AIDS on the grounds that some blacks are intravenous drug abusers.

6. An example might be a decision to screen homosexuals but not intravenous drug abusers for HIV/AIDS.

7. N. C. Andreasen, "The Amish: A Naturalistic Laboratory for Epidemiologic and Genetic Research," *American Journal of Psychiatry*, 140, no. 1 (1983): 75–76.

8. But see B. Byers, B. W. Crider, and G. K. Biggers, "Bias Crime Motivation: A Study of Hate Crime and Offender Neutralization Techniques Used Against the Amish," *Journal of Contemporary Criminal Justice*, 15, no. 1 (1999): 78–96.

9. E.g., Ky. Rev. Stat. Ann. C 214.155 (Michie 2000).

10. E.g., Fla. Stat. Ann. § 232.032 (2001); Ind. Code S 20-12-71-14 (2001).

11. *Wisconsin v. Yoder,* 406 U.S. 205 (1972).

12. D. J. Kevles, *In the Name of Eugenics* (New York: Knopf, 1985).

13. J. M. Glass, *Life Unworthy of Life: Racial Phobia and Mass Murder in Hitler's Germany* (New York: Basic Books, 1997).

14. P. A. Lombardo, "Medicine, Eugenics, and the Supreme Court: From Coercive Sterilization to Reproductive Freedom," *Journal of Contemporary Health Law and Policy,* 13 (1996): 1–25.

15. *Loving v. Virginia,* 388 U.S. 1 (1967).

16. *Skinner v. Oklahoma,* 316 U.S. 535 (1942).

17. W. L. Pierce, "Equality: Man's Most Dangerous Myth," at http://www.stormfront.orglracedifflequality.html (accessed 6 April 2002).

18. "Watson's 'Sun and Sex' Lecture Upsets Audience," *Nature Medicine,* 7 (February 2001): 137.

19. G. J. Annas, "Genism, Racism, and the Prospect of Genetic Genocide." Paper presented at The New Aspects of Racism in the Age of Globalization and the Gene Revolution, UNESCO 21st Century Talks, World Conference against Racism, Racial Discrimination, Xenophobia and Related Intolerance, Durban, South Africa, 3 September 2001, available at http://www.bumc.bu.edu/ www/sph/1w/pvl/genism.htm (quoting Craig Venter).

20. M. A. Omi, "The Changing Meaning of Race," in N. J. Smelser, W. J. Wilson, and F. Mitchell, eds., *America Becoming: Racial Trends and Their Consequences*, vol. 1 (Washington, DC: National Academy Press, 2001): 243–263.

21. M. D. Shriver et al., "Ethnic-Affiliation Estimation by Use of Population-Specific DNA Markers," *American Journal of Human Genetics,* 60, no. 4 (1997): 957–964; P. E. Smouse and C. Chevillon, "Analytical Aspects of Population-Specific DNA Fingerprinting for Individuals," *Journal of Heredity,* 89, no. 2 (1998): 143–150.

22. S. S. Lee, J. Mountain, and B. A. Koenig, "The Meanings of 'Race' in the New Genomics: Implications for Health Disparities Research," *Yale Journal of Health Policy, Law, and Ethics,* 1 (2001): 33–75.

23. *Healthy People 2010*, conference ed., 2 vols. (Washington, DC: U.S. Department of Health and Human Services, 2000).

24. L. Cooper-Patrick et al., "Race, Gender and Partnership in the Patient-Physician Relationship," *Journal of the American Medical Association,* 282, no. 6 (1999): 583–589; S. H. Kaplan et al., "Patient and Visit Characteristics Related to Physicians' Participatory Decision-Making Style. Results from the Medical Outcomes Study," *Medical Care,* 33, no. 12 (1995): 1176–1187.

25. J. Katz, *The Silent World of Doctor and Patient* (New York: Free Press, 1984).

26. J. E. Wilson et al., "Population Genetic Structure of Variable Drug Response," *Nature Genetics,* 29 (2001): 265–289.

27. L. Brewster, J. Kieijnen, and G. Van Montfrans, "Pharmacotherapy for Hypertension in People of Sub-Saharan Africa or of Sub-Saharan African Descent." Protocol of the Cochrane Hypertension Group, *Cochrane Database of Systematic Reviews*, Issue 3, 2001 (citing earlier studies).

28. American College of Obstetricians and Gynecologists, American College of Medical Genetics, *Preconception and Prenatal Carrier Screening for Cystic Fibrosis: Clinical and Laboratory Guidelines* (Washington, DC: American College of Obstetricians and Gynecologists, 2001).

29. Consensus Development Panel, "Genetic Testing for Cystic Fibrosis," National Institutes of Health Consensus Development Conference Statement, 15, no. 4 (14–16 April 1997): at 10, available at http://odp.od.nih.gov/consensus/cons/106/106_statement.htm.

30. N. A. Press and C. H. Browner, "'Collective Fictions': Similarities in Reasons for Accepting Maternal Serum Alpha-Fetoprotein Screening Among Women of Diverse Ethnic and Social Class Backgrounds," *Fetal Diagnostic Therapy,* 8, suppl. 1 (1993): 97–106.

31. See, e.g., Ark. Stat. Ann. § 20–15–302 (2000).

32. J. Tsevat et al., "Neonatal Screening for Sickle Cell Disease: A Cost-Effectiveness Analysis," *Journal of Pediatrics,* 118 (1991): 546–554.

33. Agency for Health Care Policy and Research, Public Health Service, U.S. Department of Health and Human Services, *Sickle Cell Disease: Screening, Diagnosis, Management, and Counseling in Newborns and Infants* (Rockville, MD: U.S. Department of Health and Human Services, 1993); La. Rev. Stat. S 40:1229.1 (2001), amended by Acts 1999, No. 328, S 1.

34. S. J. Teach, K. A. Lillis, and M. Grossi, "Compliance with Penicillin Prophylaxis in Patients with Sickle Cell Disease," *Archives of Pediatrics and Adolescent Medicine,* 152, no. 3 (1998): 274–278.

35. See generally P. R. Reilly, *Genetics, Law, and Social Policy* (Cambridge, MA: Harvard University Press, 1977).

36. J. P. Struewing et al., "The Risk of Cancer Associated with Specific Mutations of BRCA1 and BRCA2 among Ashkenazi Jews," *New England Journal of Medicine*, 336, no. 20 (1997): 1401–1408; T. W. Prior, "The I1307K Polymorphism of the APC Gene in Colorectal Cancer," *Gastroenterology*, 116, no. 1 (1999): 58–63.

37. S. G. Stolberg, "Jewish Concern Grows as Scientists Deepen Studies of Ashkenazi Genes," *New York Times,* 22 April 1998.

38. "Jewish Leadership Meeting on Genetics," *The American Scene* (Fall/Winter 1998), available at http://www.hadassah.org/news/pubfrm3.htm.

39. D. Harry, Coordinator, Indigenous Peoples Coalition Against Biopiracy, "Tribes Meet to Discuss Genetic Colonization," at http://www.ipcb.org/calendar/confrpt.html (accessed April 15, 2002).

40. S. Tesh, *Hidden Arguments: Political Ideology and Disease Prevention Policy* (New Brunswick, NJ: Rutgers University Press, 1988).

41. Action Group on Erosion, Technology and Concentration, "Colombian Indigenous People Negotiate to get Human Tissue Samples Back" (18 March 1997), at http://www.rafi.org/article.asp?newsid=80.

42. E. W. Clayton, "Creating a Process to Collect Human Biological Materials and Medical Records for Research from Patients in Teaching Hospitals." Abstract from presentation at A Decade of ELSI Research: A Celebration of the First 10 Years of the Ethical, Legal, and Social Implications (ELSI) Programs, printed in journal of *Law, Medicine & Ethics,* 29, no. 2, suppl. (2001): at 5.

43. 45 C.F.R. SS 46.111(1)-(2) (2001).

44. The National Action Plan on Breast Cancer in the United States was one of the pioneers in developing and pilot testing mechanisms to provide patients with these choices. See National Action Plan on Breast Cancer, National Biological Resource Banks Working Group, Sunset Report (July 1998), available at http://www.4woman.gov/napbc/catalog.wci/napbc/sunset2.htm; National Action Plan on Breast Cancer, Consent Form for Use of Tissue for Research, at http://www.4woman.gov/napbc/napbc/ consent.htm.

45. R. R. Sharp and M. W. Foster, "Involving Study Populations in the Review of Genetic Research," *Journal of Law, Medicine & Ethics,* 28, no. 1 (2000): 41–51; C. Weijer and E. J. Emanuel, "Protecting Communities in Biomedical Research," *Science,* 289 (2000): 1142–1144; M. W. Foster, A. J. Eisenbraun, and T. H. Carter, "Communal Discourse as a Supplement to Informed Consent for Genetic Research," *Nature Genetics,* 17, no. 3 (1997): 277–279; M. W. Foster, D. Bernsten, and T. H. Carter, "A Model Agreement for Genetic Research in Socially Identifiable Populations," *American Journal of Human Genetics,* 63 (1998): 696–702; M. W. Foster et al., "The Role of Community Review in Evaluating the Risks of Human Genetic Variation Research," *American Journal of Human Genetics,* 64 (1999): 1719–1727.

46. Council for International Organizations of Medical Sciences (CIOMS), "Cultural Considerations," Guideline 4, International Ethical Guidelines for Biomedical Research Involving Human Subjects, rev. ed. (January 2002), available at http://wwwcioms.ch/guidelinesjanuary 2002.htm.

47. Act on a Health Sector Database no. 139/1998, passed by the Icelandic Parliament at 123rd session, 1998–1999, available at http://brunnur.stjr.is/interpro/htr/htr.nsf/pages/forsid-ensk; Joint Statement of the Icelandic Medical Association and deCODE Genetics on the Health Sector Database (27 August 2001), available at http://www.decodegenetics.com/news/releases/older/item.ehtm?id= 17881.

48. Guideline 4, supra note 46.

25

Genetic Research and Health Disparities

Pamela Sankar, Mildred K. Cho,
Celeste M. Condit, Linda M. Hunt,
Barbara Koenig, Patricia Marshall,
Sandra Soo-Jin Lee, and Paul Spicer

Disparities in health status have increased in the United States in the last 50 years despite remarkable advances in our ability to prevent, diagnose, and treat disease.[1] The poor are the least likely to have benefited from progress in medicine, but economic status does not account completely for these disparities. Even when income and related variables are controlled for, the health status of racial and nonwhite ethnic minorities ranks lower than that of whites on numerous measures.[1] The reasons for this pattern include unequal quality of health care, education, employment, housing, and nutrition. Despite numerous studies that demonstrate the overriding importance of racial discrimination and poverty as the major contributors to health disparities,[2] several recent statements have suggested that genetic research holds considerable promise in the campaign against health disparities.[3–7] Although genetics broadly influences nearly all aspects of health, extensive research suggests that its direct contribution to the current pattern of health disparities in the United States is secondary to social and environmental influences.[1] Furthermore, overemphasis on genetics as a major explanatory factor in health disparities could lead researchers to miss factors that contribute to disparities more substantially and may also tend to reinforce racial stereotyping, which may contribute to disparities in the first place.[8]

Health Disparities and Race in the United States

Substantial evidence indicates that disparities in health status in the United States result largely from long-standing, pervasive racial and ethnic discrimination.[1]

Minorities are more likely to live in housing made hazardous by lead paint-coated walls and defective, fire-prone heating systems and to be exposed to allergens produced by cockroach and rat infestations and the indoor pesticides used to control them.[9–12] Neighborhoods where housing is most available to the minority poor are often less likely to meet Environmental Protection Agency ambient air quality standards and more likely to be located near hazardous waste sites.[13,14] Jobs open to minorities often pose serious health risks through exposure to toxic chemicals used in manufacturing or agriculture.[15,16] Psychologic stress caused by perceived racial discrimination produces higher rates of depression and a greater risk of high blood pressure among some minority populations.[17–19]

Treatment of resulting health problems and even routine preventive care can be impossible for many because of inadequate health insurance.[20] Health insurance costs pose problems to many people in the United States, particularly the elderly. However, minorities are less likely to have health insurance than whites, and among Hispanics, the number of uninsured is almost twice that of whites.[20] Much of this disparity derives from discriminatory employment practices in that minorities are less likely to have jobs that offer employer-based health coverage.[20]

American Indians and Alaskan Natives are at particular disadvantage because funds for health care in these tribes, adjusted for medical inflation and population growth, have steadily declined since the 1990s.[21] Thus, American Indian and Alaskan Native tribes have increasingly insufficient funds for even the most basic health care needs. Funding for nonreservation health care has fared even worse, with just over 1% of the Indian Health Service budget appropriated by Congress to care for urban American Indians and Alaskan Natives.[22]

Unequal treatment of minority patients extends also to inpatient services. A 1997 study that reviewed 1.7 million hospital discharge abstracts and that controlled for diagnosis, severity, age, and insurance status showed that in nearly half of the 77 disease categories, "blacks were significantly less likely than whites to receive a major therapeutic procedure."[23] Several smaller, condition-specific studies have replicated the finding that blacks are less likely to be offered and, if offered, less likely to undergo diagnostic and therapeutic procedures for heart disease and cancer.[24,25] Similar findings have been reported recently for major diagnostic categories for Hispanics[26] and for Asians for certain cardiac procedures.[27]

Shorter lives are the price that black, Hispanic, and American Indian and Alaskan Native populations pay for inadequate health care, unsafe living conditions, and high psychologic stress. The average life expectancy of white men is 74 years; of black men, 66 years.[1] Although this figure represents a gain for black men of several years since 1960, it is still lower than that reported for whites more than 40 years ago.[1] Among American Indian males, average life expectancy remains in the mid-50s, exactly where it was in 1960.[20] These inequalities are mirrored in childhood mortality data. Despite notable improvements in neonatal outcomes generally, children younger than 1 year and born to black mothers have a greater mortality rate than infants born to white or Asian mothers, and neonates born at very low birth weights (<1500 g) are three times more likely to have black than white mothers.[28]

Responses to the Health
Disparities Campaign

Alleviation of disparities in health status is a primary goal of the U.S. government, which in 2000 established the Healthy People 2010 program and earmarked substantial funds toward this effort. In 2003 alone, National Institutes of Health funding classified as supporting health disparities research was predicted to reach nearly $3 billion.[29] Among the responses to this initiative are several to identify genetic contributions to health disparities.[5–7, 30]

For example, the recent vision statement for the future of genomics by the National Human Genome Research Institute (NHGRI) named as a "grand challenge" the need to develop "genome-based tools" to address disparities in health status.[3] The statement acknowledges that social and economic factors contribute significantly to disparities but nevertheless asserts the need for extensive research to better understand the contribution of genetics. The statement also names genomics as an avenue to improve health in the third world and cites the recent mapping of the malarial parasite and malaria mosquito genome as examples of its application to third-world health problems.

NHGRI's genetically focused response to the federal health disparities initiative is consistent with its mission to promote genetics. Less predictable, however, were the responses from several other institutes that listed genetic research projects as examples of their support for the health disparities initiative. The National Institute of Arthritis and Musculoskeletal and Skin Diseases,[5] for example, highlights the importance of genetic research in all four of its research areas, citing as a rationale that these conditions, including scleroderma, lupus, and osteoarthritis, cluster in populations targeted by health disparities initiative, including blacks and Native Americans. The strategic initiative from the National Eye Institute[6] includes genetic research for three of its four research areas, explaining, for example, that glaucoma disproportionately affects blacks, and that blacks, Hispanics, Mexican Americans, Japanese Americans, and Native Americans are more likely to be diagnosed with diabetic retinopathy. Even the National Library of Medicine's list of research priorities for health disparities put genetic research at the top, above research on environment and socioeconomic status, mechanisms of disease, and epidemiologic and risk factors.[7]

Individual researchers have also characterized the importance of their work in its capacity to advance our understanding of health disparities.[31–34] Any research, including genetic research, that can help ameliorate health disparities is valuable. The problem is when researchers try to overstate the potential benefits of such research by proclaiming that it is going to significantly contribute to solving the health disparities problem. Although this research may well succeed in elucidating genetic factors that contribute to diseases associated with health disparities, the reporting of such studies all too often tends to downplay the fact that nongenetic factors are substantial contributors[35] or that the onset or severity of the disease results from a complex interaction of genetic and environmental factors.[36–40]

Most genetics researchers are, of course, presumably well aware of the importance of environmental causes of such disparities.[29,41–43] Few would seriously contend that genetic research alone is likely to be the key to the alleviation of disparities in health status. However, because this is the case, responses to the call to help alleviate health disparities that emphasize genetic research without better contextualizing their arguments about its importance require explanation.

Factors Promoting Genetic Research Proposals

There are several reasons why researchers might try to overstate the potential benefits of genetic research to alleviate and eventually eliminate health disparities. First, much genetic research depends on government funding. The U.S. government has widely publicized the Healthy People 2010 campaign and directed billions of dollars of increasingly scarce scientific research monies to health disparities initiatives. As with many similar government initiatives, such as the 1970s "war on cancer," these priorities are translated into messages that researchers should emphasize the possibility that their work will "solve" the featured health problem, even if this is an unlikely outcome.[44]

Second, characterizing genetic research as a way to help alleviate health disparities might seem more plausible in the United States because of the particular pattern of health disparities in this country. Poor health in the United States is concentrated among racial and ethnic minorities, whereas better or good health is concentrated among the majority white population. If a person's racial or ethnic identity is considered to be associated with his or her real or putative genetic ancestry, then observations of the patterns of poor and good health restricted to the United States appear to support the inference that genetic ancestry strongly influences health status. However, if genetic ancestry strongly influences health status in the United States, it should be similarly influential elsewhere. In other words, if increased rates of hypertension, diabetes, and prostate and breast cancer among blacks in the United States are strongly influenced by genetics, then individuals of African descent living outside of the United States should also have elevated rates of these conditions. Research instead shows far lower rates of these conditions.[45–50]

One explanation proposed to explain the different rates of hypertension and diabetes in black Africans and black Americans[51,52] is that new environments encountered in the African diaspora triggered expression of certain genetic variations quiescent in Africa. Even if this explanation is correct, the heterogeneity and variability of the environments encountered make it unlikely that the direction of this triggering was nearly always to confer on blacks ill health, especially considering the widely variable conditions, such as breast cancer, depression, and diabetes, that unequally affect them. Furthermore, health disparities, when examined globally rather than through an exclusively U.S. lens, do not cluster in any particular population or region, and they do not fall along stable racial or ethnic lines. Rather, they are endemic wherever poverty prevails, so that the average life expectancy among black Cubans is approximately 70 years at the same time that men in neighboring Haiti have an average life expectancy of 45 years.[53–55]

Third, the historical tendency by scientists and the press to overstate the successes and potential benefits of genetic research[56,57] may have distorted some researchers' sense of how quickly this line of research is likely to produce practical applications. For example, predictions for finding a prostate cancer gene have been scaled back considerably, with a caution that the genetic mechanisms of prostate cancer "have turned out to be remarkably difficult to unravel."[58] Recent research on asthma suggests that it results from a complex interaction of numerous genetic and environmental factors, some that protect individuals from disease and some that contribute to its development, and that each has only a small and often contingent effect in the overall disease process.[59] Even the much-heralded finding that angiotensin-converting enzyme inhibitors work less well in treating heart failure in blacks than in whites has been challenged by some scientists who have used the difficulty of determining why the finding is not as generally applicable as predicted to frame a new perspective on "therapy response" as a "complex rather than a simple phenotype."[40,60] Thus, although considerable progress has been made in understanding how genes contribute to diseases associated with health disparities, for many, the molecular genetics is still obscure and, for all, the complexity of how genes and the environment interact evades explanation.

Many geneticists recognize the need for long-term studies of gene-environment interactions, and recently NHGRT has proposed a prospective U.S. cohort study to accomplish this.[61] However, the emphasis of others on genetics as the dominant if not sole causative factor continues to require counterassertion. Some of the genetic optimism originates with media coverage of genetic findings, but recent research identifies the role played by scientists themselves in overstating the certainty and the implications of findings.[42,56,57] There continue to be far more publications that attend solely to genes than those attending to gene-environment interactions, and even the more straightforward studies often overgeneralize from findings that lack statistical significance.[62]

Thus, there exist several reasons that researchers might be inclined to overstate the potential benefits of genetic research, including the need to respond to funding initiatives, the distinctive pattern of health disparities in the United States, and the history of overoptimistic certainty in predicting the benefits of genetic research.

Pitfalls of Overemphasizing the Alleviation of Health Disparities as a Rationale for Promoting Genetic Research

Recognizing that the genetic contribution to health disparities is likely to be relatively limited is not the only reason to question the wisdom of promoting genetic research under the aegis of health disparities. First, overfocusing on genetics might divert attention from what evidence already suggests are the central causes of health disparities and might lead scientists to overlook possible actual environmental contributors.

Second, overemphasizing the potential of genetic research to alleviate health disparities fosters the misconception that disparities in health status will be easy to solve.

Standardizing access to health care and reforming attitudes toward minority patients poses a far greater challenge than introducing new treatments facilitated by genetic research. Although the idea of underlying biological causes amenable to medical intervention might be appealing, characterizing the problem in this way could send the wrong message about what kind of changes are most needed. This concern is particularly salient in light of a recent government report that depicts "health disparities" as "differences" and that highlights the scant few instances in which minority rather than white populations experience better health outcomes.[63,64]

Third, given the particular pattern of health disparities in the United States, research or policy that emphasizes a population-based genetic predisposition to disease may foster a tendency to attribute the poor health of racial and ethnic groups primarily to their genetic makeup, running the risk that those groups will be seen as inherently biologically inferior to groups who enjoy better health. Popular press coverage has already moved in this direction. For example, a recent newspaper article stated that there is "a growing mountain of research" that shows that inheritance, rather than "social, environmental and economic stresses of lower income and minority status," explains health disparities across U.S. populations, and that this acknowledgment calls for genetic research on health-disparity–related conditions such as heart disease, diabetes, and asthma.[65]

Racial labeling, even if done in an effort to better diagnose and treat patients, can reinforce racial stereotyping, and the recent Institute of Medicine report on health disparities has identified such stereotyping as a primary factor in unequal treatment of minority patients.[1] Racial stereotyping enters medical practice when conditions are linked to populations and then to the unexamined assumptions that practitioners might have about whether patients from some populations are more or less likely than those from other populations to comply with treatment regimens or to endanger the success of treatment through destructive behavior, such as drug abuse.[66] These assumptions can lead to miscommunication between practitioner and patient and to inadequate treatment.[67,68] Thus, an overfocus on genetics in the effort to alleviate health disparities could have the paradoxic result of actually exacerbating disparities.

The Genetic Contribution to Complex Diseases

Clear evidence of an easily discernible and well-understood genetic contribution to common diseases can provide valuable insights for health management, as in the cases of some breast and colon cancers. However, the question is not whether genetics has enhanced our understanding of the disease process in individuals. It clearly has. Rather the question is whether, all things considered, overfocus on genetic research is a particularly effective way to proceed with the effort to alleviate health disparities in the United States with regard to the more common, complex diseases that largely account for such disparities.

Genes undoubtedly make some contribution to disparities in aggregate group health status, but the potential genetic contribution is unknown. Geneticists recognize that the causes of most common, complex diseases consist of a complicated interaction between genes and the environment. Untangling this interaction will take a long time. For this reason, expectation for genetic research to explain health disparities must be calibrated appropriately, and those who conduct research and those who write about it should be encouraged not to overstate those expectations by promising more than genetics is likely to be able to offer. The reason to study prostate cancer genetics is not to address health disparities. It is to determine the genetics of prostate cancer.

The genetics of human health and disease and how best to alleviate disparities in health status among U.S. citizens are two vitally important areas of research. Casual observation of the particular pattern of disparities in the United States might indicate that the two are related because there are clear differences among racially identified populations in the prevalence of many common, complex diseases. But more careful reflection on the pattern of disparities globally challenges this assumption and suggests that health disparities and genetics may have little to do with each other, short of both capturing public attention simultaneously. The irony is that if we do not recognize that these are distinct, if interrelated, topics, efforts that are meant to improve the health of racial and ethnic minorities instead might inadvertently harm them, which could happen if genetic research diverts attention from productive ideas about the effects of environment on health or if it reinforces racial and ethnic stereotypes that contribute to the very discrimination that health disparities initiatives are meant to ameliorate.

It is critical that research on the genetics of human health and disease continue and bring to clinical fruition the vast storehouse of basic research that the Human Genome Project has produced. The justification for this work, however, can and should be made on its own merits and need not be the inflated claim that it will solve problems of a specific disease when we know that genes are just a small part of the problem.

Funding/Support: The works of Drs. Sankar and Cho was supported by NHGRI NIDCD grant R01 HG02189-03; Dr. Condit's work was supported by NHGRI 5R01HG002191-03; Dr. Hunt's work was supported by NHGRI 5K01HG002299-04; Dr. Lee's and Dr. Koenig's work was supported by NHGRI 1K01HG002883-01; Dr. Marshall's work was supported by NHGRI R01-HG02207-01; and Dr. Spicer's work was supported by NIEHS NHGRI 5R01ESO10830-03.

Acknowledgment: Authors are members of the Human Genetic Variation Consortium, a group of investigators convened by the Ethical, Legal, and Social Implications Research Program of the National Human Genome Research Institute to discuss common issues relating to their research on ethical, legal, and social implications of human genetic variation research.

References

1. Institute of Medicine. *Unequal Treatment: Confronting Racial and Ethnic Disparities in Healthcare.* Washington, DC: National Academy Press; 2003.

2. Geiger HJ. Racial and ethnic disparities in diagnosis and treatment: a review of the evidence and a consideration of causes. In: Smedley B, Stith AY, Nelson AR, eds.

Unequal Treatment: Confronting Racial and Ethnic Disparities in Healthcare. Washington, DC: National Academy Press; 2003.

3. Collins FS, Green ED, Guttmacher AE, Guyer MS, for the Institute USNHGR. A vision for the future of genomics research. *Nature.* 2003;422:835–847.

4. Risch N, Burchard E, Ziv E, Tang H. Categorization of humans in biomedical research: genes, race and disease. *Genome Biology.* 2002;3:2007–2012.

5. National Institute of Arthritis and Musculoskeletal and Skin Diseases. Strategic plan for reducing health disparities. Available at: http://www.niams.nih.gov/an/stratplan/strategicplanhd/strategicplanhd.htm. Accessed 4 June 2003.

6. National Eye Institute. Strategic plan on reducing health disparities. Available at: http://www.nei.gov/resources/strategicplans/disparities.htm. Accessed 11 September 2003.

7. National Library of Medicine. NLM strategic plan to reduce racial and ethnic health disparities 2000–2005. Available at: http://www.nim.nih.gov/pubs/plan/nlmplan racialethnic.pdf. Accessed 20 July 2003.

8. Lee SS, Mountain J, Koenig BA. The meanings of "race" in the new genomics: implications for health disparities research. *Yale Journal of Health Policy, Law, and Ethics.* 2001;1:33–75.

9. Berkowitz G, Obel J, Deych E, et al. Exposure to indoor pesticides during pregnancy in a multiethnic, urban cohort. *Environmental Health Perspectives.* 2003;111:79–84.

10. Istre G, McCoy M, Osborn L, Barnard J, Bolton A. Deaths and injuries from house fires. *New England Journal of Medicine.* 2001;344:1911–1916.

11. Parker D, Sklar D, Tandburg D, Hauswald M, Zumwalt R. Fire fatalities among New Mexico children. *Annals of Emergency Medicine.* 1993;22:517–522.

12. Call R, Smith T, Chapman ME, Platts-Mills T. Risk factors for asthma in inner city children. *Journal of Pediatrics.* 1992;121:862–866.

13. Hispanic environmental health: ambient and indoor air pollution. *Archives of Otolaryngology—Head and Neck Surgery.* 1996;114:256–264.

14. Soliman M, Dorosa C, Mielke H, Bota K. Hazardous wastes, hazardous materials and environmental health inequity. *Toxicology and Industrial Health.* 1993;9:901–912.

15. Shalat SL, Donnelly KC, Freeman NC, et al. Nondietary ingestion of pesticides by children in an agricultural community on the U.S./Mexico border: preliminary results. *Journal of Exposure Analysis and Environmental Epidemiology.* 2003;13:42–50.

16. Bowler R, Gynsens S, Hartney C. Neuropsychological effects of ethylene dichloride exposure. *Neurotoxicology.* 2003;24:553–562.

17. Gee GC. A multilevel analysis of the relationship between institutional and individual racial discrimination and health status. *American Journal of Public Health.* 2002;92:615–623.

18. Krieger N. Racial and gender discrimination: risk factors for high blood pressure? *Social Science and Medicine.* 1990;30:1273–1281.

19. Halpern D. Minorities and mental health. *Social Science and Medicine.* 1993;36:597–607.

20. Henry J. Kaiser Family Foundation. *How Race/Ethnicity, Immigration Status and Language Affect Health Insurance Coverage, Access to Care and Quality of Care among the Low-Income Population.* Menlo Park, CA: Henry J. Kaiser Family Foundation; 2003.

21. Henry J. Kaiser Family Foundation. *Sources of Financing and the Level of Health Spending for Native Americans.* Menlo Park, CA: Henry J. Kaiser Family Foundation; 1999.

22. Forquera R. Challenges in serving the growing population of urban Indians. In: Dixon M, Roubideaux Y, eds. *Promises to Keep: Public Health Policy for American*

Indians and Alaska Natives in the 21st Century. Washington, DC: American Public Health Association; 2001:121–134.

23. Harris DR, Andrews RM, Elixhauser A. Racial and gender differences in the use of procedures for black and white hospitalized adults. *Ethnicity & Disease.* 1997;7:91–105.

24. Merrill RM, Merrill AV, Mayer MS. Factors associated with no surgery or radiation therapy for invasive cervical cancer in black and white women. *Ethnicity & Disease.* 2000;10:248–256.

25. Schecter AD, Goldschmidt-Clermont PJ, McKee G, et al. Influence of gender, race, and education on patient preferences and receipt of cardiac catheterizations among coronary care unit patients. *American Journal of Cardiology.* 1996;78:996–1001.

26. Andrews RM, Elixhauser A. Use of major therapeutic procedures: are Hispanics treated differently than non-Hispanic whites? *Ethnicity & Disease.* 2000;10:384–394.

27. Carlisle DM, Leake BD, Shapiro MF. Racial and ethnic differences in the use of invasive cardiac procedures among cardiac patients in Los Angeles County, 1986 through 1988. *American Journal of Public Health.* 1995;85:352–356.

28. Alexander G, Kogan M, Himes J, Goldenberg R. Racial differences in birthweight for gestational age and infant mortality in extremely-low-risk US populations. *Paediatric and Perinatal Epidemiology.* 1999;13:205–217.

29. National Institutes of Health. Strategic research plan and budget to reduce and ultimately eliminate health disparities, volume 1. Available at: http://ncmhd.nih.gov/strategicmock/our_programs/strategic/pubs/VolumeI_031003EDrev.pdf. Accessed 28 December 2003.

30. National Human Genome Research Institute. Statement of programmatic interest in Native American Research Centers Health Initiative. Available at: http://www.genome.gov/10001840. Accessed 4 June 2003.

31. Burchard E, Ziv E, Coyle N, et al. The importance of race and ethnic background in biomedical research and clinical practice. *New England Journal of Medicine.* 2003;348:1170–1175.

32. Yancy CW, Fowler MB, Colucci WS, et al. Race and the response to adrenergic blockade with carvedilol in patients with chronic heart failure. *New England Journal of Medicine.* 2001;344:1358–1365.

33. Reynolds T. Study seeks to clarify genetic basis of prostate cancer in African Americans. *Journal of the National Cancer Institute.* 2003;95:1356–1357.

34. Fernandez SM Jr, Beasley TM, Rafla-Demetrious N, et al. Association of African genetic admixture with resting metabolic rate and obesity among women. *Obesity Research.* 2003;11:904–911.

35. Rotimi CN, Cooper RS, Okosun IS, et al. Prevalence of diabetes and impaired glucose tolerance in Nigerians, Jamaicans and U.S. blacks. *Ethnicity & Disease.* 1999;9:190–200.

36. Coleman AL. Glaucoma. *Lancet.* 1999;354:1803–1810.

37. Lewallen S, Courtright P. Blindness in Africa: present situation and future needs. *British Journal of Ophthalmology.* 2001;85:897–903.

38. Sommer A, Tielsch JM, Katz J, et al. Racial differences in the cause-specific prevalence of blindness in east Baltimore. *New England Journal of Medicine.* 1991;325:1412–1417.

39. Felson DT, Lawrence RC, Dieppe PA, et al. Osteoarthritis: new insights, part 1: the disease and its risk factors. *Annals of Internal Medicine.* 2000;133:635–646.

40. Mayes MD. Scleroderma epidemiology. *Rheumatic Disease Clinics of North America.* 2003;29:239–254.

41. Miller RL. Breathing freely: the need for asthma research on gene-environment interactions. *American Journal of Public Health.* 1999;89:819–822.

42. Doris PA. Hypertension genetics, single nucleotide polymorphisms, and the common disease: common variant hypothesis. *Hypertension.* 2002;39(2 pt 2):323–331.

43. Shields PG, Harris CC. Cancer risk and low-penetrance susceptibility genes in gene-environment interactions. *Journal of Clinical Oncology.* 2000;18:2309–2315.

44. Fujimura J. *Crafting Science: A Sociohistory of the Quest for the Genetics of Cancer.* Cambridge, MA: Harvard University Press; 1996.

45. Cooper R, Rotimi C, Kaufman J, et al. Prevalence of NIDDM among populations of the African diaspora. *Diabetes Care.* 1997;20:343–348.

46. Cooper R, Rotimi C, Ward R. The puzzle of hypertension in African Americans. *Scientific American.* 1999;280:56–63.

47. Glaser SL, Hsu JL. Hodgkin's disease in Asians incidence patterns and risk factors in population based data. *Leukemia Research.* 2002;26:261–269.

48. Banini A, Allen J, Allen H, Boyd L, Lartey A. Fatty acids, diet, and body indices of type II diabetic American whites and blacks and Ghanaians. *Nutrition.* 2003;19:722–726.

49. Gibson P, Henry R, Shah S, Powell H, Wang H. Migration to a Western country increases asthma symptoms but not eosinophilic airway inflammation. *Pediatric Pulmonology.* 2003;36:209–215.

50. Woodcock A, Addo-Yobo E, Taggart S, Craven M, Custovic A. Pet allergen levels in homes in Ghana and the United Kingdom. *Journal of Allergy and Clinical Immunology.* 2001;108:463–465.

51. Daniel H, Rotimi C. Genetic epidemiology of hypertension: an update on the African diaspora. *Ethnicity & Disease.* 2003;13(2 suppl 2):S53–S66.

52. Forrester T. Historic and early life origins of hypertension in Africans. *Journal of Nutrition.* 2004;134:211–216.

53. World Health Organization. Selected health indicators for Cuba. Available at: http://www3.who.int/whosis/country/indicators.cfm?country=CUB&language=english. Accessed 22 July 2003.

54. Shkolnikov V, McKee M, Leon DA. Changes in life expectancy in Russia in the mid-1990s. *Lancet.* 2001;357:917–921.

55. de la Fuente A. Recreating racism: race and discrimination in Cuba's "special period." July 1998;18. Georgetown University Cuba Briefing Paper Series.

56. Conrad P. Uses of expertise: sources, quotes, and voice in the reporting of genetics in the news. *Public Understanding of Science.* 1999;8:285–302.

57. Bubela TM, Caulfield TA. Do the print media "hype" genetic research? A comparison of newspaper stories and peer-reviewed research papers. *Canadian Medical Association Journal.* 2004;170:1399–1407.

58. Bratt O. Hereditary prostate cancer: clinical aspects. *Journal of Urology.* 2002;168:906–913.

59. Hakonarson H, Wjst M. Current concepts of the genetics of asthma. *Current Opinion in Pediatrics.* 2001;13:267–277.

60. Iacoviello L, Vischetti M, Zito F, Donati MB. Genes encoding fibrinogen and cardiovascular risk. *Hypertension.* 2001;38:1199–1203.

61. Collins FS. The case for a U.S. prospective cohort study of genes and environment. *Nature.* 2004;429:475–477.

62. Hirschhorn JN, Lohmueller K, Byrne E, Hirschhorn K. A comprehensive review of genetic association studies. *Genetics in Medicine.* 2002;4:45–61.

63. U.S. House of Representatives Committee on Government Reform-Minority Staff. *Changes to the National Healthcare Disparities Report: A Case Study in Politics and Science.* Available at: http://www.house.gov/reform/min/politicsandscience/pdfs/pdf_politics_and_science_disparities_rep.pdf.

64. Department of Health and Human Services. *National Healthcare Disparities Report.* Rockville, MD: Agency for Healthcare Research and Quality; 2003.

65. Healy M. The race factor: thousands of African Americans will donate gene samples to a unique research project that will explore the link between ethnicity and disease. Available at: http://www.latimes.com/features/health/medicine/la-he-race 8sep08.0.2737879.story?coll=la-health-medicine.

66. van Ryn M. Research on the provider contribution to race/ethnicity disparities in medical care. *Medical Care.* 2002;40(1 suppl):I140–I151.

67. Condit CM, Templeton A, Bates BR, Bevan J, Harris T. Attitudinal barriers to delivery of race-targeted pharmacogenomics among informed lay persons. *Genetics in Medicine.* 2003;5:385–392.

68. Bevan J, Lynch JA, Dubriwny TN, et al. Informed lay preferences for delivery of racially varied pharmacogenomics. *Genetics in Medicine.* 2003;5:393–399.

Further Reading

Fleck, Leonard M., "Just Caring: Do Future Possible Children Have a Just Claim to a Sufficiently Healthy Genome?" in Rosamond Rhodes, Margaret P. Battin, and Anita Silvers, eds., *Medicine and Social Justice: Essays on the Distribution of Health Care* (New York: Oxford University Press, 2002), pp. 446–457.

Institute of Medicine, *Implications of Genomics for Public Health* (Washington, DC: National Academies Press, 2005).

Jennings, Bruce, "Technology and the Genetic Imaginary: Prenatal Testing and the Construction of Disability," in Erik Parens and Adrienne Asch, eds., *Prenatal Testing and Disability Rights* (Washington, DC: Georgetown University Press, 2000), pp. 124–144.

Lee, S. S., J. Mountain, and B. A. Koenig, "The Meanings of 'Race' in the New Genomics: Implications for Health Disparities Research," *Yale Journal of Health Policy, Law & Ethics* 1: Spring 2001, 33–75.

Wachbroit, Robert, and David Wasserman, "Patient Autonomy and Value-Neutrality in Nondirective Genetic Counseling," *Stanford Law & Policy Review* 6(2), 1995, 103–111.

Index

Italicized page numbers refer to figures.